the
food
combining
bible

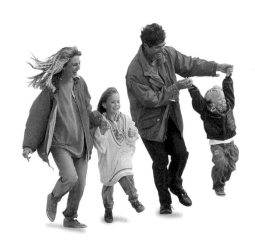

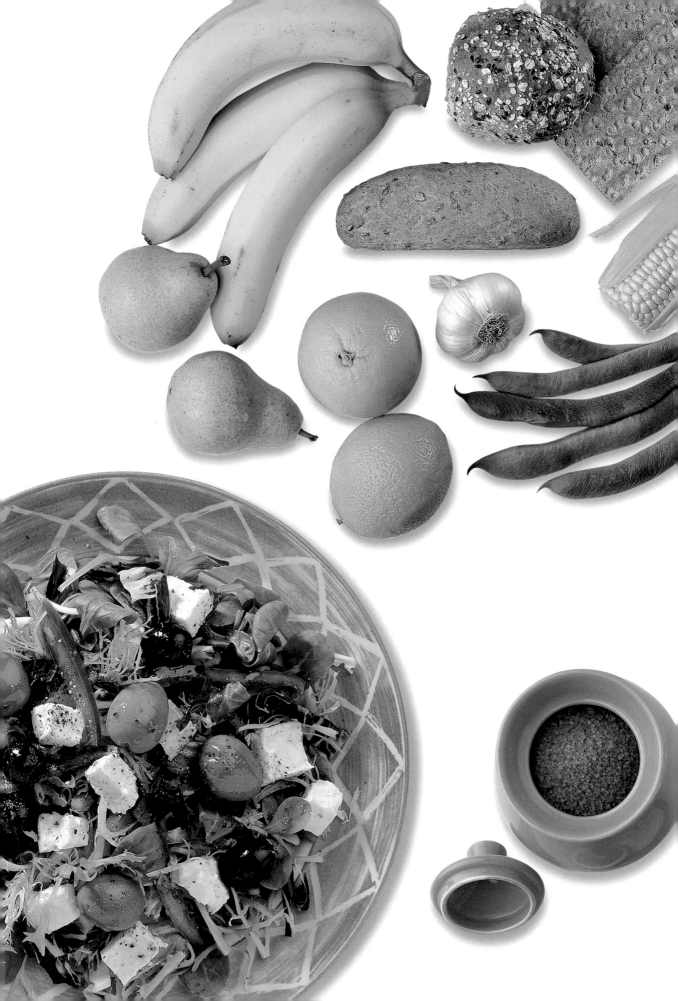

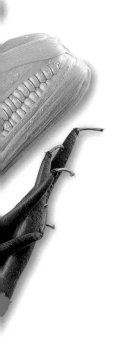

the
food
combining
bible

jan dries & inge dries

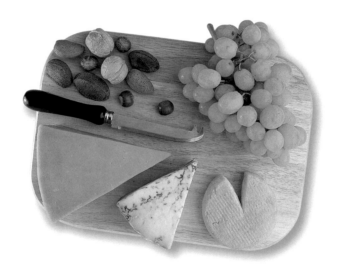

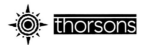
thorsons

Thorsons
An Imprint of HarperCollins*Publishers*
77–85 Fulham Palace Road
Hammersmith, London W6 8JB

The website address is: www.thorsonselement.com

and *Thorsons* are trademarks of
HarperCollins*Publishers* Ltd

First published in Great Britain in 2002 by Element
This edition published by Thorsons 2004

10 9 8 7 6 5 4

A catalogue record for this book
is available from the British Library

This book was designed and produced by
THE BRIDGEWATER BOOK COMPANY

EDITORIAL DIRECTOR Fiona Biggs
ART DIRECTOR Terry Jeavons
DESIGNER Bernard Higton
DESIGN ASSISTANT Alison Honey
PROJECT EDITOR Sarah Yelling
PICTURE RESEARCHER Lynda Marshall
PHOTOGRAPHER Ian Parsons
INDEX Indexing Specialists

ISBN 0 00 713152 6

Printed and bound in Hong Kong
by Printing Express

CONTENTS

FOREWORD

Food combining – the combining of specific foods for optimal digestive results – is a popular subject in today's world, promulgated in particular by two well-known American nutritionists, Dr Hay and Dr Shelton. All the same, it would be wrong to claim that the theory behind such nutritional harmony is generally accepted. Only very recently, in circles devoted to dietetics and health, has food combining received anything approaching the interest it deserves.

People who still cannot accept the theory of food combining tend to assume that all foods contain basically the same nutrients, and that these nutrients are subject to the digestive processes simultaneously – combining specific foods is thus a waste of time, because 'all food goes down the same way'. The same people point out that the principles on which Hay and Shelton based their work are somewhat behind the times in scientific terms, no longer corresponding to every concept of current physiological theory.

It was Jan Dries who, at least in the Netherlands, during the 1970s greatly contributed to the revival of interest in food combining, waging what almost amounted to a personal crusade in publicizing and promoting the use of these important dietary promotions. His publications, his lectures, his course studies and his private correspondence have led thousands of people over the years into the way of health by means of food combining. And, through further research undertaken during those same years, he has since come up with further significant improvements.

With no disrespect to all the highly creditable preliminary work carried out by Hay and Shelton, it would not be inaccurate to say that Jan Dries presents a completely new view of food combining. His extensive and thorough understanding of the physiology of digestion has at length furnished him with all the answers to all the questions on food combining that scientists might wish to pose.

This brilliant book is a matchless guide for anyone who is searching for better and healthier nutrition.

Jef Houben
BIOCHEMIST

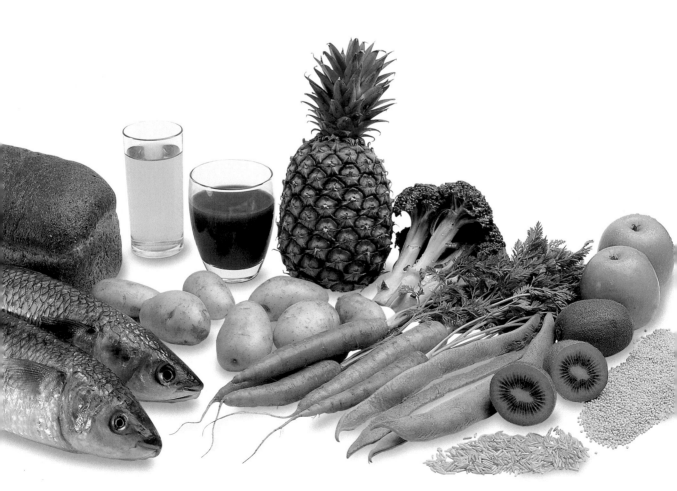

INTRODUCTION

In today's industrialized nations, news broadcasts bring home to us every day alarming reports of the state of general health: the disruption of the environment, stressful lifestyles and a lack of purposive identity. Yet the causes are well known and include the consumption of food produced and prepared by industrial methods. In Europe, North America and Australasia, humankind now enjoys immense material benefits, but ironically, must fight for the preservation of its life more than ever. The three elements essential for survival – air, water and food – correspond to the very elements most under threat in the environment.

For the last 20 years or so, considerable attention has been paid to promoting healthy foods and production. Organic farming and cultivation has been encouraged not only by consumer demand, but also by agricultural organizations and government food departments. The use of food additives has diminished rapidly and vegetarianism has become a completely acceptable way of life.

But despite all these positive developments, the food we choose is often not used to maximum advantage. Many of the people who turn to what they believe is a wholesome and nutritious diet find that they continue to experience digestive problems and other discomforts that they were hoping to eliminate, once and for all.

Food combining, in which specific foods are combined for optimal digestive results, represents the solution for everyone: it works as well for those with a conventional eating pattern as it does for those with a less conventional diet. Whatever we eat, we must always bear in mind how the human digestive system functions. If we do not, not only is the digestion disrupted, but the nutritional value we receive is minimal: we may eat plenty of food, but we do not make much use of it. This is a waste of food and energy. Moreover, it tends to clog up the intestines needlessly, overburdening the liver, and potentially causing some degree of acidosis in the tissues. Ironically, to go on eating huge quantities of food in this wasteful way is to invite any of the various deficiency conditions that are deleterious to overall health.

The simpler and more natural your eating pattern is, the less you will need to practise food combining. Those who follow a conventional eating pattern involving meat, fish, cheese, bread and so on, can benefit most from eating the recommended combinations of specific foods.

The main theme of this book is to demonstrate the value of food combining in relation to all eating patterns. The theory formerly presented by the nutritionists William Howard Hay and Herbert M. Shelton may perhaps be rather outdated, but in this book the combinations of specific foods comply fully with the most advanced scientific views of modern physiology.

The principle behind food combining can be stated very simply. Every food contains up to five nutrients: proteins, fats, sugars, starch and acids, in proportions that are specific to each particular food. Some nutrients are inert or passive in the presence of other nutrients – but some react with others, and cause disruptions in the digestive process.

The nutrient that is proportionately the greatest in quantity (the dominant nutrient) 'controls' the entire digestive process. To eat different types of food at random may result in the presence of more than one dominant nutrient, and the consequent reaction between conflicting dominants may cause anything from a mild flush to serious digestive problems and gastroenteric disorders.

Digestion relies primarily on the activity of enzymes which function within a fairly narrow range of acidity levels. Each type of food has an influence on the degree of acidity present and, in turn, can influence the digestive process for better or worse. Digestion is itself subject to circadian rhythms that are unfailingly regular in their timing, and does not respond well to random eating patterns. It is best, therefore, that a meal should comprise foods that are carefully suited to each other and that support each other as they are digested.

This book is intended to emphasize the importance of a dietary regime that takes account of the theory's combinations of specific foods. It is an attempt to familiarize the reader with the necessary structure. Above all, it contains many valuable charts, tables, diagrams and lists of information, all of which are carefully annotated and explained. Using the correct combinations of specific foods should lead to virtually perfect digestion, maximum nutritional benefits and total freedom from alimentary discomfort. As an added advantage, the body's whole metabolism should function at an optimum level, with a consistently high degree of immunity from all sorts of ailments and diseases. With this book, I hope to convince as many people as possible that food combining is necessary and a benefit for everyone and for every kind of eating pattern.

Enjoy your food!

Jan Dries

ASSESSING HOW YOU FEEL

These charts are designed as self-assessment guides, so that you can monitor the effects that the principles of food combining are having on your health. Consider the questions they pose before you start food combining, and review your progress regularly. As time passes, you should see a distinct improvement, not just in digestive health, but in the way you feel overall. However, if any symptoms continue and are severe, you should seek medical advice.

	Day 1	Day 2	Day 3	Day 4	Day 5	Day 6	Day 7
Midnight-7.00am							
Breakfast (7.00am-10.00am)							
10.00am-Noon							
Lunch (Noon-3.00pm)							
3.00pm-6.00pm							
Dinner (6.00pm-10.00pm)							
10.00pm-midnight							

KEEPING A FOOD JOURNAL

You may be under the impression that keeping a food journal is a notion confined to those trying to establish the cause of a food intolerance or following an exclusion diet, but the concept is just as useful when starting a new dietary plan of any kind. In your journal, you should aim to record everything that you eat and when you eat it. How much further you take things is up to you: you could record, for instance, how much physical exercise you are taking or even what you were thinking and feeling while you were eating. Finding out why you are eating what is just as useful as keeping track of what you are eating.

WHAT IS A FOOD CRAVING?

If you find it impossible to resist food temptations, the chances are that this is a craving, rather than actual hunger. The difference between the two is that a craving is triggered by the emotions and, as a consequence, is highly selective. You simply get the urge to eat a particular food or type of food. This condition is by no means a rare one: according to a survey carried out by a Canadian university, 97 per cent of women and 68 per cent of men experience food cravings, although generally, the older you are, the less likely they become. Researchers also believe that their occurrence may be dictated by the time of day – there is evidence to suggest that late afternoon or early evening are the prime times for food cravings. Hormones, too, are thought to play a role, particularly during pregnancy and at certain times of the menstrual cycle. To deal with a craving, you could try:

- substituting other foods
- controlling portion sizes
- giving in to the craving.

Above: Potato crisps (chips) are often a food craving.

Psychologists claim that there is logic in giving in to a craving: if you try to eat around it, you will probably end up consuming more food and calories than you would have if you had given in straight away – in the end, you are highly likely to give in anyway. If your craving is for potato crisps (chips), for instance, it is highly unlikely that either celery sticks or carrot batons will be acceptable substitutes.

LEFT: Keeping a food journal will monitor your food patterns and consumption.

HOW DO YOU FEEL IN YOUR CLOTHES?

How well your clothes fit is a useful guide to your body condition. The optimum digestion in food combining will also balance your body weight and resolve bloating.

Comfortable	☐
Restricted in movement	☐
Wish they were looser	☐
Uncomfortable	☐

HEALTH CHECK LIST

DO YOU SUFFER FROM?	NEVER	RARELY	FROM TIME TO TIME	QUITE OFTEN	OFTEN
Abdominal distension					
Abdominal pain after eating					
Aching joints					
Acne					
Allergies					
Anxiety attacks					
Bags under the eyes					
Bleeding gums					
Bloating					
Burping					
Catarrh					
Chronic tiredness					
A coated tongue					
Constipation					
Day sweats					
Diarrhoea					
Dizziness					
Dyspepsia					
Flatulence					
Fluid retention					
Food cravings					
Food intolerance					
Headaches					
Heartburn					
Hunger pangs					
Indigestion					
Insomnia					
Irritable bowel syndrome					
Joint pain					
Joint swelling					
Lack of appetite					
Low energy levels					
Migraine					
Mood swings					
Mouth ulcers					
Muscle aches and cramps					
Nausea					
The need to snack or eat meals frequently					
Night sweats					
Palpitations					
Persistent infections					
Persistent thirst					
Poor circulation					
PMS					
Recurring sore throats					
Sinus conditions					
Skin problems					
Stress					
Weight gain					
Weight loss					

CASE HISTORIES AND COMMON QUESTIONS

Thousands of people around the world have proved for themselves that good food combining not only aids digestion, but also has a beneficial influence on total health and the healing process. The case histories here are just a brief sample of *the variety of problems and conditions that food combining has helped either to cure completely or to improve dramatically. In addition, the most frequently asked questions about food combining are answered.*

CASE HISTORIES

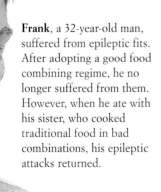

Jean, a 48-year-old woman, suffered from shortness of breath. She took medication for bronchitis, including antibiotics, over many years, but it had no effect. I noticed that her stomach and abdomen were bloated and were pushing up into her diaphragm, causing respiratory problems. By adopting the right food combinations, the swelling subsided and she was able to breathe normally.

Sarah, a 52-year-old woman, had problems with her intestines and bowels for many years. She was cured by eating small meals and correct food combinations.

Frank, a 32-year-old man, suffered from epileptic fits. After adopting a good food combining regime, he no longer suffered from them. However, when he ate with his sister, who cooked traditional food in bad combinations, his epileptic attacks returned.

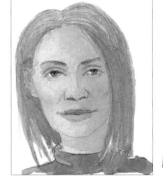

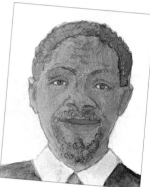

Karen, a 24-year-old woman, suffered from psoriasis. She cut all animal proteins out of her diet and ate only good food combinations. As a result, her psoriasis healed.

John, a 58-year-old man, suffered from asthma. Once he began eating food in the right combinations, his asthma disappeared. When he did not pay attention to correct food combining, the asthma returned.

COMMON QUESTIONS

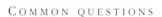

Q I understand that, in food combining, you should never mix proteins with starches, but I've read somewhere that it is important to eat one protein and one starch meal a day. Is this true? (If it is, what other foods can I combine with them without breaking food combining rules?)

A *This is not necessarily true: what is important is to make sure that, while observing the rules of good food combining, you are maintaining the proper intake of healthy nutrients across the board, which is why eating one protein and one starch meal a day is recommended by some food combining authorities. Through use of the food combining pentagon (see page 45) and combination guides (pages 96–125) later in this book, you will soon be able to sort out your own preferred* *combinations and devise an overall eating plan accordingly. The thing to do, whatever you decide, is to make sure that your diet includes plenty of salads and vegetables, since these, with a few exceptions, can be eaten freely.*

Q Many books on food combining state that the aim should be to eat one protein, one starch and one alkaline-forming meal per day. Some go further than this, though, and say that proteins are best eaten at lunchtime, while others are equally insistent on eating proteins in the evening. I'm confused.

BELOW: Fruit is best eaten on its own.

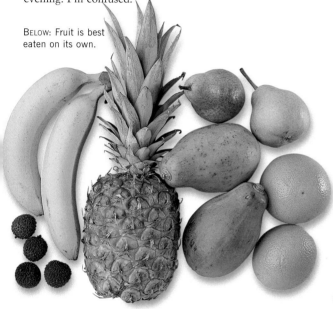

A *As you will discover as you read on, I do not support the view that some foods are alkaline – an alkaline food is a scientific impossibility. Nor do I think necessary the over-formal approach that this advice drives you towards. What you should do is plan your eating to suit your lifestyle. If you are working hard, it may be better for you to eat some starchy food first thing in the morning, to be sure of a slow, controlled release of energy that will keep you going until lunchtime. Or, as I often advise, you can start the day with nourishing fruit.*

Q It seems to be a common opinion in food combining that fruits should be kept separate from proteins and starches. Does this also mean that different types of fruit should be eaten separately or can they be combined?

A *Because fruit passes through the stomach very quickly, it is always better to eat it on its own, rather than as a dessert at the end of a protein- or starch-dominated meal, for example. If its digestion is delayed by other foods in the stomach, fermentation and indigestion, can result. However, nearly all fruits will mix happily together, although you should remember that melon is always best eaten on its own.*

FOOD COMBINING ON THE INTERNET

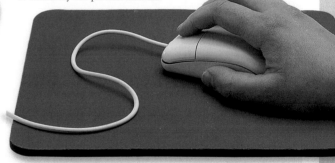

To find out more about food combining and its many possibilities, why not visit the host of useful Internet web sites devoted to health and nutrition, and discover it for yourself. When it comes to recipes, for example, there are literally hundreds of sites to try: two of the best are the low-fat vegetarian archive 'Fatfree' (www.fatfree.com), and the Mayo Clinic's 'Virtual Cookbook' which is found at (www.mayo.ivi.com/mayo/recipe/htm/maintoc.htm), where all the recipes have been analysed and tested by staff dieticians at the world-famous Mayo Clinic. You can even submit recipes of your own for Mayo makeovers.

Elsewhere on the Net, you can get in touch with and share the experiences of fellow food combiners around the world by surfing through chat rooms and bulletin boards. Remember, however, that it can be hard to tell whether the information on some web sites is from a knowledgeable, sound source, rather than a crank or someone with a nutritional axe to grind. Assess what you find out carefully in the light of your own knowledge and experience, rather than assuming that the information on the Net is necessarily 100 per cent accurate.

Q I'm confused about milk and milk products. Why is it, for instance, that food combining advises that porridge should not be eaten with milk, but can be eaten with cream?

A *The answer is simple – porridge, in which the dominant nutrient is starch, and milk, which is rich in protein, are incompatible food combinations. However, the dominant nutrient in cream is fat, and protein and fat are a permissible combination.*

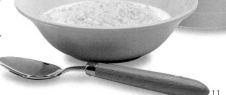

RIGHT: The fat and starch of porridge and cream are a good combination.

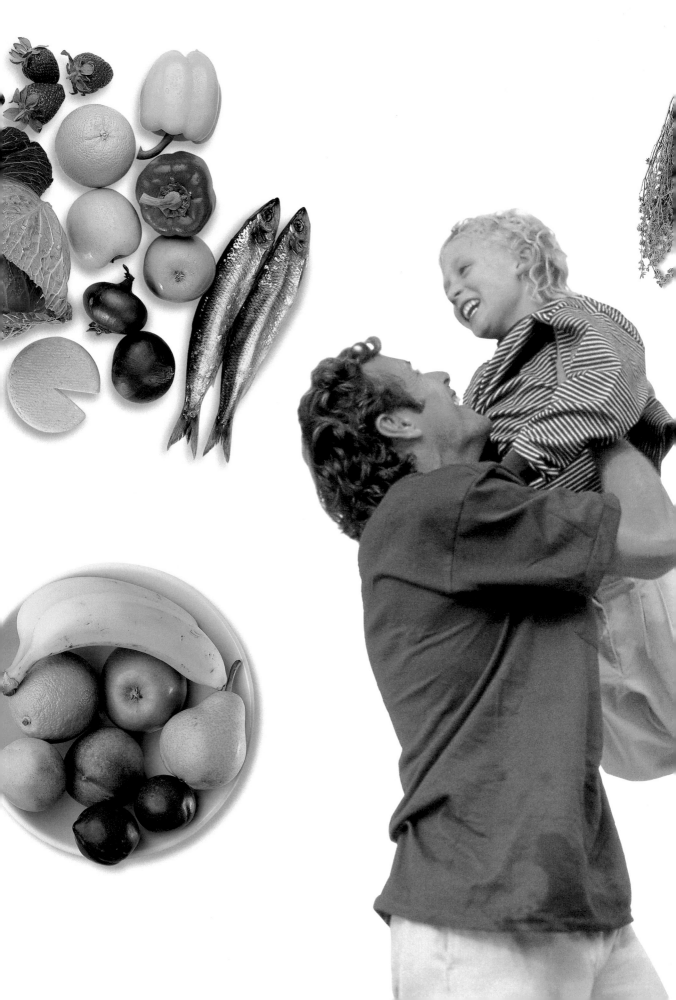

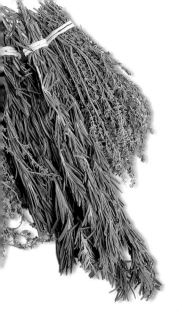

CHAPTER 1

THE IMPORTANCE OF FOOD COMBINING

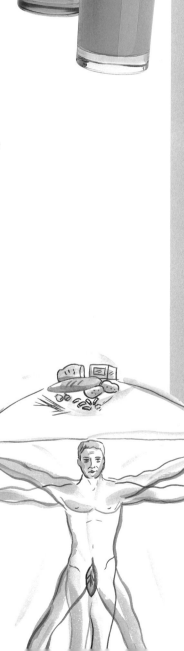

Food combining can transform your life for the better. It opens up new pathways by encouraging you to think more carefully about what you eat, why and how you are eating it, and its effects on your body. You will become healthier, fitter and happier with yourself as a result. It starts from the premise that – as Dr Herbert M. Shelton, one of the founding fathers of modern food combining recognized – 'the enzymes of the human digestive system are subject to certain restrictions. If we eat in such a way as to cause these limitations to be exceeded, we suffer digestive problems'. In the whole history of nutrition, few truer words have ever been written. Food combining puts an end to digestive problems by encouraging you to eat naturally. As you read on, you will discover that it is not a restrictive, unattractive diet. By the time you have finished this book, you will be agreeing with Shelton, that 'good food combining is no more than a way of observing these enzymatic restrictions, to the benefit of our health'.

FOOD COMBINING THEORY

Modern food combining came about largely through the work of two American doctors – William Howard Hay (1866–1940) and Herbert M. Shelton (1888–1987) – in the earlier part of the 20th century. Indeed, Hay's contribution is considered so important that food combining precepts are often referred to as the Hay Diet, and following them is known as 'Haying'. In fact, the idea goes back to at least the 1850s, when natural hygienists discovered that eating incompatible foods at the same meal could affect the digestion and absorption of valuable nutrients.

Many people suffer from acid indigestion, a distended stomach, wind (gas) in the intestines, flatulence, food allergies, obesity, constipation and other intestinal disorders. What never seems to occur to them is that one of the most likely causes of their problems is food – especially which foods they are eating together. But the food we eat, of course, is closely linked to the traditions and customs of the society in which we live. Everyone eats bread with cheese, meat with potatoes, rice with beans, a sweet dessert to finish, and perhaps a daily apple or orange. Only very recently, in circles devoted to dietetics and health for whom nutrition is the focus of attention, has food combining begun to receive the interest it deserves.

BELOW: Traditional meals can cause digestive disorders.

WHAT IS FOOD COMBINING?

Food combining means eating only foods that are suited to each other during any one meal. Some may object that this considerably restricts the choice of food, but this is a fallacious argument. All that is required, when putting together the menu for a meal, is to make choices guided by a knowledge of the anatomy and processes of the human digestive system.

Once you become familiar with the principles of food combining the choices will become so obvious and so natural to you that eating correctly will no longer require mental effort. The basic premise is to know (and preferably to

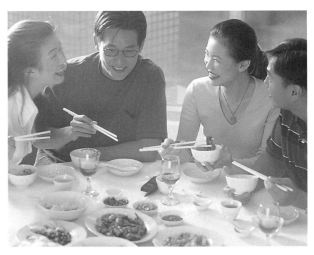

ABOVE: In food combining, compatible foods make up each meal.

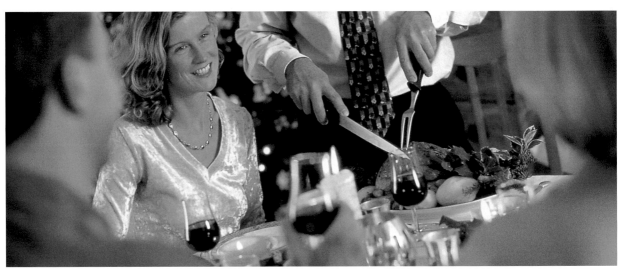

understand) why some foods can be eaten in combination with each other, and why some cannot. To achieve this, it is necessary to have some knowledge of the physiology and the process of digestion and of the chemical composition of foods. Gastroenterologists and nutritionists have a profound knowledge of these things, but anyone wanting to know how to food combine successfully should at least know how foods are classified. Some idea of these groups alone should be enough to achieve success. But it is necessary to master the principles of food combining as quickly as possible and interrupting meals to carry out calculations will itself cause indigestion. When sitting at the table, you should relax and not worry about what you are eating: it is too late, by then, to be anxious about whether the foods combine.

For that very reason, this book presents food combining in a simple and comprehensible form. The main dietary rules are easy to grasp and remember; initially, before the rules become mere second nature, there will be occasions when you may have to apply serious thought to the process – but that time will soon pass. The charts, diagrams, anecdotes and illustrations in the book should also prove helpful.

FOOD COMBINING VERSUS ORTHODOXY

The theory of food combining is not a recent innovation. In fact, Dr Howard Hay published the first book on the subject as early as 1939. In particular, Hay pointed out that a combination of high-protein and high-starch foods had appalling effects on the digestion. Between 1940 and 1950, his compatriot Dr Shelton carried out intensive research into combinations of specific foods, achieving some significant results and greatly increasing contemporary scientific knowledge of the digestive processes. Shelton discovered that different food combinations gave rise to excellent, good, problematic, or painful digestion, and he may, quite rightly, be regarded as the true pioneer of food combining. Indeed, he should be remembered as one of the most important nutritionists of all time, having published works on aspects of digestion in the 1920s and 1930s that remain classic textbooks today.

Given the work of Shelton, it is disappointing that the modern science of dietetics shows no interest in food combining. Today, medical literature is as full of references to dyspepsia caused by internal fermentation or toxic degradation (the breakdown of ingested food into substances that have some degree of toxicity) as it has ever been. In the opinion of most authorities, indigestion is seen primarily as a consequence of a reduced level of digestive enzymes, produced by the pancreas, in the small intestine. This means, generally speaking, that digestive discomfort is blamed on some form of deficiency in the digestive system itself, with no reference to possible deficiencies in the diet and the consequent result.

WHY THE EXPERTS DIFFER

That the experts hold a different view is not entirely surprising, nutritionists work empirically, judging their results on a statistical basis. Theories are not much to their liking, and even research has to be based on solid evidence. It is the results seen in real patients that count as scientific practice.

Both Hay and Shelton grounded their work on the information contained in a book by the Russian nutritional anatomist Ivan Pavlov, *The Operation of the Digestive Organs*, first published in 1902. Pavlov was the first to describe the physiology of the human digestive system in scientific detail.

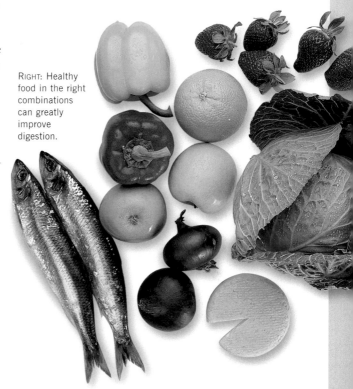

RIGHT: Healthy food in the right combinations can greatly improve digestion.

The basic principle formulated by Hay – the understanding that starch begins to ferment in the stomach once the salivary enzyme ptyalin is destroyed by gastric juice – (fundamental also to Shelton's work), is now regarded as less than scientific. The processes of the digestive system and the many enzymatic processes that contribute to it are now much better understood. If Hay and Shelton had been correct, every type of food would be indigestible: acids always surround the food in the stomach, whatever is consumed and in whatever combination.

It is certainly time for food combining to be studied in depth. The practice of harmonizing specific food types is incredibly important, and requires urgent attention. Dr Shelton, with the help of his patients, discovered quite a number of food combinations, only some of which were inaccurate. It is a pity that even the good ones were not always properly described – a failing that is directly responsible for the regrettable rejection of the whole theory until a few years ago by nutritionists, dieticians and the medical world in general.

DIETICIANS, DIETS AND DIETING

If you consult orthodox dieticians, the first thing that they are likely to do is weigh you and calculate whether you are over- or under-weight using a method called the body mass index. More often than not, they will then look at what you are eating, and how much you are eating, assuming that appropriate changes in diet and diet-related lifestyle will help to resolve your specific health problem. Often the temptation is not to take the trouble

ABOVE: Orthodox dieticians prefer to recommend changes to the diet.

to seek qualified, professional advice to sort out any dietary or diet-related problems. Instead, millions upon millions of people turn to so-called 'fad diets', which sometimes fly in the face of health commonsense and nutritional realities.

The Low Carb diet – a high protein, low carbohydrate diet, popular in the United States – is a good example, according to many dieticians. This particular diet revolves around cutting out or seriously cutting back on starchy dietary carbohydrates, such as bread, potatoes and pasta, and substantially increasing the amount of protein-rich food. General agreement among present-day nutritionists is that carbohydrates form an essential part of any healthy diet. They advise that around a third of the diet should consist of fruit and vegetables, starchy foods making up another third and the remaining third comprising other foods, including proteins. Indeed, official nutritional and dietary opinion is that there is too much high-protein food in the modern diet rather than too little. So-called 'mono-diets', such as the

FITNESS TIPS?

To start increasing your fitness level, try following these straightforward guidelines:

* Take the stairs, rather than the lift (elevator), and walk up escalators.
* Walk or cycle for short journeys, rather than relying on the car.
* Start off slowly, taking moderate exercise, rather than trying to do too much too quickly. Moderate exercise is defined as anything that raises the heartbeat, warms you up and makes you breathe more heavily than usual. You can increase the amount and type of exercise you are taking as you build up your stamina.
* Remember to do a few stretches before and after exercising. Warming up and cooling down correctly are as important a part of exercise as the exercise itself.
* Join a gym or exercise class with friends, family, children or work colleagues.
* If you are older, out of shape or suffering from medical problems, consult your doctor before starting any exercise routine or dietary regime.

cabbage soup diet, also come in for criticism. Weight loss on this type of diet can be substantial, but most of this is water, and the diet can cause nausea. The F-plan diet – the original high-fibre, low-fat eating plan – causes dehydration, because the body needs more water to soak up the extra fibre.

Even the staple orthodoxy of the body mass index is now under challenge. The British nutritionist Margaret Ashwell believes that the most important precept is where fat is stored in the body. Rather than looking at the ratio between height and weight, she has devised a system based on the ratio between height and waist measurements.

DIET, EXERCISE AND HEALTH

During the first week of any diet, the likelihood is that you will loose around 1.3 kg/3 lb of weight or more as a result of an initial loss of water from the body. Subsequently, it is healthier to aim for a steady weight loss of around 450 g/1 lb to 900 g/2 lb a week, which should come about largely through the loss of body fat.

Increasing calorie expenditure through regular exercise – you should start by aiming at three sessions a week, each lasting for 20 minutes or so – will also help to burn up fat, as well as toning the muscles and helping you to become generally fitter. The exercise does not have to be vigorous, but it is important to make it part of your lifestyle. Research studies show that people who are almost totally sedentary – that is, spend less than 30 minutes a week involved in physical activity – run almost twice the risk of premature heart disease. They also greatly increase their chances of suffering from many other diseases, from diabetes to colon cancer. Regular exercise, on the other hand, increases alertness, reduces tension, and by triggering the release of chemicals called endorphins by the brain, contributes to a feeling of wellbeing.

WHO WERE HAY AND SHELTON?

William Howard Hay was a conventional doctor who, the age of 41, found that he was suffering from Bright's disease (chronic inflammation of the kidneys), high blood pressure and a badly dilated heart. His colleagues advised him that the outlook was bleak but he analysed and changed his eating habits and as a result, his symptoms disappeared and he became healthier than he had ever been. Subsequent research led him to the conclusion that a balanced diet, eaten in the right combinations, was the key to good health. Building on

this discovery, he began to advise balancing the alkali to acid ratio of the body, and the regular and efficient elimination of waste food residues. This meant favouring vegetables, salads, most fruits and milk over all animal proteins, most nuts, all the carbohydrate foods and citrus fruits. Dr. Hay's dietary advice anticipated the views of the majority of nutritionists today. His recommendations were as follows:

THE HAY DIET

* Carbohydrates should never be eaten in combination with proteins and acidic fruits.
* Vegetables, salads and fruit should make up the bulk of the diet.
* Proteins, carbohydrates and fats should be eaten only in small amounts. Only wholegrain, unrefined carbohydrates should be used.
* Refined and processed foods should be avoided.
* There should be an interval of at least four hours between meals of different types of food.
* One meal a day should be based on starchy foods, another on protein foods, and the third should be alkaline, consisting of alkali, alkaline-forming and neutral foodstuffs.

Herbert M. Shelton ran a training college and clinic in San Antonio, Texas, from 1928 to 1981. Here, Shelton carried out intensive research into combinations of specific foods, resulting in the most comprehensive catalogue of data on the combination of foods yet available. Generally considered by food combining practitioners to be the undisputed guru of natural hygiene and food combining philosophy, Shelton's influence remains profound.

WHAT CAUSES INDIGESTION?

Indigestion is caused by excessive acid in the stomach and reflux into the oesophagus (the link between the stomach and the mouth), with heartburn and discomfort in the chest as the result. The overweight are particularly susceptible. Some foods are harder to digest, and particularly likely to trigger indigestion attacks. If you are susceptible, you should avoid:

* Alcohol, strong tea and coffee and fizzy drinks.
* Meat extracts, acidic foods such as pickles and vinegar, hot spicy foods and fried foods.
* Unripe fruits, which are rich in pectin (a substance that the stomach finds hard to digest), and cheese.

Other common triggers are stress, hurried meals, insufficient chewing, swallowing air, and long gaps between meals then bolting excessive quantities of food. The nicotine in tobacco can also spark off increased gastric acid secretion.

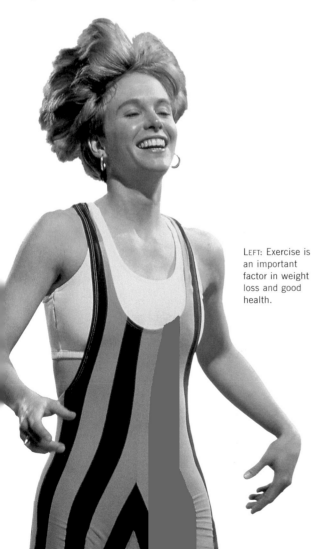

LEFT: Exercise is an important factor in weight loss and good health.

IDENTIFYING THE NUTRIENTS

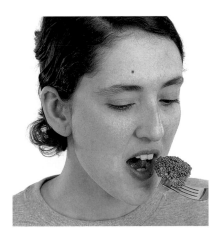

LEFT: Food combining recognizes five main nutrients.

Although food is composed of a number of substances, only five main nutrients are recognized in food combining: proteins, fats, sugars, starches and acids. The dominant nutrient out of the five in each food governs the whole digestive process: food combining shows you how to be sure that there is only one dominant nutrient in one whole meal. This avoids nutrients fighting one another, which upsets the digestive process, triggering problems such as indigestion, or worse.

Food is composed of proteins, fats, carbohydrates, vitamins, minerals, water, and a number of other factors such as roughage (dietary fibre), aromatic substances, enzymes, colourants and antioxidants. The digestive process is essentially one of analytical decomposition – that is, chemical breakdown into constituent elements – specifically into three true nutrients: proteins, fats and carbohydrates. Whether we eat an apple, a slice of bread or a steak, digestion breaks the food down into proteins, fats and carbohydrates. Protein is broken down further into amino acids, fat into fatty acids, and carbohydrate into simple sugars.

Even if only one type of food is consumed, digestion breaks down all three true nutrients simultaneously. It is completely understandable, then, that opponents of food combining are forever gleefully pointing out that Nature itself seems to cater for the simultaneous digestion of nutrients. The idea that this simultaneous digestion is Nature's way will be refuted in due course. The principle of food combining is quite simple, but other factors also play an important role. First, let us adopt a systematic approach.

THE FIVE NUTRIENTS

Carbohydrates fall into two groups: sugars and starches. The latter are actually complex sugars, which are, in their compound form, of no immediate use to the metabolism. First they have to be broken down into double sugars (disaccharides) and then into simple sugars (monosaccharides). Because complex, double and single sugars occur individually in a large number of foods, this book classifies simple and double sugars (including lactose) as 'sugars', and complex sugars as 'starches'. The total number of our nutrient groups is thus enlarged to four.

The fifth and last nutrient group comprises the acids. In food, the acids that affect digestion are free ('uncombined') acids, as opposed to bound ('conjugate') acids. The latter are released only during metabolism. Digestion converts the free acids into heat energy, and accordingly, they are regarded as nutrients. But these occur only in tiny amounts, and are normally discounted when calculating a food's calorific value.

In food combining, the following five nutrients represent our principal categories: proteins, fats, sugars, starches and acids, abbreviated where appropriate to P, F, Su, St and A. All foods contain these nutrients, in proportions that are specific to each particular food. The nutrient that is proportionately the greatest in quantity – the dominant nutrient – governs the entire digestive process. To eat different foods at random may result in the presence of more than one dominant nutrient, causing digestive disruption. Reaction between dominant nutrients may cause anything from a mild flush to serious digestive problems involving internal fermentation and gastroenteric poisoning.

NUTRIENT PROPORTIONS AND PROBLEM FOODS

Eating only one type of food (a monophagic diet) increases the overall intake of nutrients, although the proportions of the nutrients in relation to each other remains the same. The result would be identical if we were to eat several different foods of the same combinatory type. It is essential to know what the dominant nutrient is in every food that you eat. A number of nutrients can be digested during a single meal – on the condition that the proportions of nutrients mutually suit each other. These proportions are the key to food combining. Only one of the five nutrients can dominate in any one food. The crucial factor in compiling a menu for a meal is to be sure that there is only one dominant nutrient for it.

There are some foods, however, in which the dominant nutrient is not so obvious, and these present particular problems. Legumes are a classic example. Leguminous

THE FIVE NUTRIENT GROUPS

All food comprises one or more of five nutrients. It is vital to identify the dominant nutrient in a meal and to proportion accordingly.

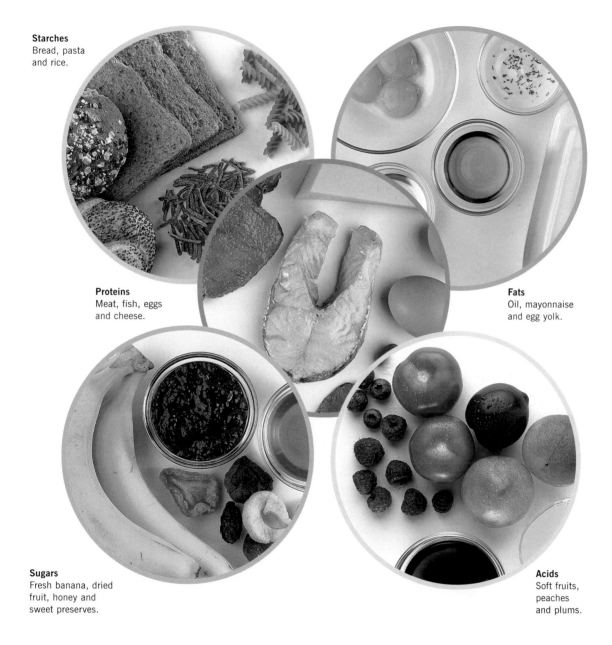

Starches
Bread, pasta
and rice.

Proteins
Meat, fish, eggs
and cheese.

Fats
Oil, mayonnaise
and egg yolk.

Sugars
Fresh banana, dried
fruit, honey and
sweet preserves.

Acids
Soft fruits,
peaches
and plums.

vegetables are remarkable in being dominated by both proteins and starches. This is, in fact, why they are so difficult to digest. Raw, they are indigestible and potentially toxic because of the fascine acid that they contain. Cooked, they tend to lie heavy on the stomach, and can cause some degree of flatulence. (The herb savory can reduce the flatulence slightly, but will not eradicate it all together). The protein-starch ratio is more favourable in cereals, but both cereals and legumes are agricultural products that were added to the menu of early humankind, although since then they have dominated human nutrition for more than 10,000 years because of their abundance and economic value.

19

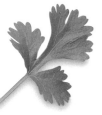

HERBS AND DIGESTIVE HEALTH

Many ancient civilizations had a keen grasp of which herbs could stimulate and improve digestion. Laxative herbs and herbs that could moderate diarrhoea, flatulence or colic were much in use. Today's recommendations by newspaper herbalists of fennel seed, anise or cumin to treat flatulence are but the latest in a tradition that goes back at least as far as the ancient Egyptians – and the Egyptians probably borrowed the idea from surrounding cultures. Similar traditions of digestive stimulation were current in the pre-Columban civilizations of South and Central America, albeit with a different selection of herbs. The conclusion is regrettably obvious. Humankind has been eating inappropriately for millennia, and has only now begun to learn about food combining.

ABOVE: Herbs have been used medicinally for centuries.

WHICH NUTRIENTS ARE DOMINANT?

The diagrams show the percentage of nutrients in some common foods. In each case, the dominant nutrient is immediately apparent. The lessons from this are obvious. If we were to eat a beef steak, some wholegrain rice, an

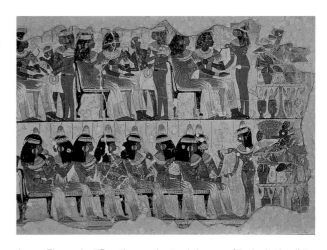

ABOVE: The ancient Egyptians understood the use of herbs in the diet.

avocado, a banana and a lemon during the same meal – actually a very presentable meal in terms of classic nutrition – we would be filling ourselves with five different dominant nutrients. No digestive system is capable of digesting such a meal properly.

The last diagram shows the dominant nutrients in the five foods. You can see at a glance how the various nutrients could fight each other, with indigestion and other digestive problems as the result.

BEEF STEAK

FAT: 4.5%

PROTEIN: 19%

STARCH: TRACE

In beef steak, the dominant nutrient is protein by a fair margin. The meat does not contain much fat, and there are just traces of the carbohydrates.

WHOLEGRAIN RICE

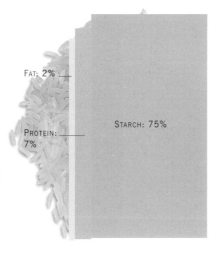

FAT: 2%

PROTEIN: 7%

STARCH: 75%

The dominant nutrient in wholegrain rice is starch. The same is true for all cereals and food products that include grain, such as bread, waffles and pasta.

AVOCADO

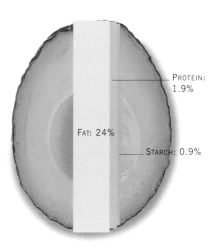

PROTEIN: 1.9%

FAT: 24%

STARCH: 0.9%

Avocado contains mainly fat, which is evidently the dominant nutrient.

CHICKPEAS (GARBANZO BEANS)

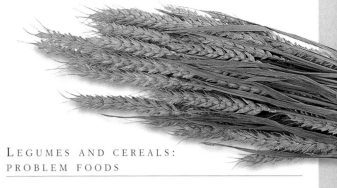

PERCENTAGES AND RATIOS

LEGUME	PROTEIN	FIBRE	STARCH	PROTEIN:STARCH RATIO
White beans	22%	1.8%	47.8%	1:2.2
Peas	23%	1.4%	60.7%	1:3.6
Chickpeas (garbanzo beans)	23.5%	3.4%	50.8%	1:2.1
Soy beans	36.8%	23.5%	23.5%	1:0.6

CEREAL	PROTEIN	FIBRE	STARCH	PROTEIN:STARCH RATIO
Millet	10.6%	3.9%	69%	1:6.5
Corn	9.2%	3.8%	65/2%	1:7
Barley	10.6%	2.1%	57.7%	1:5.4
Oats	12.6%	7.1%	61.2%	1:4.8
Rye	8.7%	1.7%	53.5%	1:6.1
Rice	7.4%	2.2%	74.5%	1:10

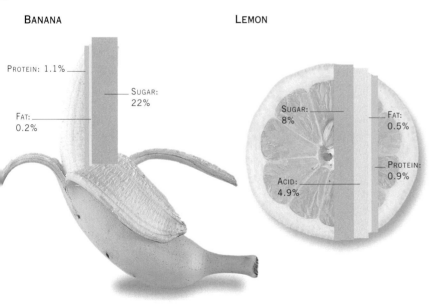

GRAINS ARE HIGH IN FIBRE.

LEGUMES AND CEREALS: PROBLEM FOODS

This table shows the percentages of Protein (P), Fibre (F) Starch (S) and Protein to Starch ratio (P:ST Ratio), in various legumes and cereals. In the legumes, there are two dominant nutrients, although in soy beans there are three. For this reason, legumes are always difficult to digest, whether eaten by themselves, or in a potentially-friendly combination. Although there are methods that can improve matters, digesting legumes requires a great deal of energy, so the final metabolic benefit is often not high either. In the percentages of nutrients in cereal products, starch is the dominant nutrient, although the protein content is relatively high – enough to hinder digestion. The chestnut is rich in starch, but is easier to digest because its protein-starch ratio, with 3.4 per cent protein against 41.2 per cent starch, is 1:12. The greater the P:St ratio, the better the food's digestibility.

BANANA

PROTEIN: 1.1%

SUGAR: 22%

FAT: 0.2%

Sugars manifestly dominate this food. The quantity of fats and protein in a banana is almost negligible.

LEMON

SUGAR: 8%

FAT: 0.5%

PROTEIN: 0.9%

ACID: 4.9%

Quantitatively, sugars are proportionately the highest nutrient in lemons. A level of 4.9 per cent acid is also very high, however. It is the acid of the fruit that has a decisive effect on the digestion – acid is the dominant nutrient.

THE DOMINANT NUTRIENTS

BEEF STEAK	PROTEIN
RICE	STARCH
AVOCADO	FAT
BANANA	SUGAR
LEMON	ACID

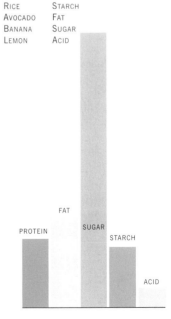

PROTEIN FAT SUGAR STARCH ACID

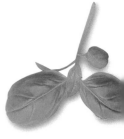

HELPFUL HERBS AND SPICES

In food combining, herbs and spices are versatile culinary additions that can live happily with proteins, starches, salads and all kinds of vegetable foods. Indeed, certain herbs are sometimes classed as vegetables: the seeds of others, when ground, are classified as spices. You can use herbs freely in cooking, because they are packed with health-giving properties. Spices, however, should be employed sparingly – in quantity, they are a source of stomach irritation, and can aggravate digestive disorders.

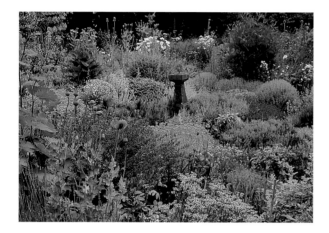

ABOVE: Use herbs freely in cooking as part of a balanced diet.

Making herbs an integral part of your diet is a sure way to boost health and wellbeing, although in purely nutritional terms the majority of herbs have relatively little value because they are consumed in such small amounts. You should also bear in mind that, despite their undoubted therapeutic properties, health experts counsel against using herbs in large quantities without obtaining proper guidance and advice. Use them regularly and in moderation as part of a properly-balanced, nutritious diet, and you will soon feel the benefits.

There are plenty of herbs to choose from, many of which you can grow for yourself. Many of the most popular culinary herbs can be grown in relatively little space. You can also combine herb plantings with those of flowers or other plants. Another alternative is to grow herbs in containers, which can be as small and basic as pots on the kitchen windowsill, or in a windowbox. As with all food, fresh is best, but to make sure that the herbs you need are available all the year round, it is

relatively easy to dry and store them. Once the drying process has been completed – it is important to start this as soon as you can after harvesting – the herbs can be stored for up to 18 months, as long as they are kept in airtight containers, out of the light. Leaves, flowers and seeds should be dried in a warm, dry, dark and well-ventilated area at a temperature of between 21°C/70°F and 33°C/91°F. If you are preserving herb roots, these need a higher temperature of between 50°C/122°F and 60°C/140°F.

HERBS FOR HEALTH

Humankind's knowledge of herbs goes at least as far back as the days of the ancient Egyptians, when priests practised herbal medicine widely as a matter of routine. There is even written evidence for this: the Ebers papyrus, which archaeologists have dated to 1500BC, lists hundreds of herbs and their uses, including many that are still common today. Other equally-ancient cultures similarly recognized the importance of herbs and their potential healing powers. In China, for instance, herbs have played an essential role in health care for thousands of years, and even today, their role in traditional Chinese medicine is of paramount importance. In India, too, herbs are an intrinsic part of Ayurvedic medicine, the origins of which go back to at least 2000BC. Herbs and their healing powers are mentioned in the *Rig Veda*, a sacred Hindu text dating from this time.

Herbs and spices are thought to aid the digestive system by stimulating the liver and gall bladder, helping to speed up the digestion, particularly of fats, and playing an important part in the elimination of harmful toxins. Specific herbs are said to have particularly useful properties. Basil, for example, is believed by herbalists and practitioners of traditional folk medicine to aid smooth digestion and ease stomach cramps. Bay, too, stimulates and aids digestion, as does chervil, and the seeds and leaves of fennel are thought to be useful in combating excessive wind (gas), nausea and vomiting. Mint, oregano, sage and rosemary are all reputed to be first-class digestive aids. Rosemary, in particular, is thought to help to soothe the digestive system and relieve symptoms of indigestion and flatulence, while sage is claimed to help in the digestion of rich, heavy foodstuffs. Parsley, for its part, is a particularly nutritious garnish, containing useful amounts of iron and Vitamin C.

COOKING WITH HERBS AND SPICES

Flavouring food with herbs or spices is probably as long-established as the art of cooking itself, as much for the flavour it brings as for reasons of health and wellbeing. Ideally when

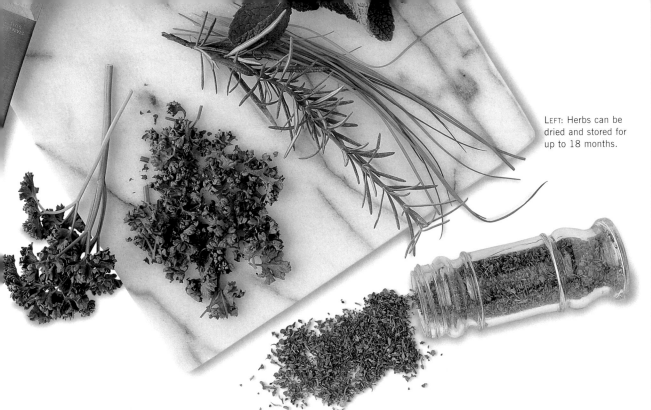

cooking with herbs, you should use the freshest varieties that you can. This is because the essential oils they contain, which are responsible for much of their savour, evaporate quickly once they have been harvested. Many of these oils are also powerful antiseptics, helping to protect the body against harmful bacteria and other micro-organisms, so it is sensible to protect as much of the content as possible. As far as spices are concerned, buy them whole and grind up as much as you need as you need it.

As you will see in many of the recipes later in this book, it is usually best to add herbs towards the end of cooking to be sure that they contribute to the perfect flavour and taste. Garlic, spices and tougher herbs, such as bay leaves, are exceptions to this rule. You should add these at the start of cooking to give their flavours a chance to permeate the food.

Adding herbs or spices to vinegars, oils or mustard can give an extra lift to dressings, garnishes and marinades. So, too, can adding salad herbs to green salads. Herbs such as dandelion, nettle, rocket (arugula) and sorrel all add appreciably to the taste. These and other salad herbs also make useful additions to soups and stews.

WISDOM FROM THE EAST

More than 700 prescriptions are commonly used by Chinese herbalists, drawing on a battery of more than 5500 herbs. The aim, as they see it, is to balance the opposing forces of *yin* and *yang* and to stimulate the flow of *qi*, the healing life energy, through the body's internal meridians, or energy channels. Similarly, ayurvedic medicine revolves around the forces of *prana*, *agni* and *soma*, which interact with the five elements and flow through energy centres in the body called chakras. Again, there is a collection of 5000 or more herbs for practitioners to draw on.

Korean or Chinese ginseng (*Panax ginseng*) has been used for centuries as a tonic by Chinese herbalists to boost the nerves and strengthen the immune system. Practitioners of traditional medicine call it an adaptogen; it affects people differently, depending on their individual needs. Taking ginseng will help to wake you up if you are tired, for instance, but will calm you down if you are tense and stressed. Siberian ginseng (*Eleutherococcus senticosus*) has similar properties.

BELOW: Fresh herbs and spices will give an extra 'lift' to your cooking.

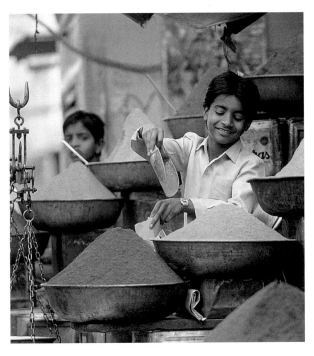

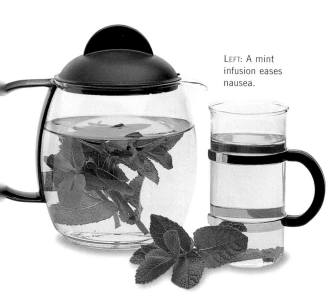

LEFT: A mint infusion eases nausea.

When you harvest herbs, you should collect only small amounts at a time and use or preserve them immediately. Always wear gardening gloves, as direct contact with some herbs can trigger an allergic skin reaction.

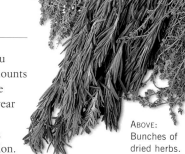

ABOVE: Bunches of dried herbs.

Leaves, flowers, fruits and seed heads should be shaken free of dirt and insects and not washed, but roots, bulbs, tubers and rhizomes should be washed thoroughly to remove soil and grit, and then drained preparatory to drying.

There are four drying methods – air-drying, freeze-drying, oven-drying and microwave-drying. Of these, air-drying is still the most widely-used preservation method. Make small bunches of herbs like thyme, rosemary and bay. Hang the bunches upside down, in a warm, well-ventilated place, until the leaves are dry and brittle. Take care not to over-do this, or the leaves will crumble when you try to remove them. Once they are dry, rub the leaves off the stems and pack them into airtight storage pots; this will avoid the risk of the dried herbs absorbing moisture from the air. Larger leaves, such as basil, and small flowers, should be laid flat on a piece of muslin (cheesecloth) spread over a cooling rack. Dill and fennel are best dried on the stem, with a paper bag tied over the seed-heads to catch the seeds as they ripen and fall.

Freeze-drying suits soft-leaved plants, such as basil, mint, chives and parsley. Pack sprigs of the herbs into labelled freezer bags and put the bags straight into the freezer. There is no need to thaw the herbs before you use them, as the leaves can be crumbled easily while still frozen. Another freezing method is to chop the herbs finely and pack them into an ice-cube tray, filled up with water and frozen. The frozen cubes can be added straight from the freezer to whatever you are cooking. Oven-drying is reserved for roots, bulbs and other underground plant parts that can tolerate a higher drying temperature. Microwave-drying is somewhat controversial because of the radiation involved in the process.

MAKING TEAS AND INFUSIONS

Food combining practitioners agree that herbal teas make a preferable alternative to ordinary tea and coffee, both of which, if relied on to excess, can have potentially damaging digestive effects. Coffee is also a potent migraine trigger. Infusions made from herb leaves and flowers are quick and simple to prepare: all you need to do is pour nearly boiling water over the herb, cover the brew and let it stand for five to ten minutes. Standard quantities are 75 g/3 oz/3 cups of fresh herb to 500 ml/18 fl oz/2¼ cups of water. If you use dried herbs, the amount goes down to 30 g/1¼ oz/¼ cup. You should also remember to take this into account while cooking – when a recipe specifies a tablespoon of fresh herbs, you will need only a teaspoon of dried ones, because their flavour is more concentrated. Infusions should always be drunk on the day they are made – they cannot be stored. Herb teas should not be mixed with milk.

POPULAR HERBAL TEAS AND THEIR EFFECTS

Chamomile
Relaxes and calms. It is believed to be helpful in relieving symptoms of anxiety and in dealing with insomnia. It is also good for any kind of digestive disorder, including stomach over-acidity, heartburn, wind (gas) and colic.

Elderflower
Eases catarrh and clears blocked or obstructed sinuses.

Fennel
May help to relieve indigestion and wind (gas), and ease bloating.

Mint
Eases nausea and lessens wind (gas).

Raspberry leaf
Soothes the digestive tract.

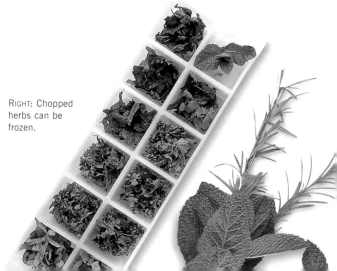

RIGHT: Chopped herbs can be frozen.

HERBS AND THEIR USES

ANGELICA
(*Angelica archangelica*)
Young angelica stalks are crystallized (candied) and used for decorating desserts and cakes: in Scandinavia, the foliage is eaten as a vegetable. Medicinally, the most useful part of the herb is the root, which should be dug up, dried and stored in the autumn (fall) of the first year of planting. Chinese angelica (*A. sinensis*) is an especially good tonic for women and, in China, is known as women's ginseng precisely for this reason. You can take angelica root as a tincture or decoction; chewing crystallized (candied) angelica is said to soothe the throat, warm the chest and stimulate the digestion.

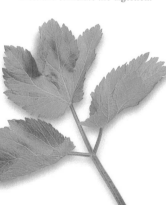

ABOVE: Angelica has many culinary and medicinal uses.

Other uses
In cooking, crystallized (candied) angelica can be used as a sweetener, as a healthier alternative to pure sugar. Note, though, that angelica should not be eaten by diabetics (it will increase the sugar level in the blood) or by pregnant women. Medicinally, decoctions or tinctures of angelica are said to relieve indigestion, strengthen a weak digestive system, and are also thought to help ease colic, cramping pains, coughs and poor circulation. The herb acts simultaneously as an antiseptic, diuretic and expectorant.

BASIL (*Ocimum basilicum*)
A restorative, warm, aromatic herb which herbalists believe improves digestion, lowers fever, relaxes spasms, calms the nervous system, and is an effective remedy against bacterial infections and intestinal parasites. Drinking basil tea may relieve nausea.

Other uses
In cooking, sweet-tasting basil leaves are used with tomatoes and form a part of many tomato-flavoured dishes, particularly in Italian cookery where they are a frequent ingredient in pasta sauces, such as pesto. Basil is also often used as a vegetable garnish and in soups and stuffing. The leaves of holy basil (*O. sanctum*), a different variety of the herb, can be added to salads and other cold dishes. Medicinally, basil is a well-known folk remedy for colds and flu, indigestion, nausea, sickness, abdominal cramps, gastroenteritis, migraine, sleeplessness and tiredness. Preparations of the herb can be applied to the skin to treat insect stings and bites, acne and other skin infections. Basil oil is used in insect repellents and some dental preparations.

ABOVE: Basil improves digestion and lowers fever.

BAY (*Laurus nobilis*)
Large, brittle bay leaves are harvested in summer and dried whole: they are an important cookery ingredient. Bay has long been regarded as a powerful antiseptic, and herbalists claim that it can relieve poor digestion, colic and wind (gas), and also stimulate lack of appetite. The essential oil is used to flavour condiments and meat products.

Other uses
In cooking, bay leaves are a widely-used flavouring for both savoury and sweet dishes, frequently added to casseroles, stews, soups, and sometimes to desserts. They are an essential part of *bouquet garni*, a classic mixed-herb seasoning widely used in French cooking to provide added flavour. Medicinally, bay can be used to stimulate and aid digestion, relieve symptoms of indigestion, and help the body to cope with related digestive problems such as wind (gas) and colic. Preparations of the leaves can be applied externally to treat dandruff, sprains and bruises, and are claimed to help to relieve the symptoms of rheumatism.

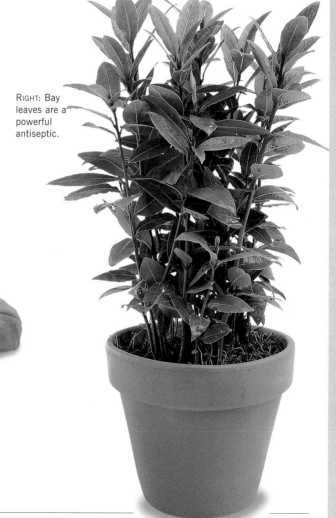

RIGHT: Bay leaves are a powerful antiseptic.

BORAGE (*Borago officinalis*)

A soothing, cooling herb that can be taken as a tisane to combat rheumatism and various respiratory infections. Its seeds are a rich source of gamma-linoleic acid, and herbal practitioners believe that the oils extracted from it can help to lower blood pressure and regulate hormone production. The leaves are gathered in spring and summer, when the plant starts to flower, and are used fresh as a salad ingredient or a garnish, or dried as the basis for infusions and liquid extracts.

Other uses

In cooking, fresh, chopped borage leaves can be added to salads, or following Italian practice, cooked as a vegetable. More frequently, they are added to long drinks as a flavouring. The flowers can be used as a garnish, although it should be noted that they turn pink on contact with acidic substances such as lemon juice and vinegar. Medicinally, borage can be used to relieve fevers, chest conditions and mouth and throat infections. Some practitioners suggest that it can treat dry skin and, used as an oil, relieve other skin complaints. It is also an ingredient in gargles, mouthwashes and eyewashes.

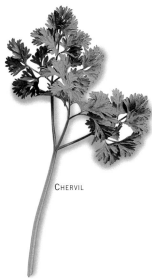

CHERVIL

CHERVIL (*Anthriscus cerefolium*)

Chervil leaves are bitter, aromatic and anise-flavoured: some people say that they taste something like parsley flavoured with a hint of aniseed (anise seed). They are a good cleansing tonic for the kidneys and liver, and generally help to stimulate the digestion. Because their delicate flavour does not withstand drying or prolonged cooking, it is best to use them fresh and raw in salads or as a garnish, or to add them to a dish just before serving it. If you do decide to try to preserve and store them, freeze-drying is a better method than air-drying.

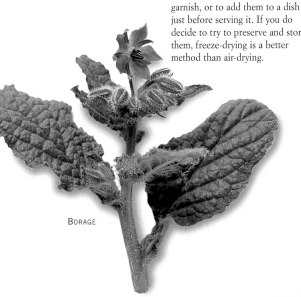

BORAGE

Other uses

In cooking, chervil is an essential ingredient of *fines herbes* and an important constituent of certain sauces. In French cookery, the leaves are often added to egg-, fish- and potato-based dishes: otherwise, sprigs or finely-chopped leaves are added to salads or used as a garnish. Medicinally, in addition to stimulating the digestion, it is thought that the herb has diuretic properties, helping to alleviate fluid retention and also relieves the symptoms of eczema, jaundice and rheumatism.

CHIVES (*Allium schoenoprasum*)

Chives are tiny, mild members of the onion family primarily cultivated for their culinary use. The leaves, bulbs and flowers of the herb are all used to add flavour to a whole medley of foods, ranging from potatoes and eggs to soups, salads and stews. Therapeutically, herbal practitioners believe that chives can ease the digestion and stimulate the recovery of the appetite with particular benefit to those recovering from illness.

Other uses

In cooking, the leaves and bulbs of chives are used to garnish and flavour soups, stews, salads, omelettes and certain sauces. The leaves are also used in some soft cheeses; the flowers can be sprinkled into and over salads as an edible garnish. Medicinally, chives encourage good digestion: Chinese chives (*A. tuberosum*), which taste of garlic as well as onion, have anti-emetic properties that improve kidney function. The chopped leaves and flower buds can be added to salads: the leaves are a frequent ingredient in Chinese cooking.

CHIVES

CORIANDER (CILANTRO)
(*Coriandrum sativum*)

Coriander (cilantro) leaves should be harvested when young and used fresh: coriander seeds are harvested when ripe and used whole or ground into a powder in cooking. Both the leaves and seeds, which have different aromas, are rich in essential oils that stimulate the workings of the digestive system, relieving indigestion and other digestive problems, at the same time encouraging the appetite. Both are used by herbalists to strengthen the urinary tract and in the treatment of urinary tract infections and disorders.

Other uses
Coriander (cilantro) is a culinary staple. In cooking, its pungent leaves are widely used to flavour food, especially in Middle Eastern and south-east Asian recipes. Coriander seeds are used as an ingredient in curries, pickling spices and Greek dishes, as a garnish, and in baking. Medicinally, coriander (cilantro) can help to relieve all kinds of minor digestive disorders: in traditional Chinese herbal medicine, it is also recommended as a possible countermeasure to food poisoning brought on by decaying matter in the gut. Eating small, fresh bunches of the leaves is said to be good for the stomach and the heart.

DANDELION
(*Taraxacum officinale*)
Dandelion is an extremely potent diuretic: it contains notably high levels of potassium, as well as beta carotene, calcium and useful amounts of iron. It is reckoned that a portion of dandelion leaves contains one and a half times the quantity of iron of an equivalent portion of spinach. Eaten young and fresh, the leaves, which have a slightly bitter flavour, make an enlivening addition to salad. Both leaves and roots are used commercially to flavour herbal beers and soft drinks (sodas), while the roots on their own are roasted and ground to make a caffeine-free coffee substitute.

Other uses
Fresh dandelion leaves can be eaten in salads: it is often the custom to blanch them before they are harvested to reduce their bitter taste slightly. You can do this by putting a flower pot upside down over the growing plant and leaving it in position for a week or so, until the leaves become white. Alternatively, dandelion leaves can be cooked like spinach; the culinary practice is to mix them with sorrel. Roots can be juiced or dried for use in teas, tinctures, decoctions and infusions. Medicinally, dandelion is said to improve liver function and the workings of the digestive system as a whole. It also has laxative and antirheumatic effects.

DILL (*Anethum graveolens*)
The leaves and seeds of this pungent, aromatic herb are widely used in cookery, especially in Scandinavian and Indian cuisine. Dill is said to calm and tone the digestive system: it relieves flatulence and is the major ingredient of the gripe water given to babies. It has been an important medicinal herb in the Middle East since biblical times.

Other uses
In cooking, sprigs of dill can be added to vinegars and pickles. In Scandinavia, chopped dill is a major ingredient of gravadlax, a form of preserved salmon. In India, dill seeds are a major constituent of curry powder. It is also widely used in soups, fish and shellfish dishes, and as a garnish, with potatoes. The oil extracted from the herb is used as an ingredient in food flavourings and patent medicines. Medicinally, dill helps to soothe indigestion and relieves colic and wind (gas).

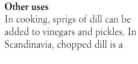

DANDELION

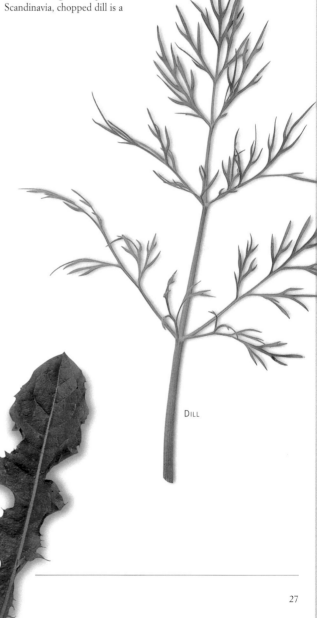

DILL

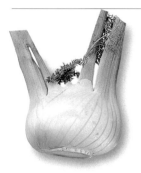

FENNEL (*Foeniculum vulgare*)

Fennel flavours vary according to strain and region: the home of sweet fennel is the Mediterranean area, while bitter or wild fennel comes from central Europe and Russia. The fronds – tasting of aniseed (anise seed) to a greater or lesser extent, depending on variety – and the seeds are widely used in cooking: the bulbous leaf bases of certain varieties can also be eaten raw in salads or cooked as a vegetable. Fennel is an aromatic, diuretic herb that relieves digestive disorders and promotes milk flow in nursing mothers. It is an antispasmodic and antidepressant.

Other uses

In cooking, fennel leaves are often added to sauces or used as stuffings for fish. The bulbous, delicately-flavoured leaf bases of the carosella and dulce varieties can be eaten raw as part of a salad, or cooked – often by roasting – and served on their own as an accompanying vegetable or added as a supporting ingredient in other dishes. The bruised or crushed seeds make a delicious herbal tea and are also used whole or ground as a food flavouring. Medicinally, both leaves and seeds aid good digestion, helping to soothe colic and bowel irritation and prevent excessive wind (gas), vomiting, nausea and sleeplessness. The oil extracted from the seeds is an ingredient of gripe water, used particularly for babies with wind (gas) or colic. When made into a mouthwash or gargle, fennel can help to alleviate gum infections and relieve sore throats. Fennel root is also said to have properties that help the body deal with urinary disorders.

FENUGREEK
Trigonella foenum-graecum)

Fenugreek is a bitter, pungent, warming herb. Its dried leaves are used as a flavouring for root vegetables in Indian and Middle Eastern cuisine: in India, the fresh leaves are also cooked as a vegetable curry. Medicinally, the herb is thought to promote good digestion, lower the level of sugar in the blood, soothe fever and, if you are breast-feeding, stimulate milk flow. It has laxative, diuretic and expectorant effects, and other powerful healing properties.

Other uses

In cooking, fenugreek seeds can be sprouted as a salad vegetable. Dried and ground seeds are used in curry powder, some spice mixtures, and pickles. They are also used as flavouring for bread, stews and fried foods, particularly in the Middle East. Medicinally, fenugreek will stimulate digestion and help to deal with digestive disorders and gastric inflammation. It features prominently in traditional Chinese and Ayurvedic medicine, where it is used to treat a multiplicity of complaints ranging from kidney-related disorders to arthritis, allergies and gout.

LEMON BALM
(*Melissa officinalis*)

Lemon balm contains a lemon-scented oil thought to have anti-viral properties, which means that teas made from the herb can be extremely good for you. In digestive terms, the herb has a soothing effect, which makes it particularly suitable for calming indigestion arising from nervous tension, and in children, excitability. The whole plant can be used fresh or dried, along with its leaves and oil.

Other uses

In cooking, fresh lemon balm leaves are used to add flavour to salads, soups, sauces, vinegars, fish dishes and game: dried leaves are a common constituent of pot-pourri and the stuffing in herb pillows. Medicinally, the herb is said to have a host of healing properties, including, as well as its digestive benefits, helping to relieve depression, anxiety, palpitations and tension headaches. Applied externally, the oil extracted from the herb can soothe herpes and other skin sores – including insect bites and stings – and relieve symptoms of gout.

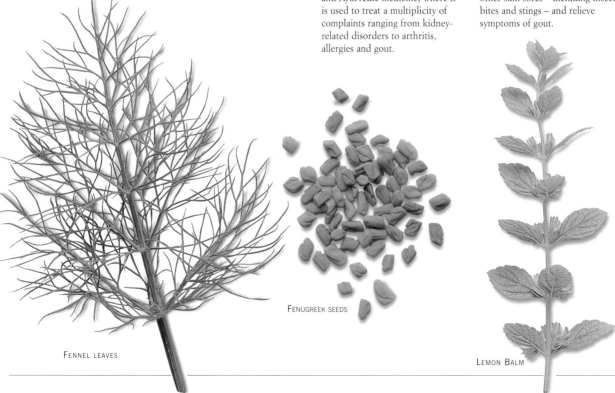

FENNEL LEAVES

FENUGREEK SEEDS

LEMON BALM

LEMON GRASS
(*Cymbopogon citratus*)

Lemon grass is one of a number of aromatic grasses: it gets its flavour from the citral it contains. The leaves and stems of the herb, which is bitter, aromatic and cooling, are used medicinally and in cooking. Medicinally, lemon grass relieves spasms and helps to soothe fever by increasing sweating; external application of its extracts can be used to treat various bacterial, fungal and parasitic skin and scalp conditions. Lemon grass oil derived from East Indian lemon grass (*C. flexuosus*) is used in food flavouring.

Other uses

In cooking, the use of lemon grass has spread from South-east Asia – particularly Thailand – into contemporary Western cookery. In Thai cuisine, the base of the plant's leaves is used fresh or as dried *sereh* powder in meat and fish dishes. An infusion of the leaves makes a good herbal tea. Medicinally, lemon grass is said to relieve digestive problems, particularly in children, and to help in the relief of minor fevers.

LEMON VERBENA
(*Aloysia triphylla*)

Lemon verbena is an astringent, aromatic herb, particularly rich in essential oils. Its leaves, which are harvested in summer, are used fresh, mainly for their oils and to make food flavouring. They are also used dried in infusions and pot pourri. In health terms, the herb has a mildly sedative effect, which makes it especially useful in relieving digestive spasms and lowering fever.

Other uses

Cooks use the fresh leaves to flavour salads and stuffings. Medicinally, it is said to relieve the symptoms of feverish colds and indigestion. Aromatherapists use its essential oils in their treatment of digestive and nervous problems, and for helping to heal skin complaints such as acne and boils.

LOVAGE (*Levisticum*)

Lovage (*L. officinale*), otherwise known as love parsley, is a pungent, bitter-sweet, aromatic herb, with a taste resembling that of celery and yeast extract. Leaves, stems, roots, seeds and oil can all be utilized – the stalks should be harvested in the spring, when they are tender and succulent. Scots lovage (*Ligusticum scoticum*), which also tastes strongly of celery, comes from a different herb family.

Other uses

The young shoots of love parsley can be blanched and eaten as a vegetable: the leaves can be used as additions to soups, salads, stews and savoury dishes. Its seeds can be added to bread and biscuits (cookies). The young leaves and stalks of Scots lovage can be eaten raw or cooked in a similar fashion. Medicinally, herbalists claim that lovage can help to cure indigestion, colic and wind (gas). Similarly, Scots lovage can help to ease digestive problems as well as uterine disorders. Its ground seeds can also be used as a condiment.

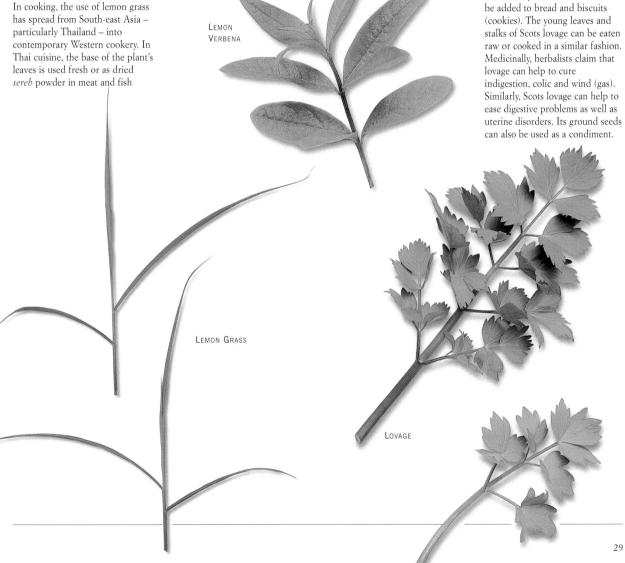

LEMON
VERBENA

LEMON GRASS

LOVAGE

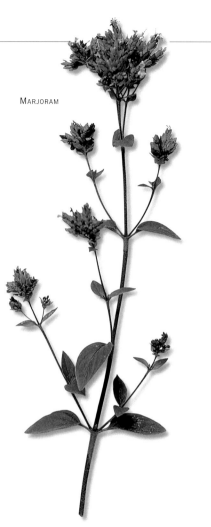

MARJORAM

MINT

MINT (Mentha)

The mint family includes many species, such as spearmint (*M. spicata*), peppermint (*M. x piperita*) and gingermint (*M. x gracilis*), which can be used fresh in fruit salads. Spearmint and peppermint are the most popular flavours. All mints contain menthol, which has antiseptic, decongestant and analgesic properties. Both spearmint and peppermint are reputed to improve the digestion: peppermint, in particular, is said to be good for the lower bowel. As well as aiding digestion, a hot infusion of mint can help to relieve symptoms at the start of a cold.

Other uses

In cooking, spearmint is the basis of mint sauce and mint jelly. It is also used as a garnish, for flavouring, and in herb teas. Medicinally, it can relieve indigestion, wind (gas), hiccups and colic. Peppermint leaves are used in salads, as a decorative constituent of iced drinks, and to make herbal tea. Medicinally, this variety of the herb is thought to ease many complaints, including indigestion, gastroenteritis, colic and irritable bowel syndrome. The oil extracted from the plant features frequently as an ingredient

in antacid preparations and mouthwashes, and is also used as a flavouring in ice cream and in other confectionery.

PARSLEY
(*Petroselinum crispum*)

Parsley is one of the few herbs that has noteworthy nutritional properties: it contains useful amounts of Vitamin C, Vitamin A and iron. It also contains a flavonoid, apigenin, which is an effective antioxidant, and helps to reduce allergic responses. It is a bitter, aromatic, diuretic herb: plain or flat leaf varieties have a stronger flavour than curly leaf cultivars. Too much parsley can be problematic in certain instances, although the small amounts used in cooking are harmless; for this reason, the herb is best avoided by pregnant women and sufferers of kidney disease.

Other uses

Parsley leaves are used as a garnish for salads and vegetables, particularly potatoes, and to flavour sauces, dressings, butter, stuffings and savoury dishes, especially fish. In digestive terms, parsley helps to promote good digestion, although to relieve indigestion it would be necessary to drink a decoction or infusion made from parsley roots or seeds. Chewed fresh, the leaves can help to clear bad breath.

MARJORAM (*Origanum*)

Marjoram is otherwise known as oregano. Its various varieties are used mainly as culinary herbs. They are rich in flavonoids and essential oils, such as carvacrol and thymol, all of which have helpful healing qualities, particularly for the digestion. Wild marjoram (*O. vulgare*) is a pungent, aromatic herb which features prominently in Italian, French, Greek and Mexican cooking. As well as using the fresh leaves, the plant can be dried for both culinary and therapeutic uses. Sweet marjoram (*O. majorana*) has a more delicate flavour; cooks prefer to use it fresh and add it towards the end of cooking. In addition to the leaves, its seeds are dried and used in condiments and meat products.

Other uses

Wild marjoram features in many strongly-flavoured dishes – other ingredients usually include garlic, tomatoes, chilli, onion and wine. Medicinally, it is good for wind (gas) and stomach upsets and indigestion: if you are pregnant, however, all varieties of the herb should be avoided. Flowers and sprigs of sweet marjoram feature heavily in meat dishes, soups, tomato and other pasta sauces. It is also a popular oil and vinegar flavouring. Sweet marjoram is also good for soothing minor digestive upsets and used as an infusion it helps the body to deal with a range of other health problems, from bronchial complaints and tension headaches to sleeplessness and anxiety attacks.

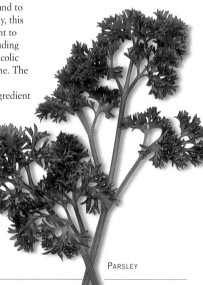

PARSLEY

ROSEMARY
(*Rosmarinus officinalis*)
Rosemary has an attractive, pervasive scent: it is almost impossible to pass by a rosemary bush without pinching a few leaves and rubbing them gently between the fingers to release their smell. Rich in antiseptic and anti-inflammatory flavonoids and phenolic acids, it is reputed to be helpful in dealing with the problems of poor digestion, and in alleviating the effects of gall bladder inflammation and gall stones and the headaches often associated with gastric upsets. In cooking, its use is widespread.

Other uses
Rosemary leaves, fresh or dried, are widely used to flavour meat, particularly lamb, and in Italian cuisine, chicken and kid. It is also used to give soups and stews added savour. Although they impart flavour, the leaves taste bitter and resinous, and should be chopped finely before you use

them, or used as sprigs that can be removed before food is served. Steeping rosemary sprigs in vinegar, olive oil or wine gives these liquids an added bite that can be employed to good effect in sauces and dressings. In health terms, rosemary is said to relieve digestive problems, especially those associated with anxiety: it will help to soothe an upset digestive system, relieving indigestion, flatulence and wind (gas). Drinking a weak infusion of the herb may help to relieve headaches, cold symptoms and neuralgia. Its antiseptic properties also make it a good throat gargle.

SAGE (*Salvia*)
In herbal folklore, sage has the reputation of promoting long life – one cup of sage tea a day is said to help maintain health in old age. There are many varieties of the herb, but the ones used most commonly in cooking are common sage (*S. officinalis*), red-topped sage (*S. viridis*) and pineapple sage (*S. elegans*), the leaves of which are used, fresh or dried, to flavour pork and other foods. The herb is thought to help the digestion work smoothly and to aid the recovery of a lost appetite.

Other uses
In Italian cooking, the leaves of common sage are an essential ingredient in authentic saltimbocca and in many liver dishes; elsewhere in Europe, they feature in cheese, sausages, as a garnish for eel, and in traditional pork and goose stuffings. Sprigs of pineapple sage can be added to cold drinks and fruit salads. According to herbal practitioners, the most appropriate use of sage is to help to make rich, heavy food more digestible. It can also help to relieve wind (gas) and combat liver complaints. Taken as a gargle, sage can ease sore throats; in the form of a tea, it will relieve attacks of indigestion.

SAVORY (*Satureja*)
Rich in essential oils, including carvacrol and thymol (which vary in their proportions from variety to variety), savory smells much the same as marjoram and thyme. Summer savory (*S. hortensis*) has been used as a food flavouring for more than 2000 years: the leaves and flowering tops of the herb can both be eaten. Winter savory (*S. montana*) can be used in the same way as its summer relative, but in this variety, the leaves and shoots of the plant are the edible parts. All varieties of savory are antiseptic, astringent and, with the exception of thyme-leaved savory (*S. thymbra*), peppery in taste. As you would expect, thyme-leaved savory tastes like thyme. The leaves of creeping savory (*S. spicigera*) are more strongly-flavoured than those of summer savory.

Other uses
In cooking, the leaves of summer savory are used to flavour pulses, sausages, stuffings and various meat dishes. They also form an essential constituent of *herbes de Provence*. Thyme-leaved savory is used in savoury breads, and to flavour meat and pulse dishes. As an infusion, its leaves can relieve digestive discomfort and clear chest congestion. Winter savory, too, is often taken in cordial form for gastric complaints. Summer savory is said to boost the digestive system as a whole, as well as helping it to cope with indigestion and other digestive disorders.

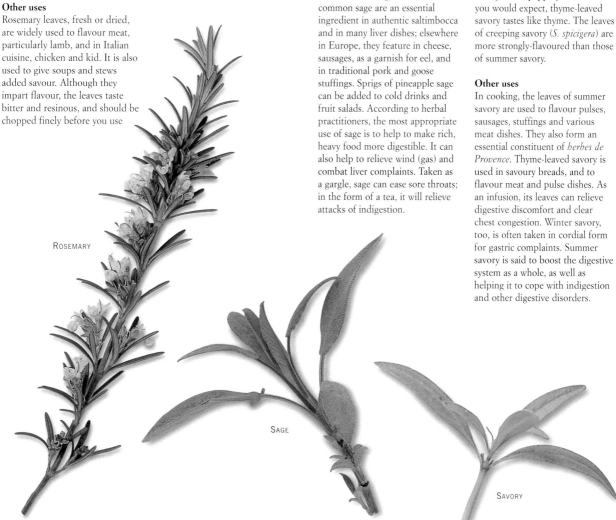

ROSEMARY

SAGE

SAVORY

SHISO (*Perilla frutescens*)

Shiso is popularly known as the beefsteak plant. Its green and purple leaves, which are used in cooking, contain a volatile oil, perillaldehyde, which is anything up to eight times sweeter than saccharin and 2000 times as sweet as natural sugar. The herb has featured in Chinese medicine since at least AD500: its stems are a traditional Chinese remedy for morning sickness.

Other uses

Shiso is a common ingredient in Japanese cooking, and its use has spread slowly to the West as cooks outside Japan become influenced by the country's culinary traditions. Shiso leaves – fresh or dried – are used to flavour raw fish, tempura, bean curd and pickles. The oil extracted from the leaves is used in many products, including sauces. Medicinally, shiso is used by complementary health practitioners to treat stomach pain, nausea, food poisoning and allergic reactions, especially those caused by allergens in shellfish. Decoctions made from the ripe, dried seeds of the herb are said to relieve constipation and its discomforts.

SHISO

TARRAGON/MUGWORT (*Artemisia*)

Tarragon is a member of the wormwood family, which includes some of the bitterest herbs known. French tarragon (*A. dracunculus*), often called estragon, is one of only two varieties that feature in cooking – the other is mugwort (*A. vulgaris*). There are frequent mentions of mugwort in classical literature: according to Roman tradition, it was planted deliberately alongside the roads that the Romans built so that legionnaires on long, forced marches could pick it and put it in their sandals to soothe their sore feet. Medicinally, French tarragon improves poor digestion and mugwort is thought to be an effective digestive tonic. In Chinese medicine, compressed dry mugwort leaf – moxa – plays a prominent part in acupuncture, and also has significant uses in Ayurvedic medicine.

TARRAGON

Other uses

In cooking, the leaves of French tarragon are used to flavour chicken and egg dishes, as well as in mustard, sauces and salad oils. Aromatherapists believe that the essential oils extracted from the herb can treat digestive and menstrual problems. Mugwort features in traditional recipes for carp and eel dishes in Germany, the UK and Spain: it is more commonly used in stuffings for duck, geese, pork and game. Medicinally, the herb relieves loss of appetite, and is said to be effective in easing dyspepsia.

THYME (*Thymus*)

Although thymes vary in their scents, the majority of them can be used to flavour food: the varieties most frequently used for this purpose are common thyme (*T. vulgaris*), lemon thyme (*T. x citriodorus*) and their cultivars. All varieties are rich in essential oils, which mainly consist of thymol. This is a powerful antiseptic. Lemon thyme, as the name implies, has a strong lemon scent; common thyme is similarly aromatic. Thyme is an essential ingredient of *bouquet garni* and features in the recipes of many classic French dishes. Ideally, slow cooking is required if its full flavour is to be retained.

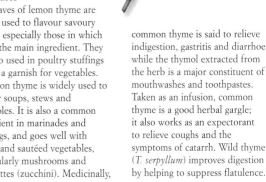
THYME

Other uses

The leaves of lemon thyme are widely used to flavour savoury dishes, especially those in which fish is the main ingredient. They are also used in poultry stuffings and as a garnish for vegetables. Common thyme is widely used to flavour soups, stews and casseroles. It is also a common ingredient in marinades and stuffings, and goes well with baked and sautéed vegetables, particularly mushrooms and courgettes (zucchini). Medicinally, common thyme is said to relieve indigestion, gastritis and diarrhoea, while the thymol extracted from the herb is a major constituent of mouthwashes and toothpastes. Taken as an infusion, common thyme is a good herbal gargle; it also works as an expectorant to relieve coughs and the symptoms of catarrh. Wild thyme (*T. serpyllum*) improves digestion by helping to suppress flatulence.

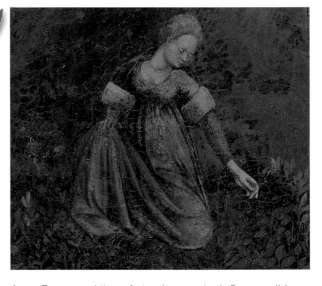
ABOVE: Tarragon and thyme feature in many classic European dishes.

SPICES AND THEIR USES

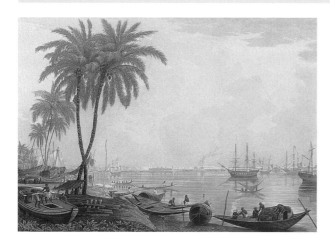

ABOVE: Allspice continues to be an important export from Jamaica.

ALLSPICE (*Pimenta dioica*)

Pungently aromatic allspice was given its name by the English botanist John Ray (1627-1705), who likened the flavour of its berries to that of a mixture of nutmeg, cinnamon and cloves. The spice is an important crop on the Caribbean island of Jamaica – hence its alternative name of Jamaica pepper. The only part of the spice used in cooking is its dark brown, unripened berries, although the fresh leaves can be used to make infusions. The fruits are also distilled to extract their oil, which is used as a commercial food flavouring.

Other uses

The dried berries, which are harvested when fully grown but before they ripen, are used whole in pickling spices and marinades. Ground, they add flavour to cakes, biscuits (cookies), puddings and chutneys. Medicinally, allspice eases indigestion, wind (gas) and diarrhoea. The powdered berries are often mixed with orthodox medicines in an attempt to make them more palatable.

CAYENNE (*Capsicum annuum var. annuum*)

Cayenne is one of the many members of the capsicum family. Some of these peppers, such as varieties of pimento, are sweet, while others, such as chillies, are extremely hot and spicy. This heated spiciness is caused by the presence of capsaicin, a bitter, acrid alkaloid, in some cultivars; capsicums lacking this alkaloid produce sweet fruit. All varieties of capsicum are rich in Vitamin C, while the pungent-fruited cultivars also have strong tonic and antiseptic properties.

Other uses

The ripe fruits of hot capsicums are dried to make cayenne and chilli powder. Paprika, which is mild in flavour, comes from the sweet red pepper varieties. The fruits themselves can be used fresh, dried, raw, cooked or pickled. Raw capsicums can be added to salads and used as garnishes; the sweet varieties rather than the hot ones are more often cooked and served as vegetables. Hot capsicums also feature in many hot pickles and

CAYENNE

chutneys and are the staples of a variety of cuisines, including those of Mexico and Central and South America, India, and South-east Asia. Some of the hottest capsicums come from the Caribbean where they are a features of traditional cooking. Medicinally, they are said to stimulate the circulation, help the body to deal with chills, and improve digestion, particularly in the elderly.

BELOW: The dried capsicum fruits are ground to make cayenne powder.

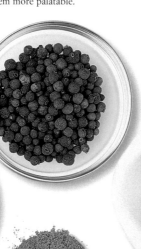

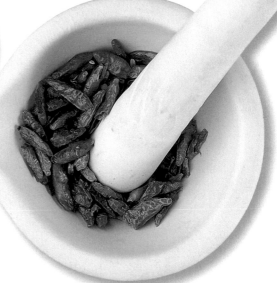

ABOVE: For culinary use the dried berries of allspice are used whole and ground. In medicine they are powdered.

CINNAMON (*Cinnamomum*)

Chinese cinnamon (*C. cassia*) is one of the oldest spices known to humanity: in China, records showing its use go back as far as 2700BC. The powdered cinnamon that comes from its inner bark is an important food flavouring. It is a pungent, sweet, hot spice, said to stimulate and improve the overall digestion. Commercially, the variety usually used in the global food industry is Ceylon cinnamon (*C. zeylanicum*). The bark and bark oil this provides is widely used to flavour meat products, baked foods, colas, pickles and ice cream. Like Chinese cinnamon, its medicinal properties improve the workings of the digestive system.

Other uses

Chinese cinnamon is used throughout western Asia to flavour curries; in South-east Asia, the equivalent is wild cinnamon (*C. iners*). In China, it is classed as one of the classic five spices – the others are anise, star anise, cloves and fennel seeds. It is used in Chinese cooking in combination with these other spices for flavouring a variety of dishes, particularly meat. Medicinally, Western herbalists believe that it combats diarrhoea, dyspepsia, flatulence and colic. In Chinese medicine, it is prescribed for poor appetite, diarrhoea and digestive complaints that are related to colds and chills.

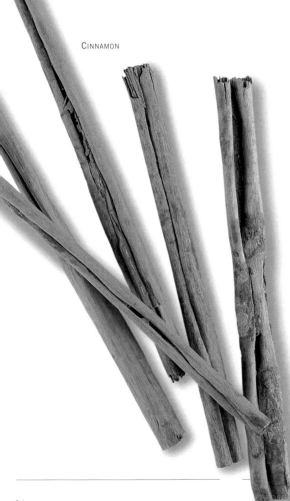

CINNAMON

CUMIN (*Cuminum cyminum*)

Since biblical times, cumin has been used widely in the Middle East and Asia: the pungent, somewhat bitter flavour of its seeds makes it an essential ingredient of curries and many other spicy dishes. Cumin is aromatic and astringent: medicinally, its properties benefit the digestive system as a whole.

Other uses

The seeds are the only part of cumin used in cooking, where they can be used whole or ground, or distilled commercially as an oil. In India, they are an important constituent of the spice mixture garam masala, and are used in couscous in North Africa and the Near East. Roasted, they add flavour to lamb-based Middle and Near Eastern dishes, and to side dishes of cucumber and yogurt. Medicinally, cumin is good for treating minor digestive complaints and in dealing with digestively-triggered migraine attacks. The spice is used in Ayurvedic medicine to promote proper liver function.

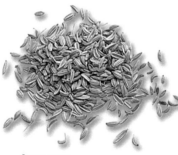

CUMIN SEEDS

GINGER (*Zingiber officinale*)

In the Ayurvedic health tradition, ginger is known as *vishwabhesaj*, or 'universal medicine', and its medicinal use is certainly widespread throughout India and China. In cooking, it is used across the world as a flavouring, and is prized for its sweet, pungent, aromatic and warming properties. The key part of the plant is the rhizome, which can be used fresh, preserved in syrup and crystallized (candied), or dried and ground to a powder for cooking, decoctions, tinctures and infusions. The spice aids digestion and is a popular folk remedy for nausea, particularly for travel and morning sickness. In natural medicine, it is used to protect against digestive disorders and to ease flatulence and abdominal pains.

Other uses

When fresh and young, ginger rhizomes are known as green ginger. They can be eaten raw, preserved and crystallized (candied), or used to flavour curries, chutneys, pickles, soups, meat and fishes dishes, and in marinades. Dried, ground ginger is used to flavour cakes, biscuits (cookies) and various sauces, while in Japanese cookery, pickled ginger – the Japanese call this *gari* – is used as a sushi flavouring. Medicinally, ginger is good for indigestion, colic and abdominal chills, although if you are suffering from a gastric ulcer of any description you should avoid it. In Chinese medicine, dried ginger root is used to treat digestive disturbances that stem from a reduction in spleen energy.

GINGER ROOT

ENGLISH (HOT)
MUSTARD

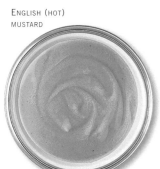

MUSTARD (*Brassica*)

Mustard's use as a condiment dates back to at least 400BC. It is a pungent, warming spice that, medicinally, is said to stimulate both the digestive and circulatory systems. In large quantities, it is a potent emetic. There are various varieties – black (*B. nigra*), white (*Sinapis alba*) and brown (*B. juncea*). Black mustard seeds are hotter than white ones. Commercially, American mustard is made from ground white seeds, English (hot) mustard uses a mixture of black and white, and French mustard is based on brown seeds. Mustard leaves and flowers can also be used in cooking.

Other uses

If you are making mustard yourself, you should always mix the ground seeds with cold water to release their full pungency. If you use hot water, or add vinegar or salt to the mixture, the mustard that results, although milder, will taste bitter. The young leaves and flowers of black mustard give an added pungency to salads; the seeds, used whole, are an ingredient of some curries and pickles. The young leaves of brown mustard can be cooked and served as a vegetable, and like black mustard, whole seeds give savour to curries and pickles – although in this instance, recipes usually call for them to be fried before use, to lessen their pungency. Medicinally, mustard features prominently in traditional folk medicine as a cure-all for rheumatism, chilblains, colds and other respiratory

infections: it can be applied in poultices, plasters and as a foot bath. The last is said to ward off flu and relieve headaches. However, it should be remembered that prolonged contact with mustard can lead to the formation of skin blisters and discomfort, especially if you have sensitive skin.

PEPPER (*Piper nigrum*)

One of the most valuable of all spices, the majority of peppers are grown for their fruits, but only *P. nigrum* is universally used in cooking. The dried, unripened fruit of tailed pepper (*P. cubeba*) features in Indonesian cuisine, while fruit clusters of Indian long pepper (*P. longum*) are used whole in curries and in the preparation of some hot pickles. Medicinally, pepper features in traditional Western medicine, Ayurvedic practice, and in Chinese medicine.

Other uses

Fruits of *P. nigrum* vary in colour depending on when they are harvested and how they are treated afterwards. If unripe, fresh and pickled, the result is green peppercorns; if dried, they become green and black peppercorns; if left until ripe and then rested for a week before drying, they become white peppercorns. Black and white peppercorns give flavour to a whole range of savoury dishes, meats, sauces, dressings, pickles and food coatings. Green peppercorns are used in creamy sauces, and dried to flavour stocks, soups and casseroles. Medicinally, pepper is regarded as a good treatment for indigestion and wind (gas) by Western herbalists. Chinese practitioners use it to deal with stomach chills and food poisoning and in Ayurvedic medicine pepper has a similar place and is used in the same way.

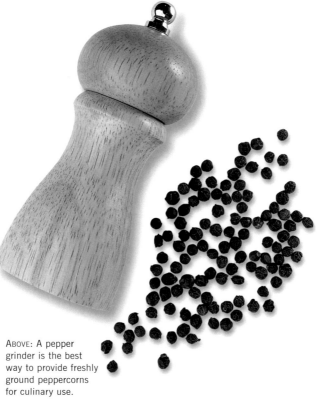

ABOVE: A pepper grinder is the best way to provide freshly ground peppercorns for culinary use.

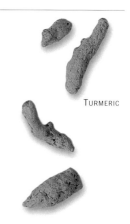

TURMERIC

TURMERIC (*Curcuma longa*)

Turmeric is one of the most popular food flavourings and colourings in Asian cooking. It is a pungent, bitter, astringent spice, which is a deep yellow colour when dried and ground. Commercially, it is a source of orange and yellow fabric dyes for wool and silk; medicinally, it is regarded as a liver tonic and helps to provide relief from digestive problems. It improves the circulation, too, and possesses marked anti-inflammatory and antibacterial properties. Wild turmeric (*C. aromatica*) is known in traditional Chinese medicine as *yu jin*. This, too, improves the digestion when taken medicinally, but it is not used in cooking.

Other uses

Turmeric's rhizomes are the useful part of the plant: they are lifted while the turmeric is dormant and then either boiled or steamed before being dried and ground into powder. In Indian cooking, turmeric is an essential ingredient of curry powder and curries. Medicinally, it is said to relieve digestive disorders and skin complaints, as well as boosting the circulation. It is also believed to help in cases of jaundice, liver complaints, menstrual problems, and combined with other herbs, in diabetes. Mango ginger (*C. amada*), another Indian variety of turmeric, can be eaten pickled or crystallized (candied).

DRINKS AND PROCESSED FOODS

Although water has no direct effects on food combining, it is important that you drink enough to be sure of good nutritional health. To meet the official recommendations, you need to drink at least 2 litres/3½pints/8¾ cups a day – less than this, and you may become dehydrated, lacking the liquid needed by the body to release the energy locked inside its cells. You must also watch your intake of processed foods, because the processes involved in their manufacture may alter their nutrient balance for the worse.

Books on nutrition often suggest that water is significant to the digestive process. Some also believe that roughage (dietary fibre) has a significant role. Water is indeed a very important constituent of the human body with a multitude of functions, yet it has no direct influence on food combining. Foods rich in water – such as fruits, berries, gourds and other vegetables, and milk – are easily digested in comparison with concentrated food sources, such as nuts, seeds, cereals, cheese and sausages. But the amount of nutrients available for digestion in watery foods is naturally much lower.

The Brazil nut, for example, has a very favourable protein-fat-sugar-starch ratio, and can be digested without any problems. 100 g/3½oz/scant 1 cup of Brazil nuts may seem a small quantity of food, but nuts are highly concentrated. The calorific value of this quantity of Brazil nuts is as much as that of 5 kg/11 lb – or 50 times the quantity – of papaya. Food rich in water is in general easier to digest precisely because it contains only a small volume of nutrients. Much less energy is, therefore, required to release the nutrients.

Water has a favourable influence on digestion (the acid-base balance), but not on food combining, although this does not apply to all foods rich in water. After all, meat and fish also have a high water content.

FIBRE AND ROUGHAGE

Much the same is true of roughage, which, properly defined, is the indigestible remains of foods that are capable of swelling in the presence of liquids, and are sticky and glutinous. Roughage – to which plant fibres such as cellulose, pectin, and a number of other substances belong – is inert in the digestive processes of the stomach and small intestines. In the large intestine, however, it swells so as to occupy the complete cross-section of the alimentary canal, and, thanks to its stickiness, defecation can occur easily and smoothly.

Important as it may be for this purpose, roughage does not influence food combining. However, some roughage should always be a significant presence in the diet in order to maintain defecatory regularity.

PROCESSED FOODS

The processing of foods may change the proportions of the nutrients within them – sometimes for the better, sometimes for the worse. Rice has a protein-starch ratio of 1:10. During

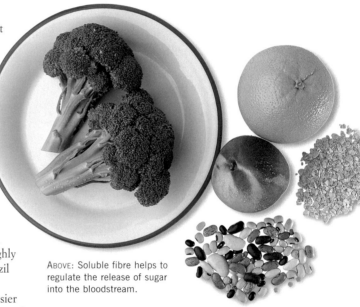

ABOVE: Soluble fibre helps to regulate the release of sugar into the bloodstream.

WHY FIBRE IS GOOD FOR YOU

Although dietary fibre has no direct effect on food combining, it is an essential constituent of a healthy diet. The official recommendation is to eat at least 18g/⅝oz of fibre a day, but some nutritionists advise eating far more than this to be sure of digestive health and regularity. There are two types of fibre – soluble and insoluble – with many foods, particularly wholegrains, containing both. Soluble fibre slows down the absorption of carbohydrates, helping to regulate the release of sugar into the bloodstream. For sources of this form of fibre, you can look to most fruits, vegetables, pulses and oats. Insoluble fibres, which aid the excretion of body wastes, include rice, bran, nuts, fruit peel and some vegetables with their skins.

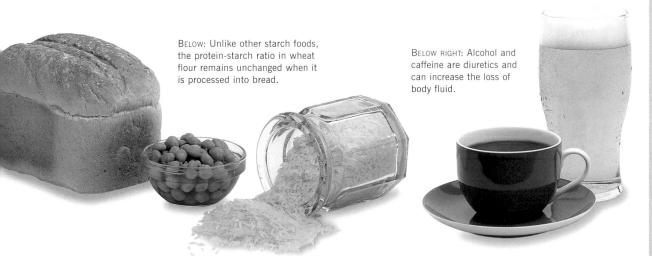

BELOW: Unlike other starch foods, the protein-starch ratio in wheat flour remains unchanged when it is processed into bread.

BELOW RIGHT: Alcohol and caffeine are diuretics and can increase the loss of body fluid.

cooking, a great deal of water is absorbed into the rice and a new, more favourable ratio of 1:12 results.

In bread, on the other hand, the protein-starch ratio remains unchanged. But in starch on its own, as in potato starch, corn starch, rice starch, and so on, the protein-starch ratio is subject to major changes. Such starch is processed industrially as a commercial food ingredient, and the industrial processing generally produces unfavourable ratios. Industrially-processed food products have an unfavourable ratio, more often than not.

Raw and unprocessed food is generally easier to digest than processed food, but their good properties may have no effect on food combining. Cooked foods may be eaten in combinations that give excellent results, and raw foods eaten in combinations that give appalling results, and vice versa. It is a fallacy, by the way, that cooked – that is, boiled – food digests more easily than raw food. The food may have so little goodness in it after cooking that there is nothing to be digested, and it will pass virtually straight through the digestive tract, untouched by the digestive process.

WHAT SHOULD YOU DRINK?

When you drink, water, diluted juices, raw juices or all three are better for you than alcohol or strongly-caffeinated drinks such as coffee and colas. Alcohol and caffeine are diuretics: if you rely on them too heavily to quench your thirst, you will find that you may be losing more water from your body in your urine than you are actually absorbing, and dehydration can result. If you become dehydrated, you will feel tired and lethargic, and lack concentration. To deal with this, what you need to do is recharge your liquid levels. You should try to drink before and between meals, but avoid drinking too much when you eat or immediately after you have eaten, as this can have counterproductive effects on food digestion. Keep a supply of still mineral water or filtered water by you and sip it throughout the day. Above all, try

to avoid the temptation to turn to caffeinated drinks when you feel that you need a quick energy surge. The effects of such drinks are short-lived and their nutritional content is minimal. Snacking on a piece of bread or a banana is infinitely preferable, because both are sources of slow-release carbohydrate, which supplies energy that will keep you going for much longer.

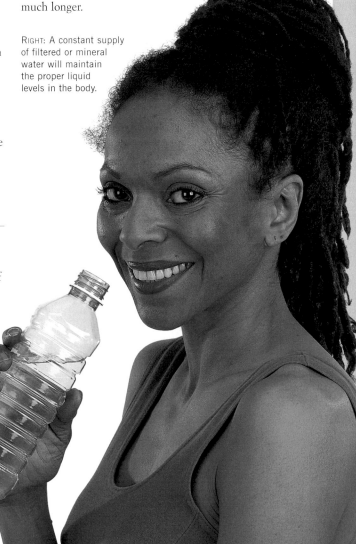

RIGHT: A constant supply of filtered or mineral water will maintain the proper liquid levels in the body.

JUICING FOR HEALTH

Nutritious, natural and easy to prepare, juices made from raw fruits and vegetables are a potent addition to the food combining armoury. If you make them a part of your daily diet, you will find that the vitamins and minerals they contain will help to stimulate mind and body, helping you to beat debilitating tiredness and fatigue. Put at its simplest, juicing is a straightforward, delicious way of maximizing your intake of all the nutritional goodness of fruit and vegetables.

ABOVE: Delicious juice drinks can be extracted from fresh fruit and vegetables.

By making the drinking of fresh fruit and vegetable juices an integral part of your food combining programme, you will be helping Nature guarantee your optimum intake of vitamins, minerals and the other essential nutrients required for good health. Every time that you drink a glass of fresh juice, you can bank on it containing virtually the same amount of nutrients, although not so much fibre, as if you were eating the fruit or vegetable from which the juice is made.

There is nothing particularly new, novel or quirky about this concept: it has been around in nutritional circles for quite some time. Since the 19th century, naturopaths have been prescribing fresh juices and raw foods to help their patients boost their health. German and Swiss pioneers led the field with what is known as the *Roehsaft Kur* (the fresh juice cure). This is still a staple today at health clinics around the world. What is changing today is the way in which nutritionally-aware people perceive food, how they eat it, and what they should do to be certain that they are making the most of all the goodness it contains.

WHY JUICING IS GOOD FOR YOU

Unlike ready-made juices, homemade juice is packed full of concentrated goodness – it has nothing added to it, and nothing taken away. You can be certain that it contains many of the vitamins and minerals we need to keep us healthy and well, including beta carotene, Vitamin C, potassium and phosphorus. It is also rich in powerful antioxidants, which help the body to deal with potentially harmful free radicals. Even more importantly, such juices are easy to digest, as well as possessing remarkable cleansing and restorative powers. Contrast this with cartons or bottles of orange juice. This is often pasteurized, a process that food combiners believe can alter the nutritional values of the juice. In addition, commercially made juices may contain additional acids, additives, sugar, and on occasion, pulpwash produced during the manufacturing process by soaking the fruit skins in water.

Fresh is undoubtedly best as far as juicing is concerned, since you can count on all freshly-juiced fruit and vegetable juices having certain things in common. The pure water they contain means that the body has one less set of impurities to contend with once it starts to digest the contents of the juice. In addition, fruits contain acid, which can help to remove toxins from the digestive tract, while the chlorophyll green vegetables contain also has cleansing properties. Once they have been digested, fruit and vegetable juices all become alkalinizers, thus helping to keep the body's all-important acid-base balance in check.

Nor should the pulp produced by the juicing process be forgotten. This is the more fibrous, solid fruit or vegetable content that is separated out of the liquid by the juicer and is equally good for you. The American food combining authority Wayne Pickering advised that we should chew our liquids and drink our solid foods, so the pulp should not be ignored and discarded. Either eat it on its own, or combine it with other foods.

BELOW: Homemade juices from fresh fruits and vegetables are pure and easy to digest.

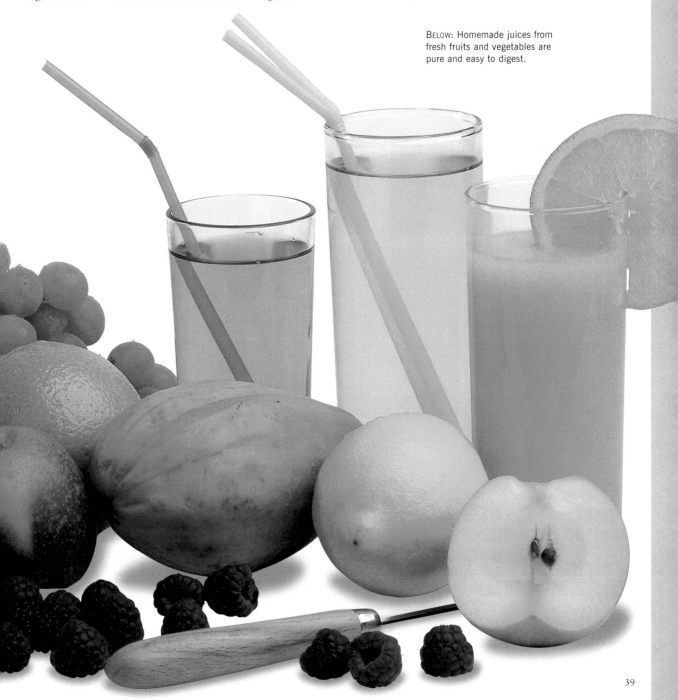

JUICING FOR DIGESTION

Juicing will help to keep you fit and healthy; it can also help to deal with health problems, if they arise. Drinking fresh juices helps to keep the digestive organs healthy and well-toned. Improved digestion also allows the body to absorb more beneficial nutrients. For indigestion, pineapple and papaya juices are excellent standbys: pineapple contains bromelain, an enzyme which helps to balance acid and alkaline levels in the digestive system, while papaya contains papain, which helps to break down protein, taking some of the burden off the stomach enzymes. To relieve an upset stomach, try soothing garlic juice. Apple juice is a good cleanser.

HOW MUCH, WHEN AND WHAT?

Juicing experts advise that, when you start juicing, you should drink no more than three glasses of concentrated juice a day, upping the amount to six glasses as you get used to what you are drinking. In any event, you should dilute dark green vegetable juices and dark red ones by four parts juice to one part milder juices or still water, as, in their neat form, they can have unpalatable effects. Remember, too, that it makes sense to drink both vegetable and fruit juices, rather than sticking to one of them exclusively, as this will maximize the nutritional benefits. Drinking an excessive amount of fruit juice, in any case, will overload your system with fructose, the form of sugar contained in all fruit – a rapid rise in blood sugar levels is the probable consequence. Nor should you mix vegetable and fruit juices together in the same glass – if you do, you may well suffer from an attack of flatulence as a result. The exception to the rule is apple juice, which can be mixed happily with any vegetable juice.

How long you can leave the juice once you have made it is a matter of dispute. Purists advise always drinking it immediately after it has been juiced. Otherwise, they say, the juice will oxidize very quickly indeed, and all its goodness will be lost. Certainly, such juices should always be drunk the same day, although to combat the oxidizing problem you can store them in airtight containers in a refrigerator until you are ready to drink them.

What can you juice, and what can you combine with what? There is a host of possibilities from which to make a selection. Some of the best vitamin and mineral sources are as follows. For beta carotene, which the body turns into Vitamin A, the best fruit and vegetables to juice are apricots and carrots. For the B vitamins, you can try avocado and banana – because neither of these will juice well on their own, they will need to be blended with other ingredients. Kale is a particularly good source of Vitamins B_1, B_2, B_3 and calcium; Brussels sprouts contain noteworthy amounts of Vitamin B_6, folic acid and zinc. Blackcurrant is rich in Vitamin C, iron, phosphorus, potassium and sulphur. Broccoli is a good source of Vitamin B_5 and magnesium. For delicious juices that are all equally healthy, try combining apples, pears and kiwi fruit, carrot and apple, or blackcurrant, kiwi fruit and orange.

When planning your juice combinations, you should not forget that the basic rules of food combining still apply. As with fresh fruit, it is better to consume fruit juice on its own, preferably on an empty stomach. Also, melon juice is always better drunk uncombined, rather than mixed together with other fruit juices.

CHOOSING A JUICER

If your food processor has a juicing attachment, you can use this to start with, but, as you progress, it is well worth investing in a purpose-built juicing machine. The difference between the two is simple. A blending attachment purées pulp and juice together, while a juicer separates out the two. The main types of juicer available are: centrifugal juicers, which work by grating their contents and then spinning this rapidly to separate the juice from the pulp; masticating juicers, which extract a greater amount of juice; and hydraulic juice presses, which are the most efficient – and expensive – of the three.

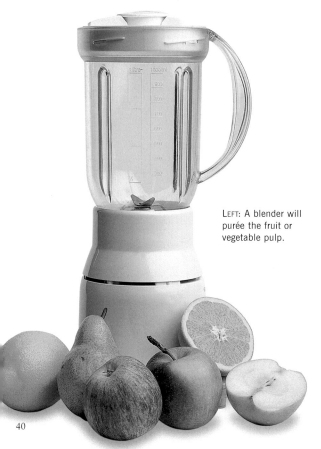

LEFT: A blender will purée the fruit or vegetable pulp.

JUICING REMEDIES

The quantities in the juices described here make approximately one glass of juice. Vary the juice combinations for maximum benefits, remembering that you should drink no more than a maximum of three glasses of juice a day.

FOR INDIGESTION

½ papaya
½ peach
50 ml/2 fl oz/¼ cup still water
or
2 thick slices of pineapple
1 mango
or
2 large carrots
1 clove garlic

PEACH AND
PAPAYA

FOR CONSTIPATION

½ medium watermelon
125 ml/4 fl oz/½ cup
still water
or
6 large spinach leaves
4 tomatoes
3 thick slices cucumber

WATERMELON

FOR DIARRHOEA

1 apple
125 ml/4 fl oz/½ cup still water
or
2 large carrots
125 ml/4 fl oz/½ cup still water

FOR IRRITABLE BOWEL SYNDROME

1 pear
125 ml/4 fl oz/½ cup still water
or
2 celery sticks (stalks)
125 ml/4 fl oz/½ cup still water

PEAR

FRESH
CARROTS

FOR NAUSEA AND VOMITING

1 grapefruit
1 teaspoon freshly
ground ginger
125 ml/4 fl oz/½ cup
still water
or
½ head of fennel
1 teaspoon freshly
ground ginger
125 ml/4 fl oz/½ cup
still water

FENNEL

Right: Fresh juices
have many medicinal
benefits.

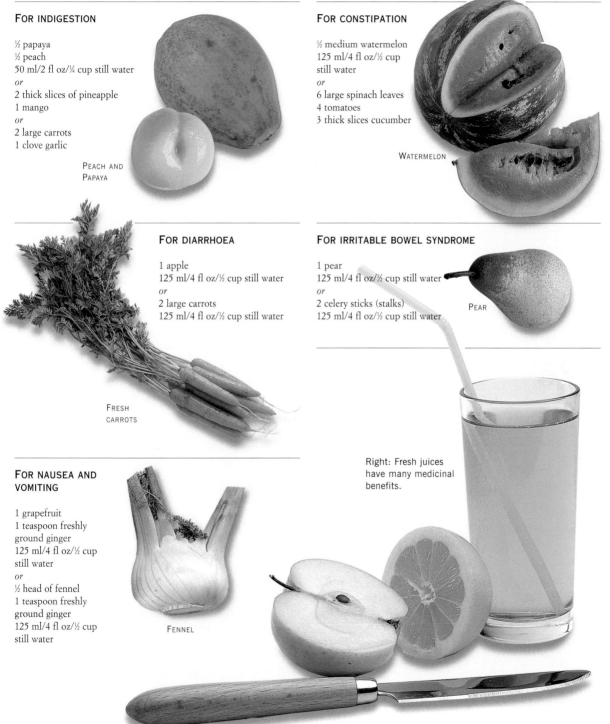

THE ACID-BASE BALANCE

Even though, as you will see later, there is no such thing scientifically as a truly alkaline food, there are foods that diminish acidity, and these are effectively alkaline. Keeping the correct balance between acids and alkalis is particularly important

if the digestive and metabolic systems are to function as they should. In ideal circumstances, by far the majority of the foods we eat should be alkalizing, and the amount of acid-forming foods we consume should be reduced substantially.

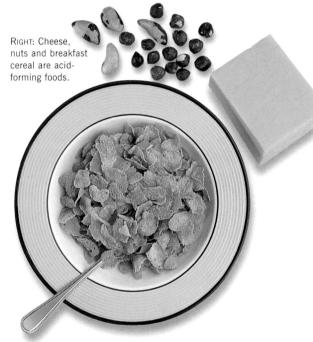

RIGHT: Cheese, nuts and breakfast cereal are acid-forming foods.

At the beginning of the 20th century, Professor Ragnar Berg (1875–1956) published a study that divided all foods into two basic groupings: 'concentrated foods' and 'unconcentrated foods'. The distinction is readily made because it corresponds fairly well with the distinction between high- and low-calorie foods. But, in Professor Berg's work, the distinction was not so obvious: the principle behind his classification was whether the foods contained metallic elements or non-metallic elements.

Foods that contain a high proportion of non-metallic elements, such as sulphur, phosphorus and chlorine, are acid-forming – that is, during the metabolic process, these elements are responsible for the formation of acids. Foods that diminish acidity and are effectively alkaline tend to contain many metallic elements, such as potassium, sodium, magnesium, iron and calcium. These foods also tend to contain a lot of water, but not very much protein. Acid-forming foods, on the other hand, generally contain a fair amount of protein, but only a small amount of water, and the non-metallic elements are normally found in the protein.

THE BALANCE IN THE BODY

The acid-base balance has considerable influence on the digestion, and it is thus appropriate to discuss it briefly here. On the pH scale of acidity/alkalinity, human blood varies between 7.3 and 7.5, so is slightly alkaline (neutral = 7.0). Professor Vincent, the founder of the diagnostic method known as 'Bio-electronics', believes that for excellent health, the blood ideally should be neutral.

To maintain a constant acidity/alkalinity value, the body's acid-base balance makes use of three major mechanisms: the blood (through substances in it known as buffers), the lungs (through respiration, to remove carbon dioxide) and the kidneys (through the filtration of acids and alkalis in liquid wastes). The buffers in the blood neutralize excess acids, preventing acidosis. Depending on its severity, this may result in tiredness, nausea, and an increase in the breathing rate. Sometimes, it causes a distinct aroma of acetone on the breath, which smells like nail-varnish remover.

The body's acid-base balance has considerable influence over the metabolic processes as well. As we have seen, foods rich in water are easily digestible. The low proportion of nutrients in relation to the water in such foods corresponds to the ideal ratio between metallic and non-metallic elements.

ACIDIC, ALKALIZING OR NEUTRAL?

If we eat too much acid-forming food, digestion is problematical, even if the foods otherwise combine well. Acid-forming foods that have a high calorific value include meat, fish, cheese, bread, cereals, nuts, leguminous vegetables and fruit seeds and stones (pits). Alkalizing foods include fruits, berries, non-leguminous vegetables (including gourds), potatoes and other root vegetables, milk and milk products such as skimmed (skim) milk, yogurt and buttermilk.

Some authorities have presumed that there must also be neutral foods, in which metallic and non-metallic elements work to neutralize each other. Such combinations do not occur in Nature, although there are some foodstuffs, such as edible oils and household sugar, which contain neither metallic nor non-metallic elements. Soft drinks (sodas) contain only water and sugar, to which flavourings and colour have been added.

DEALING WITH CONSTIPATION

Food combining authorities say that constipation is a physical sign that the acid-base balance has been upset, since it often results from an excess of acid in the system. To help your body to deal with the problem, you should:

* Make sure that you are eating wholemeal (whole-wheat) bread.
* Eat plenty of fresh fruit and vegetables.
* Base your breakfast around a bowl of plain bran.
  Muesli (granola) is to be avoided, as it is a bad food combination.
* Drink at least 2 litres/3½ pints/8¾ cups of water a day.

If this does not work, taking a dose of a gentle laxative such as Epsom salts can help to relieve the problem in the short term. You should avoid relying on any laxative for too long, however, as this will overstimulate the bowel, with counter-productive results. A dietary response is by far the healthier solution.

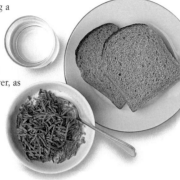

ACIDIC OR ACID-FORMING?

The Danish nutritionist Dr Nolfi and other experts who were not aware of the theory of food combining, but who were intimately concerned with the effects of food on the acid-base balance, derived results that only rarely showed any differences from those expected in food combining. The acid-base balance has a critical effect on digestion and metabolism, and therefore ultimately on overall health. Interestingly, Dr Hay – unlike Dr Shelton – made a thorough study of this. Yet it was Dr Shelton who recommended the consumption of large amounts of (alkalizing) vegetables when eating preparations of (acid-forming) cereals. He was evidently, if unconsciously, seeking to make sure of a good acid-base balance for his patients.

So that no one can misunderstand, it should be emphasized that there is a great deal of difference between acidic food and acid-forming food. Acidic food has an acidic taste – sour, or sour within sweet – whereas acid-forming food is quite different, and may taste of something else altogether. It should also be stressed that although meat and fish contain a lot of water (perhaps around 75 per cent by volume), they are acid-forming foods. The water content of meat and fish is lower only after they have been smoked or dried. Acid-base balance depends not on water so much as on the ratio of metallic to non-metallic elements.

Milk is one of the alkalizing foods, but milk products, such as hard or semi-hard cheese and cottage cheese are acid-forming foods. The protein content of milk is 3.3 per cent. In cottage cheese and hard cheese, such as Cheddar, Cheshire and Emmenthal, it is between 12 and 18 per cent, and in semi-hard varieties such as Edam, Gouda and Port Salut, it is between 25 and 28 per cent.

Cooking food may cause a slight change in the way that the food affects the acid-base balance, but the change is so small that it can be ignored.

MAINTAINING THE ACID-BASE BALANCE

Various internal mechanisms help to keep the body's acid-base balance regulated. If we did not rely on these mechanisms at all, we would have to eat a diet comprised of 80 to 90 per cent alkalizing foods, and only 10 to 20 per cent acid-forming foods. In conventional diets, the ratio between the two is more like 55:45. To help your body to maintain the balance, you should:

* Eat frequent small meals instead of one or two large meals.
* Chew your food thoroughly before you swallow it.
* Try not to rush through your food, and eat in a relaxed environment.
* Avoid any foods that trigger problem symptoms.
* If you smoke, stop.
* Cut down on stimulants, such as coffee, tea and alcohol.
* Substitute paracetamol for aspirin.
* Avoid foods that are rich, fried, high in fat or spicy.
  Additives, such as monosodium glutamate (MSG), can also affect digestion adversely.

In an ideal diet, between 80 and 90 per cent of what we eat should be alkalizing, and only 10 to 20 per cent acid-forming.

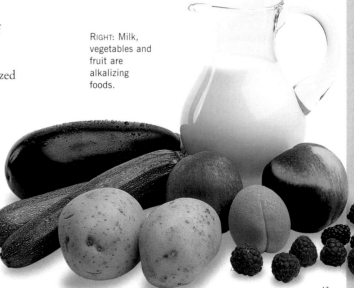

RIGHT: Milk, vegetables and fruit are alkalizing foods.

THE NUMBER OF POSSIBLE COMBINATIONS

Despite initial appearances, food combining is not so hard as it might seem, so if what you have read so far strikes you as over-complicated, do not let this deter you. There is no need to weigh portions or count calories – nor is there any restriction on quantities, apart from obvious commonsense. All you have to do is ascertain which foods combine together successfully in digestive terms and which do not. Nor is the diet a limited one: within combinations, there are hundreds of different recipes from which to choose.

LEFT: Fruits can be eaten in any combination, with the exception of melon.

Anybody who buys a five-digit combination lock relies on the fact that there are almost countless possible combinations, although there are only five original digits to make these combinations. A thief would have to search for the correct combination among all those possibilities. Fortunately, the possible combinations of foods that harmonize with each other are not so numerous and may be systematized.

REDUCING THE POSSIBILITIES

All of the five dominant nutrients – proteins, fats, sugars, starches and acids – may be combined as pairs with each other in foods, so there are 15 possible combinations (discounting combinations that are of the same nutrient, or merely an inversion of a combination already counted). Combinations of three, four and five nutrients are also possible. Taking into account all of these variables, there is a total of 246 combinations, good and bad, many of which occur in industrial food products.

Food combining theory reduces the combinations to a manageable total of ten, four of which are good and six of which are bad. They may be schematized in the form of

a pentagon (see diagram opposite). This is not the only way in which the theory may be schematized, but it does provide an outline that is fairly easy to memorize and use. To remember the pentagon and how it works is to have all you need to know about food combining immediately to hand and removes the need to consult lists or diagrams.

WHAT THE PENTAGON MEANS

Using the pentagon, you can learn which groups of food combine well, and which combinations should be avoided. Put at its most basic, you will see that starchy and sugary foods should never be combined with foods in which protein and fat are the dominant nutrients. Many food combiners also believe in another golden rule – that fruit should be eaten separately from both proteins and starches. What this means in practical terms is that once you adopt food combining principles, you will be increasing the amount of fruit, salads

RIGHT: Meat and fish are both protein foods.

BELOW: A baked potato with butter is a starch and fat combination.

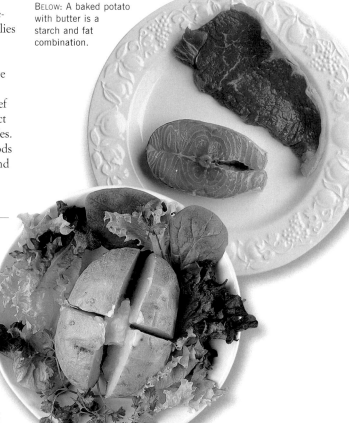

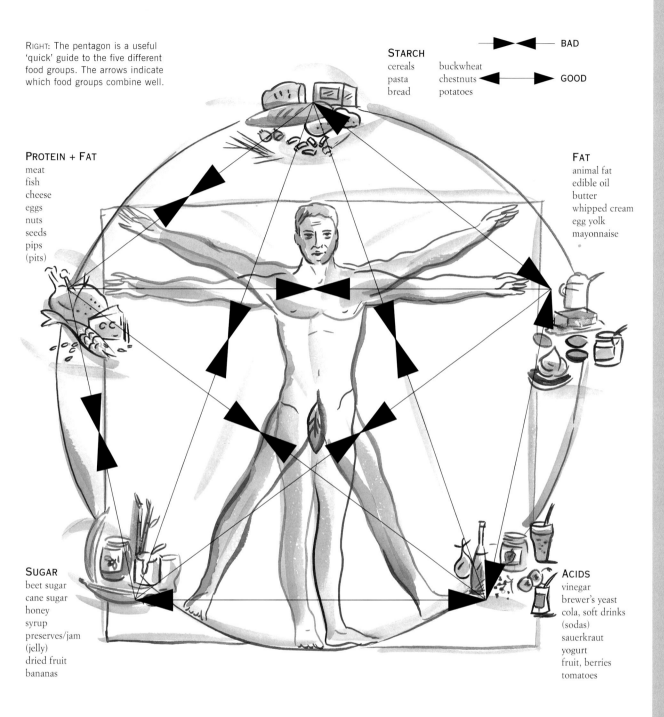

RIGHT: The pentagon is a useful 'quick' guide to the five different food groups. The arrows indicate which food groups combine well.

STARCH
cereals   buckwheat
pasta   chestnuts
bread   potatoes

BAD

GOOD

PROTEIN + FAT
meat
fish
cheese
eggs
nuts
seeds
pips
(pits)

FAT
animal fat
edible oil
butter
whipped cream
egg yolk
mayonnaise

SUGAR
beet sugar
cane sugar
honey
syrup
preserves/jam
(jelly)
dried fruit
bananas

ACIDS
vinegar
brewer's yeast
cola, soft drinks
(sodas)
sauerkraut
yogurt
fruit, berries
tomatoes

and vegetables you eat and reducing your intake of processed and refined foods. As well as helping the digestive and metabolic processes overall, this will help to preserve the equally important acid-base balance.

This does not mean that you will have to give up all your favourite foods. What it does mean is that you must rethink what foods to combine, and when you should eat a particular

food. Combining fish with brown rice and vegetables is not a good combination, since fish is protein-dominated and rice is high in starch. Instead, you could enjoy the fish with a salad, and eat the brown rice with the vegetables at the next meal. Or, instead of meat with a baked potato – a classic bad food combination – eat the meat separately, with a salad or a suitable side-dish, and save the potato for later

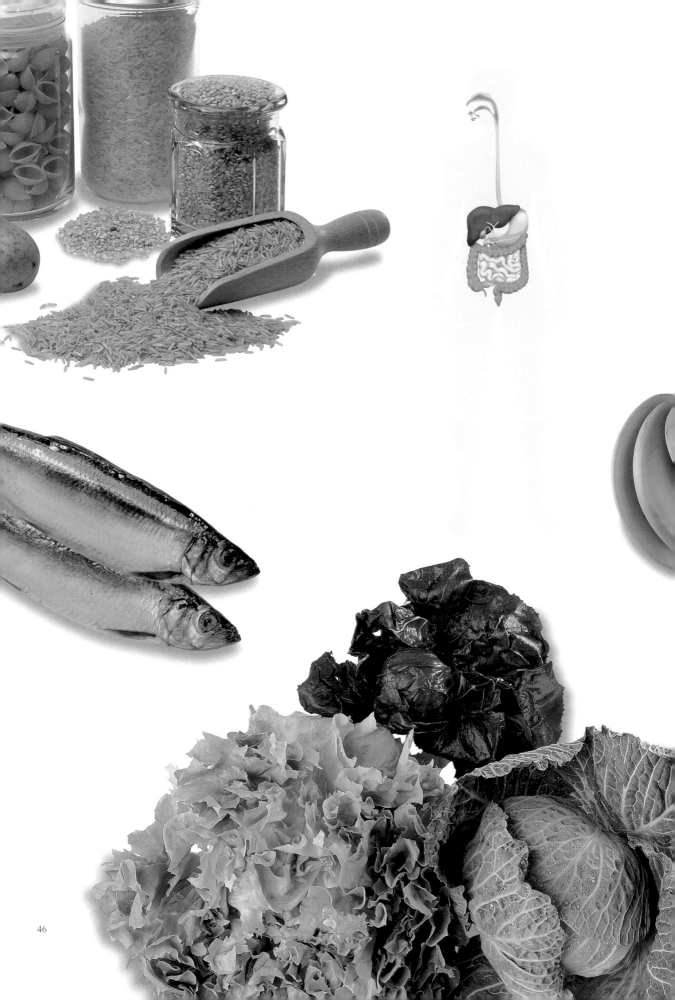

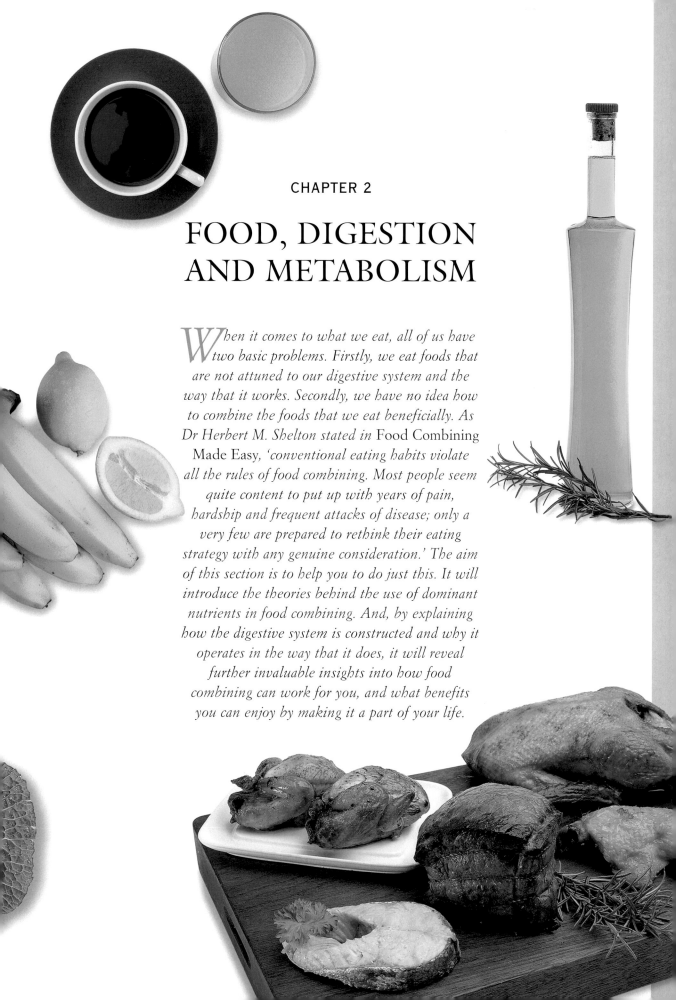

FOOD, DIGESTION AND METABOLISM

*W*hen it comes to what we eat, all of us have
two basic problems. Firstly, we eat foods that
are not attuned to our digestive system and the
way that it works. Secondly, we have no idea how
to combine the foods that we eat beneficially. As
Dr Herbert M. Shelton stated in Food Combining
Made Easy, 'conventional eating habits violate
all the rules of food combining. Most people seem
quite content to put up with years of pain,
hardship and frequent attacks of disease; only a
very few are prepared to rethink their eating
strategy with any genuine consideration.' The aim
of this section is to help you to do just this. It will
introduce the theories behind the use of dominant
nutrients in food combining. And, by explaining
how the digestive system is constructed and why it
operates in the way that it does, it will reveal
further invaluable insights into how food
combining can work for you, and what benefits
you can enjoy by making it a part of your life.

The Choice of Food

When you think about what you are eating you must ask yourself the following questions: How much do you eat? When do you eat your meals? How do you combine one food with another? How do you prepare and eat it? Your first step should be to go back to the fundamentals. Firstly, *get rid of any notion you might have that humans are complete omnivores – able to eat anything and everything at will. Secondly, having set the goal of a healthy, revitalized digestion for yourself, you can ascertain exactly what part food combining can play in helping you to achieve this.*

Before looking at the classification of foods and the physiology of human digestion, it is advisable to look at the choice of food. By this, I mean how to choose foods that are in harmony with the anatomy and functional physiology of the digestive system.

Are we omnivores?

It is notable that in the animal world, each species has its own eating pattern. Biologists distinguish between carnivores (meat-eaters), herbivores (plant-eaters), granivores (seed- and grain-eaters) and fructivores (fruit-eaters). The digestive system of a carnivore is completely different from that of a herbivore: a dog, fox or cat digests in a totally different manner from that of a cow, rabbit, or goat. Granivorous creatures, such as chickens and other gallinaceous birds, have a beak, a crop, a glandular stomach, a muscular stomach, a pancreas with three outlet ducts and lengthy intestines (guts) with tiny follicles (cavities). Their digestive system is focused entirely on the processing of starch in grains and seeds. Primates are mostly fructivores, surviving by consuming berries and nuts: their very specific digestive system is able to derive surprising amounts of energy from small quantities of food.

Humankind, on the other hand, is supposed to be omnivorous, eating everything and not caring two hoots about the choice of food. That choice is determined, in industrialized countries at least, by advertising, price, taste, fashion and culinary expertise, among other factors. Nutritionally, however, this is far from the whole picture.

Where humankind stands

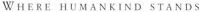

The health of human beings has never been uniformly excellent, as we have already discussed. To a great extent, the history of gastric ailments mirrors the history of agriculture. To be more accurate, it could be said that the history of indigestion runs parallel with the history of inappropriate food combining. Humans just pile all the food together and swallow it down with no thought for their digestive systems: naturally enough, the results are painful and debilitating, and people remain susceptible to all kinds of disease.

It is generally agreed by palaeontologists that humans are herbivorous – plant-eaters – by nature, but became omnivorous by teaching themselves to eat other things, almost like learning a skill. So today we eat meat, fish, cereals, milk, fruit and nuts in addition to vegetables. And most of us eat them all at the same time. Despite the millennia of evolution and cultural development, humans have no single characteristic that places them well

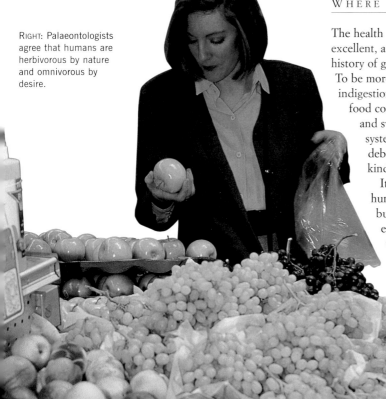

RIGHT: Palaeontologists agree that humans are herbivorous by nature and omnivorous by desire.

Below: The digestive systems of the various species can be totally different. A dog or cat which is carnivorous has a very different digestive system from a rabbit and the digestive system of gallinaceous birds is different again. Despite cultural development, humans have no single characteristic that places them solely among the carnivores, the herbivores or the granivores.

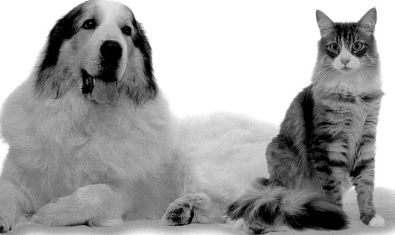
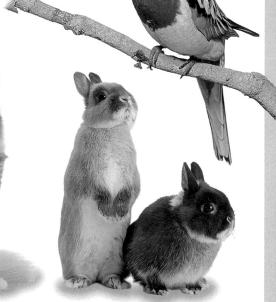

and truly among the carnivores, the herbivores or the granivores. To eat meat, humans often require a toothpick: unlike a dog's teeth, human teeth are rather too close together for comfortable meat-eating. Humans cannot digest grass at all – indeed, many people have severe problems digesting raw vegetables. And, in spite of 10,000 years of agriculture during which grains and cereals have formed a predominant part of the diet, humans have still not developed a beak, a crop or a dual stomach.

THE DUAL PROBLEM

What we do have is a dual problem. Firstly, we eat foods that are not attuned to our digestive systems, and secondly, most of use have no idea how to combine foods properly. This book, of course, is concerned to rectify the second problem, bearing in mind Dr Shelton's dictum that all the foods we eat should be combined in a useful way. The theory of food combining can be applied to all eating patterns. It is in the interests of every single person to combine foods appropriately, whether he or she is a conventional meat-and-fish eater or a vegetarian. The more natural the eating pattern, the easier it is to combine foods harmoniously. A fructivore, who may eat nuts as well as fruits and berries, gains little from food combining. On the other hand, people with conventional eating habits benefit from it the most.

The one great advantage of food combining is that it can be applied to almost all eating patterns. It is not just for health freaks and vegetarians – and certainly not only for people who are weak or ill. Everybody can benefit from it.

TRYING OUT FOOD COMBINING

Anyone who really makes an effort with food combining should achieve constantly perfect digestion. There is no need to resort to forceful persuasion on the subject: it should be enough for you to test out the combinations for yourself. After a meal consisting of appropriately combined foods, you should leave the table feeling satisfied rather than bloated, heavy or fatigued, with nothing else to remind you that, in fact, you have just eaten.

As long as the digestive processes are operating at an optimum, body weight will automatically regulate itself: weight will be gained or lost until the ideal weight is attained. Acid indigestion, bloatedness and flatulence will be gone forever. There is a good chance, too, that anyone suffering from a food allergy will discover that he or she is no longer allergic: many food allergies result from the presence of toxic substances in the intestines that only arise because of inappropriate food combining. Residues of undigested proteins can be particularly toxic, for example. Pressed against the intestinal wall, they can pass into the bloodstream and cause an allergic reaction throughout the body.

INTESTINAL PROBLEMS

The normal intestinal bacteria ('flora') depend for their life and function on the ingestion of food. Occasionally, food residues can cause certain bacteria to increase rapidly and disproportionately, disrupting the floral balance. If these residues originate from starch, fermentation occurs, causing

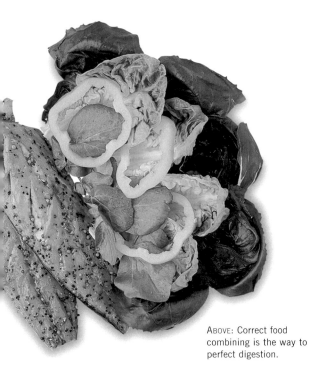

ABOVE: Correct food combining is the way to perfect digestion.

the formation of lactic acid and substances known as short-chain fatty acids. These fatty acids then irritate the intestinal wall, sensitizing it in a way that quite frequently leads to diarrhoea and an 'upset stomach'.

Disruption of the normal floral balance can have even more serious consequences if the causative factor is protein residues. Peptides and amino acids in undigested proteins can be converted into nitrogen compounds called amines by unusually disproportionate amounts of intestinal flora. Amines are both unpleasantly pungent and toxic – whereas odourless intestinal gas caused by fermentation is not especially serious, pungent intestinal gas can be dangerous. The protein residue damages the intestinal wall by causing it to secrete fluid and protein as nourishment for the intestinal flora. The amines may pass through the intestinal wall, eventually, and travel on in the bloodstream all the way up to the brain.

A number of disorders are primarily the result of the dysfunction of the intestines: diarrhoea caused by the presence of toxic substances in the intestines is usually the result of a combination of protein and starch. In all too many people, the large intestine is a disgustingly smelly duct, partly clogged with faeces at all times. Constipation, which is extremely common, can lead to acidosis, eventually, and even poisoning of the tissues and the consequent contamination of adjacent organs. The majority of people in industrialized countries have intestines that are subject to acidosis and poisoning to some degree. Medication does not help much – only good food combining can really improve the condition.

WHAT FOOD COMBINING CAN DO

Using appropriate combinations of foods is the way to perfect digestion, through which the body purifies itself by eliminating toxic substances and by not allowing the production of further toxins. It restores the floral balance in the intestines, and the regularity of daily bowel movements. A clean intestine means less activity by the liver and potential relief to intestinal surface tissues. Sometimes, even sleeping disorders can be traced back to the effects of poorly-functioning intestines: food combining therefore may contribute to a good night's sleep after years of insomnia. Obesity should disappear, as should any feeling of bloating or distension in the stomach and intestines, replacing it with a sense of wellbeing and even improving confidence in your appearance and self-esteem.

Thousands of people who have applied these simple dietary rules have been amazed that food combining has been able to change their lives so radically and so immediately. Basic health can certainly be said to depend on combining appropriate foods, and although not all health problems can be solved so easily, recovery from just about any ailment or disorder can be assisted through the use of food combining. To do justice to the process, particular attention must be paid to maintaining a good acid-base balance, the correct choice of foods, and to exercising moderation in the quantity of food or drink we consume in the course of a day.

ABOVE: Fruit should always be eaten separately from other foods.

To apply beneficial combinations of food – and to avoid potentially disastrous ones – the dominant nutrient of each food must be established. As I have already outlined, there are up to five nutrients in every food – proteins, fats, sugars, starch and acids. In most foods, only one of these nutrients is dominant, but when two or three vie for supremacy, the food is not easily digestible, even if eaten by itself. Combining this type of food with others usually makes it even more difficult to digest. Successful combining requires a thorough awareness of nutrient classifications, which are discussed in detail on the following pages.

FOOD CLASSIFICATIONS: PROTEINS

Proteins contain a very large number of constituent elements, unlike carbohydrates or fats – they consist of compounds of 20 amino acids. The numbers of different proteins that can be built up from these amino acids is quite high.

The digestion of protein is initiated by enzymes produced in the stomach, the pancreas and the wall of the small intestine. Protein digestion always results in waste products or acids, because the process is naturally difficult. The proteins thus require particular attention in relation to food combining.

At this point, it is enough to say that three types of protein are distinguishable – animal protein, lactoprotein (dairy protein) and vegetable protein. Later in this chapter, you will see how each of these types of protein has its own process in human digestion.

HOW MUCH PROTEIN DO WE NEED?

For many years, it was thought that animal protein was vital to life. This opinion was quite understandable, given that vegetable protein and lactoprotein contain none of the essential amino acids found in animal protein. Debate over the body's daily protein requirements still continues. For too long, the sole consideration was body weight, but now we know that other factors in protein digestion are much more important. Heat changes the properties of a protein by altering its structure, destroying the protective jacket of water around the protein molecule. It is important for us to combine proteins in the correct way in order to improve our digestion of them, which is already problematic.

The usefulness of protein in food is determined by the presence of eight 'essential' amino acids. We cannot produce the eight essential acids by ourselves, however – they must be supplied in the food that we eat.

The need for protein depends both on digestion and on the quality of the protein: good food combining can reduce the need for protein, thereby drastically reducing the waste products. This is a measure of how important food combining can be in relation to high-protein food.

HIGH-PROTEIN FOODS

In nature, protein occurs only in the presence of fat. In meat and fish, the proportions of protein and fat are relatively quite different, with protein predominant by far. In concentrated dairy products, such as hard and semi-hard cheese, the proportions are closer to each other. And in nuts, fruit seeds and stones (pits), the fat content usually exceeds the protein content. Nonetheless, all of these are rich in protein. The fat content can also be increased by cooking: fish dishes can be cooked in oil, for example. Similarly, the fat content can be reduced by using low-fat dairy products or lean meat, and so on.

BELOW: Animal protein is no longer considered vital to life.

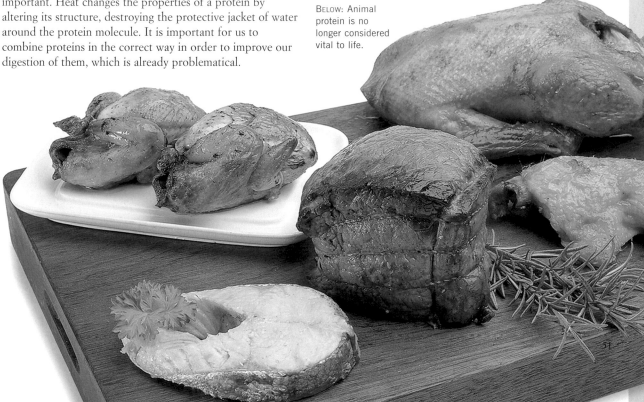

To be considered high-protein, a food must consist of at least 10 per cent protein. All meat and fish contain a lot of protein, even when they are relatively fatty. Exceptions are cod liver oil (6 per cent), bacon (4.1 per cent) and kidney lard (1.2 per cent), which are not so much high-protein foods as high-fat foods. In terms of lactoproteins, only milk products in concentrated form are regarded as high-protein. For convenience, however, eggs are also classified within the lactoprotein group.

Another exception among vegetable high-protein foods is the coconut. It is actually a low-protein nut, containing only 4.2 per cent protein. Coconut flakes contain 5.6 per cent protein and 62 per cent fat – so it is a high-fat food. Dried mushrooms, on the other hand, are rich in proteins, but water added during cooking reduces the protein content. The same is true of cocoa powder, which is also high-protein, although when it is processed into the form of chocolate or chocolate milk, the protein content is no higher than 10 per cent.

WHY OUR BODIES NEED PROTEIN

The body can manufacture most of the 20 different amino acids commonly found in animal and plant proteins for itself, but as I have already stated, can obtain eight of the essential acids required for life only from the food we consume. These eight acids are: isoleucine, leucine, phenylalanine, valine, threonine, methionine, tryptophan and lysine, plus histidine for children, since they cannot as yet make enough to cover their body needs. Like the other amino acids, each one of these is made up of carbon, hydrogen, nitrogen and oxygen – the four elements vital for life – while the proteins created by the different amino acid combinations each have their own function. Collagen and keratin, for instance, give hair and skin their strength and elasticity, while myoglobin and haemoglobin are the essential oxygen-binders of the muscles and blood. We also need proteins in order for the body to create the enzymes it needs. These play a key role in triggering energy release, in making digestion possible, in the excretion of body wastes and in the production of the hormones, which keep the body working efficiently, and antibodies, which help it to fight infection. Nutritionally, food is classed as either a high-quality or low-quality protein source, depending on whether its proteins contain all, or only some, of the different amino acids the body needs. Meat, poultry, fish, eggs and soy beans are all considered high-quality protein sources; low-quality proteins include nuts, pulses, bread, rice,

RIGHT: A wide variety of foods are high in protein.

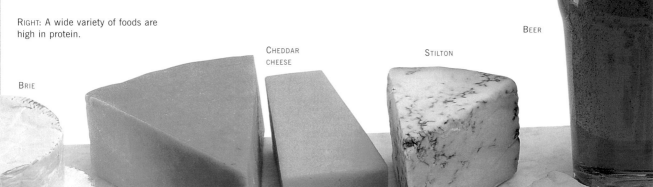

BEER

CHEDDAR CHEESE

STILTON

BRIE

pasta and potatoes. Here, food combining has an important role to play, since correct combining of low-quality protein sources means that what is scientifically regarded as a 'complete protein' can be created. Successful vegetable combining in dishes like dhal, for example, can give the combination as high a quality of protein as meat, with the added bonus of lacking the undesirable saturated fats with which most animal protein is naturally combined.

HOW MUCH PROTEIN TO EAT

Nutritionists currently recommend that men should eat 55 g/ 2 oz of protein a day: women need around 45 g/1½oz. Put another way, this means getting no more than 10 to 15 per cent of your daily calorie intake from protein, with 35 per cent coming from fat and the remainder from carbohydrates. It is important that you maintain these percentages if you are to meet your body's energy needs. If you do not, the body breaks down body proteins instead, and uses these to meet its energy requirements. Eating protein to excess is equally, if not more, counterproductive, since the body lacks the ability to store it for later use. Instead, the liver converts the excess into glucose and by-products such as urea which have to be excreted, putting an extra strain on both the liver and the kidneys. Excess protein in the body also leads to the production of acidic urine. This, too, has the potential to be damaging, since it involves a loss of calcium, which increases the risk of osteoporosis developing in the bones. Controlling the amount of protein you eat is also important, if you need to watch your weight. High-protein foods are rich in fats and calories: eating too much of them can lead to unwelcome weight gain.

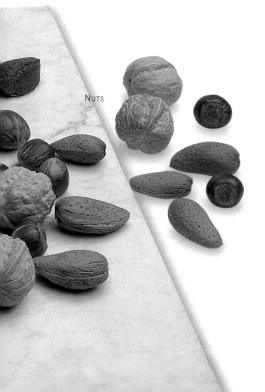

NUTS

WHICH FOODS ARE RICH IN PROTEIN?

Protein is essential for life, even though modern nutritionists believe that, in industrialized countries at least, people are eating excessive amounts of it, particularly of the animal variety. The tables below are an accurate guide to the quantities of protein contained in specific high-protein foods.

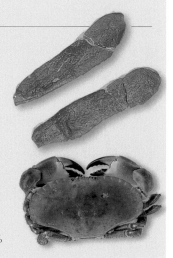

ANIMAL PROTEIN

Veal	22%
Beef	21.3%
Pork	21.1%
Rabbit	20.9%
Chicken	20.6%
Lamb/mutton	20.4%
Dried fish	20–79%
Game	20–22%
Goat meat	19.5%
Fish products	16–21%
Poultry	15–24%
Freshwater fish	15–20%
Seawater fish	15–19%
Meat products	11–29%
Crustaceans	9–18.6%

LACTOPROTEIN

Powdered egg yolk	46.2%
Powdered buttermilk	38.6%
Powdered skimmed milk (nonfat dry milk)	35.3%
Powdered egg white	31.1%
Powdered whole milk (dry milk)	25.5%
Egg yolk	16.1%
Hen's egg	12.9%
Cottage cheese	11–13%
Egg white	10.9%
Hard/semi-hard cheese	9.2–32.2

VEGETABLE PROTEIN

Dried brewer's yeast	48%
Peanut butter	47.8%
Soy flour	43.4%
Rye germ	42%
Soy beans	36.8%
Wheatgerm	28%
Peanuts	26%
Seeds	20–36%
Dried legumes	19–23.9%
Pips (pits)	13–27%
Nuts	13–19%
Baker's yeast	1.1%

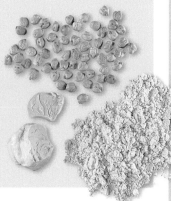

FOOD CLASSIFICATIONS: FATS

Nutritionally speaking, there are so-called 'bad' fats and 'good' fats. Eating too many bad (saturated) fats can be harmful, but good (unsaturated) fats play an important part in preserving good health and helping to protect the body against disease. The temptation is to consume too many saturated fats, and not enough beneficial unsaturated ones. As far as food combining is concerned, because protein and fat are already combined, more often than not, it is essential to check which is the dominant nutrient in the combination.

Fats, or lipids, include most substances that are insoluble in water, and are present in all cells. Most foods contain some fats, which are almost always found together with protein. To absorb fats from ingested food and to digest them and metabolize concentrated forms, the body makes use of two indispensable fluids – bile (occasionally known as hall) and pancreatic juice. The digestion of fats begins in the duodenum, the first section of the intestine after the stomach, and is comparatively separate from the rest of the digestive process. Only people who suffer from dysfunction of the gall-bladder, which secretes bile, or from a diseased liver, tend to have any problems digesting fats.

FATS IN COMBINATION

Fat combines readily with starch – a combination that retards the activity of the stomach. This is a property that, in turn, can prove useful in digesting some combinations of food, but may cause difficulties with others.

Because fat and protein are ordinarily found together in foods, it is always necessary to check which is the dominant nutrient in any one food. Protein always tends to dominate, whereas fats tend to be comparatively subordinate.

Consuming a large quantity of fatty food in which the protein proportion is higher than 10 per cent, however, runs the risk of creating a poor food combination if the food is eaten in combination with starchy foods.

Egg yolk contains 16.1 per cent protein and 32 per cent fat. In theory, protein should be the dominant nutrient, because the protein content is higher than 10 per cent, although the fat content is double that of the protein by volume. In practice, however, things are somewhat different. Egg yolk is always used in small amounts. One egg yolk contains about 3 g/¹⁄₁₀ oz of protein and 6 g/¹⁄₅ oz of fat. If one egg yolk is incorporated into a meal, the effect is virtually negligible.

SUNFLOWER OIL

CORN OIL

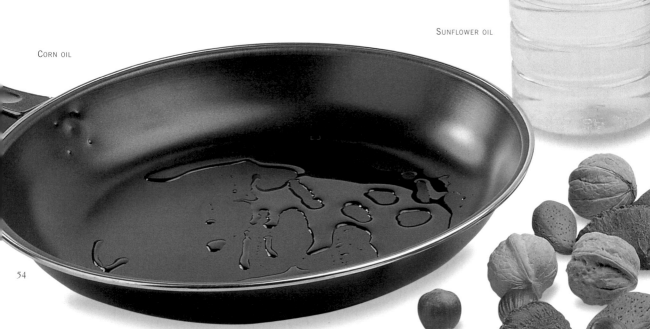

WHERE FATS COME FROM

In food combining terms, fats are classed according to their origins – animals, milk or vegetables. This table lists common sources of fat under these three headings, in order of the percentages of fat they contain. Eating too many fats and oils of any kind may prove harmful to health, but it is a mistake to exclude them from the diet totally. Not only are they a rich source of the calories that the body needs to meet its energy requirements: they also contain important nutrients – essential fatty acids – and help to make food tasty and palatable. The two whipped cream percentages highlight the difference between standard and commercially-produced low- or reduced-fat versions.

ANIMAL FATS

Cod liver oil	99.9%	Kidney lard	94.4%
Melted lard	99.7%	Bacon	65%
Beef fat/dripping	96.5%		

VEGETABLE FATS

Corn oil	99.9%	Groundnut (peanut	
Safflower oil	99.9%	oil)	99.4%
Soy oil	99.9%	Walnut oil	91.5%
Palm oil	99.8%	Coconut oil	90%
Sunflower oil	99.8%	Mayonnaise	80%
Cottonseed oil	99.7%	Margarine (all kinds)	80%
Olive oil	99.6%	Coconut flakes	62%
Linseed oil	99.5%	Avocado	24%
Sesame oil	99.5%	Black olives	17%
		Green olives	13.3%

MILK FATS

Butter	83.2%
Whipped cream (standard)	40%
Egg yolk	32%
Whipped cream (low-fat)	10%

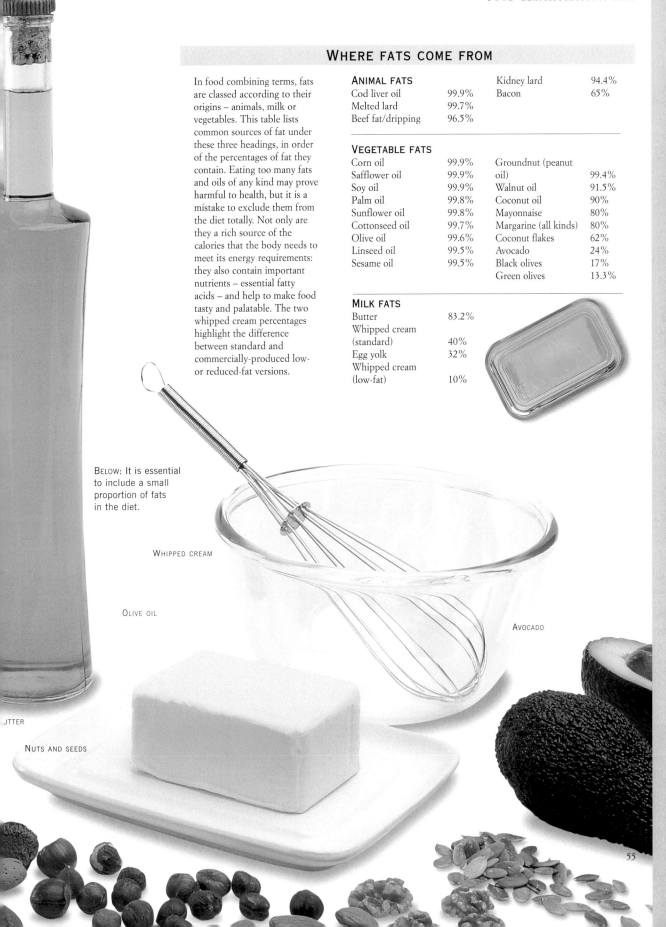

BELOW: It is essential to include a small proportion of fats in the diet.

WHIPPED CREAM

OLIVE OIL

AVOCADO

BUTTER

NUTS AND SEEDS

GOOD FATS AND BAD FATS AT A GLANCE

In health terms, fats are defined additionally in terms of the type of fatty acids they contain. Fatty acids are made up of carbon, hydrogen and oxygen, their classification varying depending on the proportion of hydrogen they contain. As the name implies, a fat is classed as saturated when its molecules hold the maximum amount of hydrogen.

Monounsaturates hold a little less, and polyunsaturates hold the least. In the main, so-called trans fats are artificially created by the hydrogenation process involved in the making of margarine and other processed foods such as biscuits (cookies), pies, crisps (chips) and cakes: they also occur naturally in meat and dairy products.

FATTY ACID	FOOD SOURCE	ROLE	GOOD OR BAD
Saturated 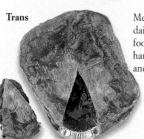	Butter, hard cheese, cream, hard margarine, solid cooking fats, fatty meat products, biscuits (cookies), cakes, chocolate, pastries	Adds flavour to food. Excessive amounts can lead to obesity, heart disease, atherosclerosis and can contribute to the causes of various types of cancer.	Bad
Trans 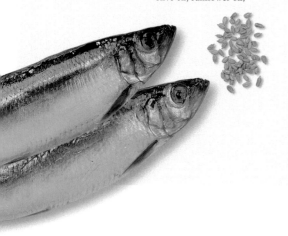	Meat and meat products, dairy products, processed foods, commercially-hardened margarines and other cooking fats.	In processed foods, have been linked to increased risks of heart disease. Frying food in commercially-hardened fats can turn good fats into bad fats. Use pure vegetable oil instead.	Bad
Monounsaturated	Olive oil, rapeseed oil avocados, nuts and seeds.	Use to replace bad fats, as they have no negative health effects. Many also contain polyunsaturates as well.	Good
Polyunsaturated	Fish oils, oily fish, walnuts, rapeseed oil, olive oil, sunflower oil,	Omega-6 fatty acids needed for healthy cells and to help regulate various body functions. Deficiencies can lead to blood clots and skin problems, and impair the workings of the immune system. Omega-3 fatty acids are needed in infancy for healthy development of the brain and retina of the eye. They help educe inflammation and tendency of blood to clot and protect against heart disease, arthritis, psoriasis and various other medical conditions. Sunflower oil is also particularly rich in Vitamin E, which is thought to have antioxidant properties.	Good

FAT GROUPINGS

Fats, in the same way as proteins, are grouped according to whether they are animal-, vegetable- or milk-based. For food combining, there is no need to make a further distinction between them but to promote overall good health, it is important to know more about them – in particular, which types of fat medical authorities believe can be good for you and which they have identified as potentially damaging.

Modern medical science has demonstrated conclusively that foods rich in saturated fat will boost blood cholesterol levels and increase the risk of developing serious health problems, such as obesity, atherosclerosis and cancer of the breast, pancreas and the bowel. This is why official guidelines state that saturated fats should contribute a maximum of 10 per cent of the daily fat intake, with trans fats – fats artificially produced by food manufacturers through a process called hydrogenation – making up no more than 2 per cent. The balance of fats should come solely from unsaturated forms.

There are two types of unsaturated fats: monounsaturates, found in vegetable oils, such as olive, corn and safflower oil, and polyunsaturates: the richest sources of which are oily fish, such as mackerel, herrings and sardines, and some vegetable oils – notably those derived from soy and rapeseed. Unsaturated fats contain fatty acids – omega-9 in monounsaturates and omega-6 and omega-3 in polyunsaturates – which are all important for health: both omega-6 and -3 are classed as an essential dietary constituent. When converted by the body into gamma-linolenic acid (GLA) and then into prostaglandins, these fatty acids help to reduce the risk of heart disease and circulatory disorders: a lack of these can weaken the body's immune system.

Adults need around 4 g/⅛ oz of omega-6 fatty acids daily, with an upper daily limit of 25 g/1 oz). Exceeding this may be harmful to the body. The body needs slightly less of the omega-3 fatty acids – you would meet the recommended quota by eating a single serving of oily fish or a handful of walnuts, which are also rich in fatty acids, on a daily basis.

CHECK THAT LABEL

Carefully check the labels on any processed food products that you suspect may contain large amounts of hidden fats. It is a legal requirement to specify the polyunsaturated, monounsaturated and saturated fat levels in all pre-prepared food. However, more general claims can often be confusing, and even misleading. 'Reduced' fat, does not necessarily mean the same as 'low' fat. In this context, reduced, according to food regulators, means that there should be a reduction of 25 per cent or more in overall fat content in an average serving, but this can still allow for an awful lot of fat in the food. Terms such as 'light' (or 'lite') should also be viewed sceptically unless they are backed-up by scientific verification.

HARMFUL foods
Hard margarine and solid cooking fats.
Biscuits (cookies), cakes, chocolate and pastries.
Fatty meat and meat products.
Full-fat dairy products, including hard cheese, butter and cream.

HELPFUL foods
Wholemeal (whole-wheat) bread, Granary (multigrain) bread, rye bread.
Rolled oats and cereal containing cooked bran.
Oranges, apples, pears, bananas and other fresh fruit, dried apricots, figs and prunes.
Sweetcorn (corn), mangetouts (snow peas), garlic, onions, haricot (navy) beans, red kidney beans, broad (fava) beans and similar vegetables.

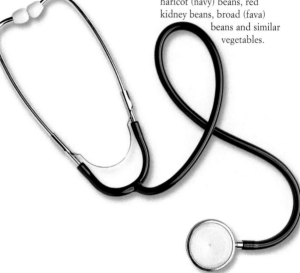

WHAT IS CHOLESTEROL?

There are two types of cholesterol – dietary cholesterol and blood cholesterol. The former is contained in food, while the latter, which is manufactured by the liver, is essential, in the correct amounts, for the proper functioning of the body's metabolic system. Problems can arise if the blood cholesterol level rises unduly, because if the level stays high, or climbs higher, heart disease is the likely result. Scientists have shown that there is not necessarily a link between the amount of cholesterol in the food you eat and the level of cholesterol in the blood, although obviously, if you have a raised blood cholesterol level, it would make sense to reduce the former. What certainly does influence cholesterol levels, however, is the amount of saturated fats and trans fats you are consuming on a daily basis. Medical research indicates that, if you cut right back on saturated- and trans-fat consumption, the blood cholesterol level can be lowered by as much as 14 per cent. The list above shows you what foods are thought to help in lowering blood cholesterol down to normal levels and keeping it that way. It also indicates which types of food contribute to raising it and keeping it raised.

FOOD CLASSIFICATIONS: SUGARS

Together with starch, sugars are one of the main types of energy-providing carbohydrates, but as far as food combining is concerned, this is where the similarity ends. Because most sugars can be digested and turned into glucose quickly, they are an almost immediate energy source. However, the

drawback is that the energy boost you receive does not last for very long and you can feel more tired afterwards than you did before. Sugars are not nutrient-rich either, containing very little 'food-value' which is why the calories they contain are often referred to as 'empty' calories.

Although sugars and starches are both carbohydrates, they behave very differently in combination with other foods, and will be discussed separately. This section, therefore, concerns foods in which sugars are the dominant nutrient.

   Although sugars are speedy providers of energy because the body finds them extremely easy to digest, convert and absorb, they are not great sources of vitamins, minerals, fibre and other healthy nutrients. It is therefore important, nutritionally, to make sure that sugar-rich drinks and snacks are not eaten to the exclusion of other more health-beneficial foods – especially by children. Sugar, it should be noted, has a suppressant effect on the appetite, which can add to nutritional problems.

There is also a proven link between the excessive consumption of foods rich in refined sugar and tooth decay. This happens because the bacteria already present on the teeth quickly break down the sugar to form an acid that attacks and destroys tooth enamel.

SUGAR VARIETIES

As far as food combining is concerned, sugars are subdivided basically into milk sugars and vegetable sugars, although fruits rich in sugar must also be taken into consideration. Honey, for its

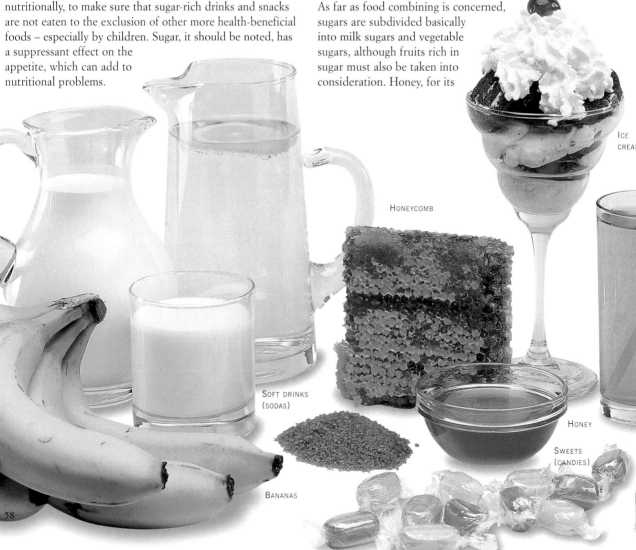

ICE CREAM

HONEYCOMB

SOFT DRINKS
(SODAS)

HONEY

SWEETS
(CANDIES)

BANANAS

part, is believed to be a vegetable product, despite being produced through the agency of bees. Some people refuse to eat honey on ethical grounds, but purely from the point of view of nutrition, it is an excellent food.

A number of fruits have a sugar content of more than 12 per cent. In these fruits, sugar is the dominant nutrient, although a different grouping is made in the section in this book about acids. This is because some fruits that are rich in sugar also contain large amounts of acid. Milk sugars generally have a low sugar content: they are included really only for interest. Milk is a nutritious food, but it is difficult to combine with other foodstuffs.

INTRINSIC AND EXTRINSIC SUGARS

Conventional nutritionists have another means of distinguishing between the types of sugar. They divide the various types, which themselves are defined according to their degree of sweetness, into 'intrinsic' and 'extrinsic' sugars. The difference between the two is simple and straightforward – intrinsic sugars are contained within the cell walls of plants, extrinsic sugars are not. Examples of intrinsic sugars include fruit and sweet-tasting vegetables, such as beetroot (beet) in its natural, unprocessed state, and carrots. The sweetest form of sugar is fructose, found in fruit and honey, followed in descending order by sucrose, glucose, maltose and lactose.

These foods, on the whole, are good for you because of the other, more valuable nutrients that they contain. Beetroot (beet), for instance, is rich in potassium, which helps to regulate the heartbeat and maintain normal blood pressure and nerve function. It is a good source of folate and contains some Vitamin C. Fresh, raw beetroot (beet) juice is such a concentrated vitamin and mineral resource that it is considered a perfect tonic for convalescents. The vegetable is believed by some medical researchers to contain various valuable anti-carcinogens. However, the one drawback of such foods,

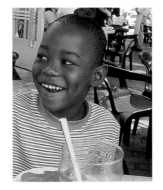

LEFT: In the modern diet sucrose accounts for 30 per cent of the carbohydrate intake.

although a minor one, is worth noting. Not only does the sugar in them act as an appetite suppressant: the fibre that they contain helps to make people feel full.

Extrinsic sugars include table sugar, or sucrose – which is the main constituent of sugar cane and sugar beet – syrup, molasses, and lactose, the sugar found in milk and its derivative products. Because these types of sugars are thought to put the teeth at most risk of damage, the official viewpoint is that they should not exceed more than 10 per cent of the total daily calorie intake. This is not the figure mirrored in the typical modern diet – at least, not in the industrialized world, where sucrose accounts for 30 per cent of the daily carbohydrate intake in the average adult diet, with lactose and a mixture of other sugars trailing way behind with figures of 10 per cent each.

SUGAR AND HEALTH

With the exception of the proven link between extrinsic sugars and an increased incidence of tooth decay, the health jury has yet to return a clear verdict on whether or not sugar is definitely bad for you. Although sugar has suffered a bad press, health-wise, over the years – eating excessive amounts of it have been linked, in theory, to an increased risk of heart and kidney disease and to the onset of non-insulin-dependent diabetes – there is still insufficient clearcut scientific evidence to clinch such claims. Some health experts even argue that there is no hard-and-fast connection between eating large amounts of sugar and the incidence of obesity, pointing out that reputable research indicates that, in fact, thin people eat more sugar than overweight people.

Because sugar, in itself, does not contribute anything other than energy to bodily well-being – its vitamin, mineral and fibre content is minuscule, if present at all – it should not be a major dietary constituent. White sugar, for instance, has 90 per cent of its vitamin and mineral contents, which are already low, removed by the refining process. Provided that you do not eat more than a moderate amount of it, however, eating it is still acceptable nutritionally in conjunction with a well-balanced and well-combined dietary mix of vitamins, minerals, fibre, fat, protein and other forms of carbohydrate. The one exception is milk, which can be a problem for people with lactose intolerance, because their bodies are deficient in lactase, the enzyme required to digest milk sugar.

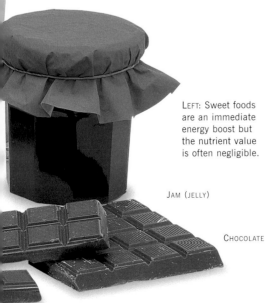

LEFT: Sweet foods are an immediate energy boost but the nutrient value is often negligible.

JAM (JELLY)

CHOCOLATE

WHICH FOODS CONTAIN THE MOST SUGAR?

When it comes to food combining, although sugar is classed, along with starch, as a carbohydrate, it is important to ascertain how much sugar specific foodstuffs contain. You need to find out whether or not sugar is the dominant nutrient: if it is not, as is sometimes the case with fruit, despite surface appearances, this knowledge may well have an effect on the planning of good food combinations. The following tables show the percentages of sugar in a variety of common food sources, split into the sugar families that food combiners favour.

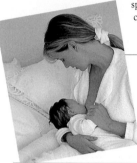

Milk sugar (lactose)

Breast milk	7.1%
Cow's milk	4.8%
Goat's milk	4.8%
Sheep's milk	4.7%

Vegetable sugar

Industrial sugar	100%
Brown cane sugar	98%
Honey	91%
Sweets	84-97%
Soft drinks (sodas)	82%
Preserves	80%
Jam (jelly)	63%
Apple syrup	60%
Maple syrup	60%
Fruit cordial	57%
Chocolate	54%

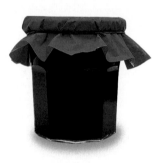

Fruits rich in sugar

Sweetened canned fruit	60%	Greengage	13.5%
Fruit concentrate	57%	Passion fruit	13.4%
Dried fruit	55%	Fresh fig	12.9%
Banana	23%	Mango	12.8%
Bilberry (wild)	19.6%	Sweet cherry	12.7%
Rose-hip	19.3%	Nectarine	12.4%
Bilberry (cultivated)	19%	Cactus fig	12%
Grape juice	17.1%	Honeydew melon	12%
Lychee	17%	Redcurrant juice	12%
Grape	16.8%	Plum	11.9%
Mirabelle plum	15.5%	Pomegranate	11.6%

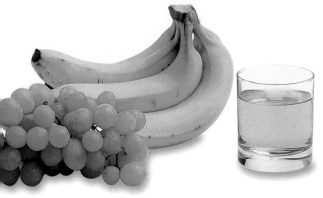

Just because you cannot see sugar listed among the ingredients on a food or soft drink (soda) label does not mean that it is not there. Look out also for sucrose, lactose, maltrose (the sugar contained in sprouting grains, malted wheat and barley and malt extract), fructose, honey, molasses, glucose, dextrose, corn syrup and invert syrup. All of these sugars have little, if any, nutritional value: they are a source of 'empty' calories, good for a quick energy burst, but nothing more, and are potentially harmful to the teeth into the bargain. Most sweetened soft drinks (sodas), in particular, are packed with sugar: a can of regular, non-diet cola, for instance, contains 21 g/¾ oz on average – just over four teaspoons. Some other drinks are almost equally guilty with a sugar content ranging from a single teaspoon to four or more a glass. The table shows the calories and amounts of sugar contained by some popular soft drinks (sodas), measured by the can or glass. A teaspoon of sugar weighs about 5 g/⅙ oz.

Nor are the low-calorie, sugar-free soft drinks that you can substitute for sugar-laden ones the complete answer to the problem. Some experts on nutrition – food combiners in particular – have their doubts about the effects of the artificial sweeteners that many of these drinks contain, the argument being that there is some evidence that, if relied on in excess, these can also affect blood glucose levels adversely and, just like

DRINK	CALORIES	SUGAR
Regular cola	86	21g
Rosehip syrup	77	21g
Lemonade	42	11g
Tonic water	50	11g
Lime juice cordial	58	10g
Orange drink	36	10g
Diet orange drink	3	1g
Diet cola	0.9	No sugar

real sugars, stimulate sugar craving. There is certainly a dispute as to whether the 'isotonic' drinks specifically produced for sportspeople are positively good for you, as is often claimed. In addition to boosting energy, such drinks are also designed to help to replace the valuable electrolytes (mineral salts) that the body looses as it sweats. However, the caffeine usually contained in such drinks is a diuretic as well as an energy booster, and is more likely to encourage dehydration rather than replenish fluids. Some sports drinks also have added sugar, and claim that this helps the body to absorb the water in the drink far more quickly than through drinking water alone, but the amount of sugar added can be anything from around 5 per cent to as much as 18 per cent of the content.

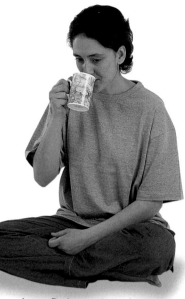

ABOVE: Replacement sweeteners are used as an alternative to sugar.

ARTIFICIAL SWEETENERS: WHAT THEY ARE AND WHAT THEY DO

There are two main types of artificial sweeteners – 'bulk' sweeteners and 'intense' sweeteners. Examples of bulk sweeteners include mannitol, sorbitol, xylitol and hydrogenated glucose syrup. These have around the same calorific value as true sugar, and are used as a replacement for it in many processed foods. Intense sweeteners, used mainly in diet soft drinks (sodas), desserts and as domestic alternatives for sweetening tea and coffee, include acesulfame K, aspartame and saccharin. Take care not to use too much of these, because they are at least twice and sometimes four times as sweet as the sugar they are replacing. Saccharin, too, can leave a bitter aftertaste, although aspartame tastes much the same as genuine sugar. Some health authorities dispute exactly how good for you these sugar alternatives really are. Although they are virtually calorie-free, there have been claims that aspartame, in particular, can trigger blurred vision, headaches, and in some instances even symptoms of hyperactivity, but to date, such claims have not been backed by reliable scientific evidence. Equally, claims that artificial sweeteners trigger the urge to eat more have been discounted by most experts.

SUGAR, DIABETES AND DIET

Blood sugar levels are controlled by a hormone known as insulin. When the organ that produces insulin (the pancreas) malfunctions, it causes diabetes – a metabolic disorder. In diabetics, the pancreas stops manufacturing insulin, or fails to make enough of it. The condition can also occur if, for whatever reason, the body is unable to use insulin, even when the pancreas is producing it effectively. What causes the pancreas to malfunction is actually unknown.

The condition takes two forms: insulin-dependent diabetes, in which insulin production ceases completely (this usually starts in childhood, although it can strike at any age), and non-insulin-dependent diabetes, in which the body's cells fail to respond to insulin (much more common among older people, primarily those aged over 40 who are unfit and overweight). The condition cannot be caused simply by eating too much sugar or the wrong type of food. Diabetes is on the increase, particularly in the industrialized world: statistics show that, since the mid-1980s, the number of diagnosed cases has tripled. This, however, could be merely the tip of the iceberg, because for every confirmed case of non-insulin-dependent diabetes, it is likely that at least one other case remains undiagnosed. Although the effects of the condition can be mitigated, both types of diabetes are incurable. If you suffer from insulin-dependent diabetes, you will have to inject yourself with insulin for life: depending on its degree of severity, non-insulin-dependent diabetes may be treated by diet alone, or by a combination of tablets and diet, although it may prove necessary to inject insulin at a later stage. If you are diagnosed as a diabetic, following a healthy diet is a vital factor in controlling the disease, regardless of type. A dietician will advise you to:

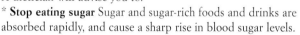

ABOVE: Injected insulin is vital for some diabetics.

* **Stop eating sugar** Sugar and sugar-rich foods and drinks are absorbed rapidly, and cause a sharp rise in blood sugar levels.
* **Eat regularly** This is important – it maintains the correct balance of sugar in the bloodstream.
* **Increase fibre intake** Fibre promotes slower absorption of sugar from foods. You should eat wholemeal (whole-wheat) bread and high-fibre cereals, pulses – peas, beans and lentils – and plenty of vegetables and salads.
* **Reduce fat intake** Cutting back on fat is particularly important in achieving an ideal body weight. Cut the fat off meat, use less butter and margarine – grill (broil) rather than fry, use oil (preferably extra virgin olive oil) eat less cheese, nuts only in moderation, drink semi-skimmed (low-fat) milk and avoid cream.
* **Reduce salt intake** Use only a small amount in cooking, and do not add more salt at the table. Meat and yeast extracts are very high in salt, and should be used sparingly.
* **Moderate your drinking** Alcoholic drinks are particularly high in calories and can upset diabetic control. Keep within the recommended maximum number of units in any one day: three units for men and two units for women. Drink red wine, rather than white wine, and avoid spirits, beer and lager completely.

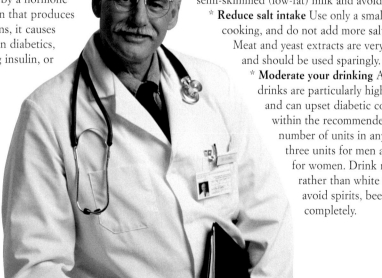

RECOMMENDATIONS FOR THE DIABETIC DIET

FOODS TO BE AVOIDED

Sugary food
Sugar, glucose, sorbitol, sucron, sweets (candies), chocolate, standard jam (jelly) and marmalade, honey, treacle (molasses), syrup, lemon curd, sweet mincemeat, marzipan.

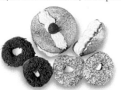

Starchy foods
Cakes, sweet biscuits (cookies), pastries and tarts, sweetened desserts, canned spaghetti, canned ravioli, sausage rolls, Cornish pasty, pork pie, rissoles, meat pie, dumplings, batter, canned and packet soups.

Fatty foods
Fried foods, lard, dripping, standard salad dressing and mayonnaise, cream, evaporated and condensed milk, cream, cheese, fatty meat such as belly (side) pork and breast of lamb.

Drinks
Standard sparkling drinks, sweetened fruit juices and drinks, malted milk drinks.

FOODS TO EAT IN MODERATION

Poultry
Chicken and turkey without skin.

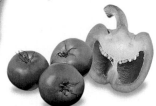

Lean meat
Pork, lamb, beef.

Offal (variety meats)
Kidney, liver.

Fish
All varieties

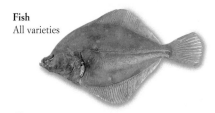

Cheese
Low-fat cheeses (24 per cent to 26 per cent fat maximum)

Eggs
Two to three a week

FOODS TO EAT FREELY

Vegetables
All vegetables and salads.

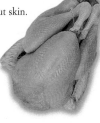

Fruit
Grapefruit, lemon, melon, rhubarb, gooseberries, blackberries, black and red currants, raspberries, and up to three pieces of all other fruits a day.

Drinks
Tea, coffee, mineral water, diabetic and sugar-free drinks, sugar-free fizzy drinks (sodas), tomato juice, unthickened vegetable soups.

A DIABETIC MEAL PLAN

Breakfast
Whole-grain cereal or porridge.

Mid-morning
Tea, coffee or a low-calorie drink.

Lunch
Lean meat, poultry, fish or pulses; vegetables or salad.

Mid-afternoon
Tea, coffee or a low-calorie drink.

Evening meal
Lean meat, poultry, fish, eggs, cheese or pulses; vegetables or fruit.

Bedtime
Tea, coffee or a low calorie drink; a firm banana.

The table above shows which foods and drinks diabetics should avoid, which they can eat freely and which can be eaten in moderation. It is also important for diabetics not to let their blood sugar levels fall too low. This may cause a condition called hypoglycaemia, the symptoms of which are weakness, confusion, irritability, sweating, seizures and even loss of consciousness. At the first sign of such an attack, eating something to give the body an instant sugar boost is the essential first response. The conventional meal plan was prepared for a 52-year-old man with recently-diagnosed non-insulin-dependent diabetes. However, food combiners would query the positioning of fruit in this meal plan, placing it at the end of the meals, or preferably, on its own for breakfast, or as part of the two between-meal snacks. Nor should vegetables be starch-dominated if they are combined with food that is rich in protein. The banana at bedtime should certainly stay, as this helps to keep the body supplied with a trickle of energy through the night.

FOOD CLASSIFICATIONS: STARCH

Starch is what is known as a complex carbohydrate, accounting, in the average diet, for around half of the total carbohydrate intake. Conventional nutritionists argue that, ideally, complex carbohydrates should provide the body with two-thirds of the calories it needs each day, *but food combiners are not so confident that the accepted view is totally correct. Although there is a number of starch-rich foods to choose from, the fact remains that it is almost impossible to combine them well with other foods and particularly with proteins.*

Starch belongs to a group classified as polysaccharides, or complex sugars: it is the most important form in which saccharides (sugars) are found in plant cells. It is present in large quantities in the seeds of grasses, such as buckwheat, and in chestnuts, carrots, tubers, root crops, stalks, and sometimes in fruits and leaves.

Many of the starch-rich parts of plants are important sources of nutrition for humans and animals, and are of major economic significance as a result. These include potatoes, wheat, corn, rice, oats, barley, rye, buckwheat, leguminous vegetables, soy, cassava (from which tapioca is derived), arrowroot and sago, from the pith of a variety of palm.

PROBLEMS IN COMBINATION

Starch is important to conventional nutrition. A substantial proportion of all the world's agricultural production for human and animal consumption consists of starchy foods. Most books on nutrition, too, emphasize the importance of starch as a source of energy. From an economic viewpoint, this makes good enough sense, but from a purely nutritional angle, differing opinions on the value of starch foods are beginning to make themselves heard.

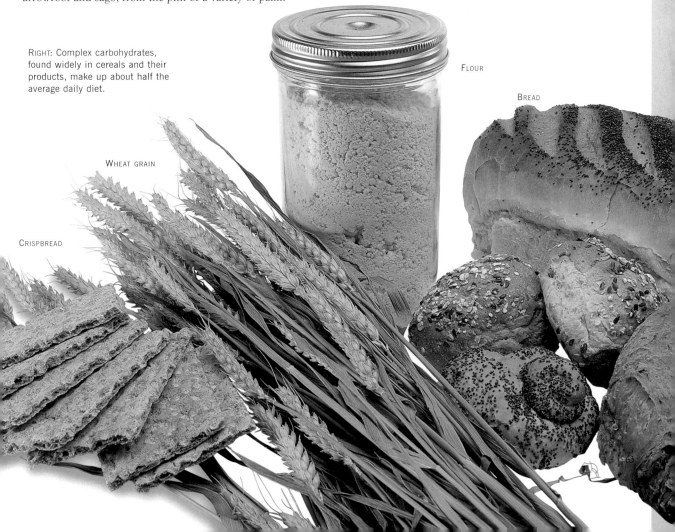

RIGHT: Complex carbohydrates, found widely in cereals and their products, make up about half the average daily diet.

FLOUR

BREAD

WHEAT GRAIN

CRISPBREAD

An analysis of the results of food combining leads directly to the conclusion that foods rich in starch are extremely difficult to combine with other foods, and that all such combinations tend to cause a plethora of digestive problems. Indeed, the first axiom of classic food combining is that starch-rich or sugary foods should never be combined in the same meal with foods in which protein is the dominant nutrient. Similarly, fruit should be eaten separately from proteins and starches.

The reasons for keeping starch-rich foods and foods rich in protein well apart should be obvious. The human body simply was not designed to digest more than one concentrated food at a time with any degree of efficiency. Starches and proteins, in particular, are treated entirely differently by the digestion and, if eaten in combination, either – or both – may not be digested properly as a result. The obvious consequences are attacks of gas, bloating, flatulence, abdominal and intestinal discomfort and, sometimes pain, which on occasion can be extremely severe. In other words, poor combining has led to all the signs and symptoms of a classic indigestion attack.

MAKING SURE OF GOOD DIGESTION

The golden rule is that poor digestion is a result of inadequate absorption: the body is failing to ingest some of the nutrients it needs with obvious effects on its energy levels and its ability to maintain itself in peak condition. Nor is this all.

A shortage of vital nutrients through poor digestion and continual strain on the digestive system has the potential to compromise the workings of the immune system, reducing the ability to fight off infections and illnesses. In certain circumstances, it may even increase the long-term risk of developing a degenerative disease.

Observing food combining commonsense will alter your eating habits for the better and make it easier for your digestive system to be sure that your body is getting all the vital health-sustaining nutrients it requires, when and how it needs them. A healthy body works long and hard to keep itself that way, so you should be encouraging the process, rather than hindering it. If the digestive system becomes overloaded and overstressed, it will eventually clog up with unwanted waste products, which will sap your vitality and drain your energy reserves.

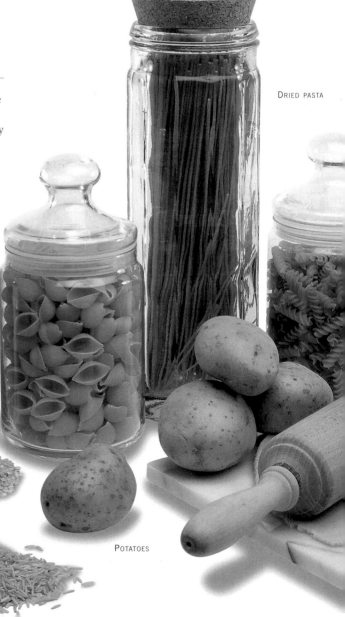

DRIED PASTA

RICE

POTATOES

WHY THE BODY NEEDS STARCH

This is not to say that we should turn the clock back to the days when starchy carbohydrates, such as bread, pasta, potatoes and rice, were generally considered by old-school nutritionists and dieticians to be stodgy, fattening, second-rate foods. This is far from the case. Although food combining experts are opposed to the combination of starch-rich foods with protein-dominated ones, and as explained later, have raised considerable doubts about other problematical food combinations, they do not question the fact that complex carbohydrates should form an important part of any healthy-eating plan. There are two reasons for this: not only are starch-rich foods an important energy resource, but the way in which they are digested means that they can provide energy over a longer period than, for example, simple sugars, and the foodstuffs which contain them.

HOW STARCH IS DIGESTED

The main difference between the body's digestion of simple sugars and complex carbohydrates lies in the time it takes for these substances to be broken down, and consequently, what the body does with the results. Generally, simple sugars are converted directly into glucose, an energy source that the body can use instantly because it is absorbed straight into the blood. Complex carbohydrates, on the other hand, take longer to break down. By the time they have been digested fully, the body's immediate energy needs tend to have been satisfied by the glucose it has already processed. The body, therefore, turns the complex carbohydrates into glycogen, a form of sugar it can store in the liver and the muscles, ready to be turned into glucose when the need arises.

Technically, glycogen and glucose are 'interconvertible': if the body has enough glucose, carbohydrates will be converted into glycogen; if there is a glucose shortage, glycogen will be turned into glucose to make up the deficiency. The rate at which carbohydrates are digested helps to maintain a healthy

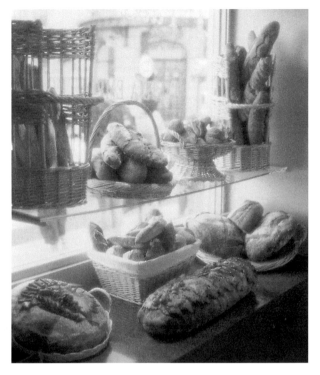

ABOVE: Starch-rich foods are an essential energy source and help to balance glucose in the blood.

balance between the levels of glucose in the blood and the state of the glycogen reserves, always assuming that you are eating enough carbohydrates in roughly the right proportions in the first place. This is why it is such a bad idea to cut right back on the amount of complex carbohydrate you eat to try to lose weight, a method frequently advised in old-fashioned diet books. The body reacts by draining all its glycogen reserves, which then are not replenished fully because of the dietary cut-backs that have been imposed. Living off glycogen reserves will work for a short time, but you will soon start to feel the effects as they run down and the muscles are starved of the energy they need. Muscles normally contain enough glycogen to fuel between 90 minutes and two hours of intensive physical activity: after a bout of intensive exercise, their uptake of glucose can be increased by a factor of three or four. It is far better, modern nutritionists agree, to cut back on fat intake instead.

POTATO CRISPS (CHIPS)

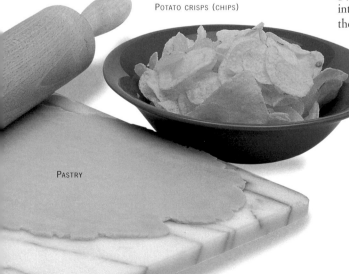

PASTRY

LEFT: Complex carbohydrates should form part of any healthy-eating plan.

HOW MUCH STARCH?

Starch is present exclusively in vegetable foods, with the exception of an animal starch known as glycogen, a sort of precursor of glucose stored in organs, such as the liver, the heart and the tongue, and in the muscles. As a constituent in food, amounts of glycogen are so small that they can be ignored in food combining.

Although the different kinds of starch combine freely, the table below distinguishes between the various farinaceous (starchy) foods,

to provide a better insight into their great variety. If you want to widen food combining possibilities still further, starch ceases to be a dominant nutrient in a particular food if its content is less than 4 per cent, although you should remember that you can still create a false combination by distorting food-to-food ratios unfavourably. This is why, when planning meals, it is best not to take chances and accidentally create unfortunate combinations.

GRAINS

White rice	78%
Wholegrain rice	75%
Millet	69%
Corn	65%
Oats	61%
Wheat	60%
Barley	58%
Rye	54%

FLOUR

Rice flour	79%
Cornflakes	74%
Barley flour	72%
Wheat flour	72%
Popcorn	68%
Cornflour (cornstarch)	65%
Rye flour	65%
Oatmeal	61%
Puff pastry	37%

BREAD

Crispbread	66%
Rusk	61%
Wholemeal (whole-wheat) rusk	58%
White	48%
Rye	45%

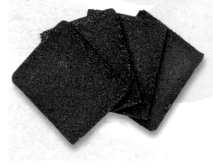

PASTA

Spaghetti	75%
Noodles	65%
Wholewheat noodles	64%

SEEDS

Buckwheat	71%
Buckwheat flour	71%
Chestnut	41%

INDIVIDUAL STARCHES

Corn starch	86%
Rice starch	85%
Tapioca starch	85%
Potato starch	83%
Wheat starch	83%

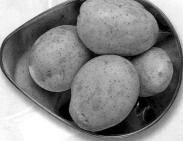

VEGETABLES RICH IN STARCH

Potato crisps (chips)	53%
Potato chips (French fries)	35%
Potato croquettes	20%
Raw potato	15.4%
Boiled potato	14%
Horseradish	11.7%
Ginger	11%
Mashed potato	11%

VEGETABLES LOW IN STARCH

Garlic	6%
Green beans (pods)	5%
Pumpkin	5%
Winter radish	4.1%
Jerusalem artichoke inulin, a starch substitute	4%
Kohlrabi	4%
Chicory (Belgian endive)	3%
Asparagus	2%
Chinese leaves (cabbage)	2%
Blanched celery	1%
Endive (chicory)	1%
Mushrooms	1%
Parsley	1%
(Bell) Peppers (red and green)	1%
Radish	1%
Parsnip	0.5%
Celeriac (celery root)	0.4%

STARCH-FREE VEGETABLES AND HERBS

Aubergine (eggplant)	Lamb's lettuce
Broccoli	(mâche)
Brussels sprouts	Leek
Cabbage (red and white)	Lettuce
Carrots	Nettle
Carrot tops	Onion
Cauliflower	Purslane
Chervil	Rhubarb
Courgette (zucchini)	Salsify
Cucumber	Shallot
Dandelion	Swede
Garden cress	(rutabaga)
(land cress)	Tomatoes
Garden sorrel	Turnip
Fennel	Watercress
Finocchio/Florence fennel	
Gherkin (cornichon)	

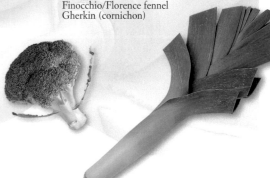

EVERYDAY FIBRE SOURCES

Although fibre has little, if any, purely nutritional value, there is no doubting the fact that an adequate fibre intake is vital to good digestion. Both types of fibre – soluble and insoluble – have their own important roles to play in regulating blood sugar levels and speeding up the passage of food through the system. Dieticians recommend that you eat at least 18 g/⅝ oz of high-fibre food a day, unless you have been warned by a doctor that you cannot tolerate a high-fibre diet – this caution applies in particular to sufferers from diverticular disease, certain types of irritable bowel syndrome and inflammatory bowel disease. The table shows the most important fibre sources.

SOLUBLE FIBRE

Barley
Brown Rice
Beans
Oats and oat bran
Pulses
Many vegetables and fruits
(e.g. carrots, grapes and oranges)

INSOLUBLE FIBRE

Fruit skins
Nuts
Rice
Wheat and corn bran
Wholegrain breads and cereals
Many vegetables and their skins
(e.g. green beans and potatoes)

SOLUBLE AND INSOLUBLE FIBRE

Dried fruit
Fresh fruit (usually ½ soluble, ½ insoluble:
e.g. apple peel is insoluble cellulose,
apple flesh is rich in soluble pectin)
Most grains (⅔ soluble to ⅓ insoluble)
Oatmeal, barley and legumes
(65 per cent soluble)
Most vegetables (⅔ soluble to ⅓ insoluble)

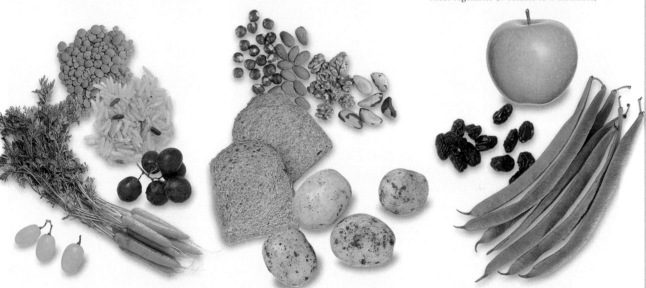

STARCH AND FIBRE

Eating plenty of starchy foods has an added bonus: many of them, particularly fresh fruit and vegetables, are also rich in dietary fibre. Although this has almost no nutritional value in itself, it is a vital dietary constituent, since it encourages efficient, effective digestion. There are two main types: soluble fibre, which is found in most fruit and vegetables, pulses and oats, and insoluble fibre, found in foods such as wheat, rice and nuts. Some foods, notably wheat bran, wholegrains and dried fruit, contain both.

Soluble fibre slows the rate at which glucose is absorbed into the bloodstream, helping to control blood sugar levels and keep them stable. It also helps to reduce blood cholesterol levels by binding with the cholesterol that is contained in bile, a liquid secreted by the liver to help to break down fats. Some of this cholesterol stays combined with the fibre and is excreted as waste, rather than being reabsorbed into the blood. This reduces the risk of contracting heart disease.

Insoluble fibre, or 'roughage' as it is sometimes popularly termed, increases stool bulk, speeding up the passage of food residues through the digestive tract. This helps to keep the intestines in good order, reducing the risk of intestinal conditions such as bowel cancer, diverticular disease and gallstones. It certainly helps to prevent constipation, and may help to prevent the build-up of harmful carcinogens.

Yet another bonus is that both types of fibre are filling, which means that you are less likely to fall victim to snacking on sugary and fatty refined foodstuffs.

HOW MUCH FIBRE?

Eating plenty of fibre-rich food and drinking at least 2 litres/ 3½ pints/8¾ cups of water a day is a healthy way of giving the digestive system a much-needed boost, according to modern nutritionists. The more fibre you eat, the more water the digestive tract can absorb, with a desirable increase in faecal bulk as a result. Most experts recommend eating at least 18g/⅝ oz of fibre a day – the current average in the industrialized world is 40 per cent less than this. Some, however, go much further than this, arguing that at least 35 g/ 1½ oz of fibre a day is needed to be sure of good digestive health. A food is considered to be a good source of fibre if it provides at least 2.5 g per serving.

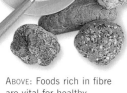

ABOVE: Foods rich in fibre are vital for healthy digestion.

There is a slight risk, however, in such a dramatic increase in fibre intake. Eating too much fibre can restrict children's absorption of calcium, which they need for bone building and strengthening; in women it may restrict the absorption of iron. There is also a possibility of zinc deficiency. This is especially the case if you are eating lots of bran and brown rice, because of the phytic acid they contain. The simple solution is to make sure that the fibre you eat comes from a variety of foods. This will help to prevent any potential adverse effects. If you suddenly switch to a high-fibre diet, you may experience some flatulence and digestive discomfort, at least initially. Dieticians advise building up the fibre intake gradually, starting by upping the amount of soluble fibre you consume. They also say that you should drink more water than you think you need, particularly between, rather than with, meals.

LOW STARCH, NO STARCH

While some vegetables are starch-rich and therefore calorie dense, others are mostly composed of water. They are also a great source of Vitamin C, folate, beta-carotene, minerals and fibre, and contain practically no fat of any description. If you are watching your weight – or want to vary what you eat while maintaining the rules of good food combining – these non-starchy vegetables are the ones to choose. In percentage terms, a starch level of less than 4 per cent means that the starch content can be discounted the purposes of food combining.

Regularly eating a selection of cruciferous vegetables, such as pak choi (bok choy), broccoli, Brussels sprouts, cabbage, cauliflower, kale, radishes, turnips and watercress, is

particularly to be encouraged. All of the vegetables in this family are proven cancer-fighters – particularly helpful in protecting the body against cancer of the colon or rectum. They are also rich sources of calcium, iron and folate. Other deliciously healthy vegetables you can eat without worrying about accidentally creating a bad or problematic food combining mixture include asparagus, chicory (belgian endive), mushrooms, (bell) peppers and tomatoes, as well as a wide variety of greens.

HOW WE KNOW WHEN IT'S TIME TO EAT

When your body needs to eat, its response is to trigger the release of neurotransmitters – chemicals that transmit information to your brain cells. Scientists now believe that one neurotransmitter in particular, Neuropeptide Y (NPY), is thought to respond when the body needs carbohydrate. Their theory claims that NPY is released from the hypothalamus when glycogen and blood glucose levels are lowered. As the NPY levels increase, so does the desire for sweet and starchy food, which is why, for instance, favourite morning foods include cereal, bread, biscuits (cookies), bagels and fruit. If you skip breakfast and lunch, the cravings get worse until you are read for a carbohydrate binge. Satisfying the need turns off the supply of NPY and triggers the action of another brain chemical, serotonin. When the serotonin level goes up, the NPY level decreases, telling your body that you have had enough food and can stop eating.

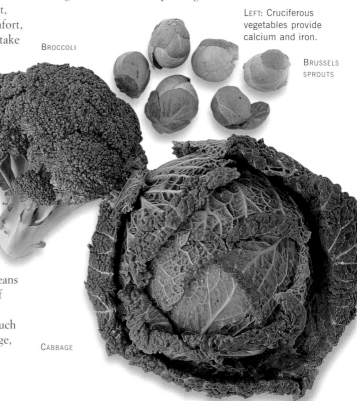

LEFT: Cruciferous vegetables provide calcium and iron.

BROCCOLI

BRUSSELS SPROUTS

CABBAGE

FOOD CLASSIFICATIONS: ACIDS

You will find that many food combiners, taking their cue from Dr Hay and Dr Shelton, talk a great deal about acidic and alkaline foodstuffs, and the importance of veering towards the alkaline in the food that you eat and reducing the acid. As you will discover, I believe that much of *this argument is scientifically unsound. For good digestion, it is important that the body's own acid-base balance is kept in kilter, to maintain a constant acidity/alkalinity value. This job largely falls to substances in the blood known as buffers.*

WHERE HAY WENT WRONG

The traditional food combining argument first proposed by Dr Hay runs more or less as follows. Firstly, he assumed that alkaline-forming foods definitely exist, and that nearly all protein-rich foods and foods rich in starch are acid-forming. For improved digestion and good health, Hay believed that we ought to eat far more alkaline-forming food, cut back on the acidic proteins and starches, and never eat starch and protein together. The best way to make sure of this, he argued, was to plan out a day's eating that included one protein, one starch and one alkaline meal per day, thus keeping what he understood to be the three key dietary constituents separate, as far as possible. Hay concluded that we should eat four times the amount of alkaline foods as acidic ones, to maintain what he perceived as the ideal 80:20 alkali-to-acid ratio within the body. He did his best to establish this ratio scientifically by measuring the amounts of alkaline and acidic elements excreted through the skin, lungs, bowel and kidneys. Through this, he discovered that the body lost more than four times the amount of alkaline elements as acidic ones.

Many of Dr Hay's precepts have stood the test of time and are perfectly valid today – notably, his statement that 'it is not how much we eat, but how much we can fully digest, absorb and metabolize, that counts'. There are all sorts of good reasons, too, for not combining protein-rich foodstuffs with foods in which starch is the dominant nutrient, as you will see when you come to the chapter on good, bad and problematic combinations. However, there were occasions on which he fell into scientific error. Hay's belief in alkaline-forming foods – and the beliefs of other food combiners who accept his views uncritically – would be acceptable if such things actually existed. Scientifically speaking, they do not.

The definition of acid-alkaline neutrality, in scientific terms, is a pH of 7. The higher on the scale you go, the more alkaline the substance or substances involved. The lower you go, the greater the amount of acid they contain. As I will explain later, no food has a pH value of 7 or over: foods always have a greater or lesser degree of acidity. What happens to what we eat once it is inside the body is a very different matter.

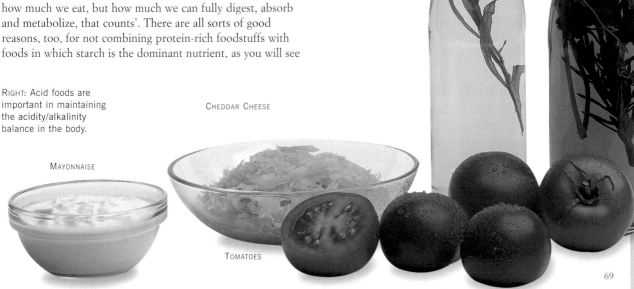

RIGHT: Acid foods are important in maintaining the acidity/alkalinity balance in the body.

MAYONNAISE

CHEDDAR CHEESE

TOMATOES

VINEGAR

DEGREES OF ACIDITY

In these pages, we will discuss those foods which contain acids that have an effect on food combining. The acids involved are known as free acids. If we eat too much acid-forming food, digestion is problematic, even if the foods combine well otherwise.

A distinction must be made between the degree of acidity – the pH value – and the acid content, which is the constituent proportion of acids expressed as a percentage by volume. A high degree of acidity gives a low pH value; a low degree of acidity gives a high pH value. Acids can damage the salivary enzyme ptyalin and slow down the production of gastric juice – but they usually have a corresponding number of beneficial properties.

The tables opposite distinguish between individual acids, acidic drinks, lactic acid products and acids in fruits. Apart from tomatoes, vegetables contain few acids, on the whole. Their degree of acidity varies from pH5 to pH6.6.

WINE: PROS AND CONS

Health authorities differ over whether drinking wine in moderation is good or bad for you. It has been suggested, for instance, based on research in France, that drinking red wine reduces the risk of heart disease. Research also indicates that red wine contains substances that lessen the clotting tendency of the blood – an advantage if you are suffering from clogged arteries and are considered a stroke risk. Red

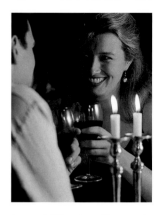

ABOVE: A little wine with a meal can aid digestion.

wine, some believe, can also act as an antioxidant. However, these views are by no means universally accepted. The French research figures have been challenged, while some substances in wine are now suspected of causing cancers of the mouth and throat. There are also elements in wine – notably the histamine in red wine – that can trigger asthma attacks, migraine and allergic reactions. What is clear, though, is that drinking a little wine with a meal can aid digestion, and makes it easier for the body to absorb any iron contained in the accompanying food.

RIGHT: The degree of acidity in foods is defined by its pH value.

SPARKLING MINERAL WATER

LEMONADE

LEMONS

BEER

BLACKBERRIES

INDIVIDUAL ACIDS BY pH VALUE

The pH value of vinegar is established by the amount of acetic acid it contains: a typical proportion is 5g/⅛ oz of acetic acid per 100 ml/3½ fl oz/scant ½ cup of water (or whichever other liquid is used). The acid gives the vinegar its characteristic flavour; it also makes it an extremely effective preservative. Excessive consumption of any food or food product containing lactic acid should be avoided. If the acid builds up in the muscles of the body, cramps can result, either during or immediately after physical exercise. All the acidic drinks listed here should be drunk only in moderation, for various nutritional and health reasons.

ACIDS

	pH value
Vinegar	1.8
Wine vinegar	2.2
Cider (apple) vinegar	2.4
Brewer's yeats	4.5

ACIDIC DRINKS

	pH value
Cola	1.9
Wine	2.1
Fizzy lemonade	2.5
Bitter lemon	2.6
Tonic water	2.6
Fizzy orangeade	2.7
Beer/lager	2.9
Port	3.2
Sparkling mineral water	4.0
Instant coffee	4.9
Tea (brewed)	5.4

LACTIC ACID PRODUCTS

	pH value
Liquid with cocktail onions	2.7
Vegetables containing lactic acid	3.2
Sauerkraut	3.4
Liquid with sweet-sour gherkins (dill pickles)	3.7
Live organic yogurt	3.9
Live yogurt	4.0

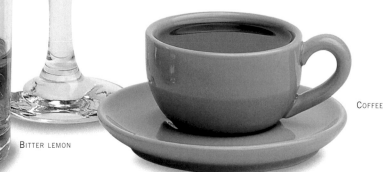
WINE
BITTER LEMON
COFFEE

ACIDS IN FRUITS

This table shows how the acidic nature of fruit varies, from mildly acidic through semi-acidic and to acidic. Some of the fruits listed in the last category may surprise you slightly, but remember that in some instances, in terms of taste, their acid content can be masked by the sugars that they contain. The pH values for the mildly-acidic fruits range from pH3.6 to pH3.9; for semi-acidic fruits, from pH3 to pH3.5; and for acidic fruits from pH2 to pH 2.9. This table lists acid content – acid as a percentage of volume.

MILDLY ACIDIC FRUITS

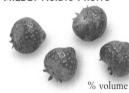

	% volume
Papaya	0.20-0.50
Pear	0.20-0.50
Cherry	0.20-0.60
Mango	0.20-1.20
Pomegranate	0.40-1.00
Apple	0.40-1.20
Banana	0.45
Plum	0.50
Strawberry	0.50
Grape	0.70
Peach	0.70
Guava	0.80
Orange	0.80
Pineapple	0.80
Sweet sloe	0.80
Quince	0.95

Raspberry	1.30
Kiwi fruit	1.60
Gooseberry	1.60
Fairly sharp grape	1.60
Fairly sharp orange	1.60
Blackberry	1.80
Morello cherry	1.80
Rowan berry	2.00
Grapefruit	2.10
Redcurrant	2.50
Cowberry	2.60

SEMI-ACIDIC FRUITS

	% volume
Elderberry	1.20
Apricot	1.30
Bilberry	1.30

ACIDIC FRUITS

	% volume
Sour cherry	3.00
Rose-hip	3.10
Whitecurrant	3.10
Blackcurrant	3.30
Whitebeam	3.30
Passion fruit	3.40
Sour sloe	3.50
Cranberry	3.80
Sea-buckthorn	3.80
Lemon	4.90

VITAMINS: THE KEY TO GOOD HEALTH

Vitamins, one of the major nutritional discoveries of the 20th century, are what are known as organic dietary compounds. Unlike carbohydrates, proteins and fats, they are not energy-providers, but are essential for health, because the body simply cannot operate without them. Although only small amounts of vitamins are required, they are vital as the trigger for enzyme functions, which in turn promote other activities, from growth and muscle function to protection against disease.

ABOVE: Vitamins are vital to maintaining a healthy body.

Because the body is unable to manufacture most vitamins for itself, to maintain good health it is vital to make sure that the food you eat contains enough of them. The World Health Organization and other international and national health agencies have devised a system to help you with this, based on lists of recommended daily allowances (RDAs) or reference nutrient intakes (RNIs). This system specifies the minimum healthy levels of daily vitamin intake: the recommendations, however, are only an average, with individual requirements varying, according to age, sex and circumstances. Babies, children and teenagers, for instance, all have specific vitamin requirements, and the elderly, ill and convalescent may have unusually high requirements for certain vitamins.

Nutritionists divide vitamins into two categories, depending on whether they are soluble in fat or in water. Vitamins A, D, E and K are fat-soluble. Unlike water-soluble vitamins, they can be stored in the body, but because they are insoluble in water, the body cannot get rid of any excess by excretion in the urine. This means that an excessive intake can be damaging to health. Vitamin C and the complex of B vitamins are water-soluble. With the exception of Vitamin B_{12}, they cannot be stored by the body, which means that a daily intake of the right amounts is a health priority.

LEFT: Fresh vegetables are a source of vitamins.

VITAMIN A: ESSENTIAL FOR GOOD EYESIGHT

Vitamin A, often referred to as retinol because of the vital part it plays in maintaining good eyesight, has several important tasks. It is needed for growth, to protect the lining of the respiratory, digestive and urinary tracts, and to make sure of normal embryonic development. The adult RDA is 700 mcg for men and 600 mcg for women, although, if you are breastfeeding, you need slightly more than this. Children, in contrast, need slightly less.

Vitamin A has two main food sources. Retinol itself is present in large amounts in liver, and can also be found in egg yolk and dairy products. Artificial forms of it are used to enrich margarine. An excessive intake of retinol can be dangerous, however, particularly if you are pregnant or trying to conceive; in early pregnancy, it can damage the foetus. The beta carotene in plant foods is a safer Vitamin A resource. Although you need to eat more of such food in order to secure adequate supplies of the vitamin, beta carotene has an added plus – it is also a powerful antioxidant, helping to protect the body against certain cancers. Carrots, in particular, are an excellent beta carotene resource, as are red (bell) peppers, mangoes, cantaloupe melons and leafy greens, such as spinach.

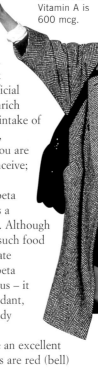

BELOW: For women the RDA of Vitamin A is 600 mcg.

THE B VITAMINS: A COMPLEX OF EIGHT

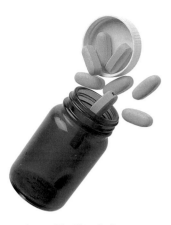

ABOVE: The Vitamin B group consists of 8 separate vitamins.

Originally, there was thought to be only a single B vitamin. Eight separate B vitamins have now been identified scientifically, all of which, with the exception of Vitamin B_{12} and folate, help the body to release and utilize the energy it receives from food.

Vitamin B_1, or thiamin, helps to convert carbohydrates, fats and alcohol into energy, and prevents the build-up of toxic by-products. If left unchecked, these by-products could lead to heart damage and problems with the nervous system. The suggested adult RDA is 1 mg daily for men and 0.8 mg for women. Good sources include potatoes – especially the skin – pork, eggs, some nuts, brown rice and beans. Some breakfast cereals are artificially enriched with it.

Vitamin B_2 is also known as riboflavin. It is a vital constituent of the body's energy-releasing process, so the need for it is determined by the amount of energy the body is using. The RDA is 1.3 mg for men and 1.1 mg for women, although pregnant and breastfeeding mothers need more, as do children during growth spurts. Milk is an excellent source, although its vitamin content is quickly destroyed if left exposed to sunlight. Other sources include poultry, liver, eggs and dairy produce.

Niacin helps in the metabolization of carbohydrates and fats, the formation of neurotransmitters, the proper functioning of the digestive system and healthy skin maintenance. Good sources of niacin include liver, lean meat, the white meat of poultry, pulses, dried beans and nuts. The body can convert proteins containing the amino acid tryptophan into niacin; sources of tryptophan include milk, eggs and cheese. RDAs are 17 mg for men and 13 mg for women.

Pantothenic acid is present in all animal and vegetable foods, particularly wholegrains, nuts and dried fruit. Nutritionists recommend between 3 mg and 7 mg daily for good health, regardless of age or sex.

Vitamin B_6, or pyridoxine, is a trio of related compounds that helps the body to break down proteins and release energy from them. Foods rich in proteins, such as chicken, fish and pork, are the best sources; other important sources include potatoes, brown rice, nuts, soy and other dried beans, and wholegrains. B_6 is also one of the few vitamins that the body can manufacture for itself, in the gut. On average, adult men need 1.4 mg and women 1.2 mg.

Vitamin B_{12} plays a vital part in healthy cell growth and division, the formation of red blood cells and the making of

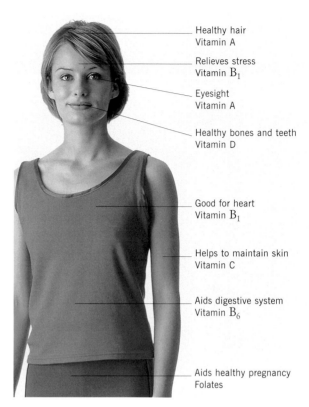

Healthy hair
Vitamin A

Relieves stress
Vitamin B_1

Eyesight
Vitamin A

Healthy bones and teeth
Vitamin D

Good for heart
Vitamin B_1

Helps to maintain skin
Vitamin C

Aids digestive system
Vitamin B_6

Aids healthy pregnancy
Folates

ABOVE: Vitamins promote growth and muscle function and give protection against disease.

DNA, RNA and myelin (the sheath that protects nerve fibres). You need only a tiny amount of it daily – the RDA is 1.5 mcg, which can come from any animal protein; eggs and dairy products are alternative sources. However, Vitamin B_{12} cannot be absorbed by the body unless a special form of glycoprotein, known as intrinsic factor, is present. The body manufactures this in the stomach.

FOLATES AND BIOTIN

Folates, a group of compounds derived from folic acid, are needed for DNA and RNA formation, cell division and protein synthesis. Without folates, for example, the body cannot produce the iron-containing protein haemoglobin – a vital constituent of red blood cells. Liver, leafy greens, nuts, pulses, mushrooms and wholemeal (whole-wheat) bread are all good sources of folate. The usual adult RDA is 200 mcg, although some experts advise that, if you are trying to conceive, you should double this to 400 mcg a day, continuing the dose through early pregnancy. In pregnancy, liver, although a source of folate, should be avoided because of its high level of Vitamin A.

ABOVE: Green leafy vegetables

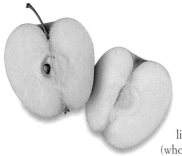

ABOVE: All fruit and vegetables contain biotin.

Biotin is what is known as a coenzyme. It is found in small amounts in all animal and plant foodstuffs: good sources include liver, kidney, wholemeal (whole-wheat) bread, grapefruit, dried beans, bananas, egg yolk and mushrooms. It helps in the formation of fatty acids and so is an essential ingredient for good digestion, although the body needs only very small amounts.

VITAMIN C: DOES IT CURE THE COMMON COLD?

Although there is no scientific evidence to confirm the popular belief that taking large amounts of Vitamin C cures colds, the vitamin is certainly vital for good health in many other ways. It helps to improve the body's ability to absorb iron and also has antioxidant properties. Above all, it is a vital link in the production of collagen, the protein that maintains healthy skin, bones, teeth and gums, and assists in healing wounds and burns. Vitamin C also produces noradrenaline, the neurotransmitter that helps to regulate the blood flow, and serotonin, which aids sleep promotion.

Unlike most other animals, humans are unable to make their own Vitamin C, so a regular intake from food is essential. Because the vitamin is easily destroyed by processing and cooking, fresh, raw fruit and vegetables are the best sources. Citrus fruits, blackcurrants, strawberries, kiwi fruit and guavas are among those with the highest content; (bell) peppers, green vegetables, potatoes and tomatoes are also rich in the vitamin. The usual adult RDA is 40 mg a day for men and women, although, if you smoke, this doubles to at least 80 mg a day

Adequate Vitamin C is extremely important. Any major Vitamin C deficiency, if left unchecked, will lead to tiredness, loss of appetite, and an increased risk of contracting potentially harmful infections. In extreme cases, it can cause scurvy. However, megadoses of the kind suggested to prevent colds are inadvisable. In the long term, these can trigger headaches, stomach upsets, sleep disorders and kidney stones.

VITAMIN D: THE 'SUNSHINE' VITAMIN

The absorption of calcium and phosphorus by the body relies on Vitamin D. Its nickname arose because the body can synthesize it in the skin through the action of ultraviolet rays. Food sources include oily fish and egg yolk; in artificial form,

it is a common constituent of breakfast cereals and margarine. In the body, it is converted into a hormone in the kidneys which controls the amount of calcium absorbed by the body and regulates calcium and phosphorus levels in the bones and the blood.

Because, in normal circumstances, all the body's Vitamin D needs can be satisfied by sunlight, no RDA has been officially set, although if you are pregnant or confined indoors, an intake

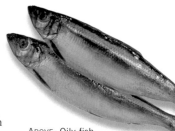

ABOVE: Oily fish

of around 10 mcg daily is recommended. Eating a small can of sardines is enough to meet this requirement. However, too much Vitamin D can cause kidney damage, so if you are taking it in the form of a vitamin supplement, it is important to monitor the dosage carefully.

VITAMIN E: PROTECTING AGAINST POLYUNSATURATES

The main role of Vitamin E, which consists of powerful antioxidant compounds, is to limit the body damage caused by polyunsaturated fatty acids when oxidation takes place inside the cell membranes. It also helps to maintain enzyme function, protect lungs and other tissues from pollutants, and keep red blood cells healthy. Good sources of Vitamin E include vegetable oils, some margarines, nuts, seeds, wheat germ and some vegetables. The RDA is a minimum of 4 mg for men and 3 mg for women, although if you are eating a diet high in polyunsaturates, you should increase your Vitamin E intake accordingly. The healthier alternative, however, is to cut back on the amount of polyunsaturates in your food.

VITAMIN K: A VITAL BLOOD-CLOTTING FACTOR

This vitamin is essential to the formation of substances called glycoproteins, which promote blood clotting, and to other proteins needed to maintain healthy tissues and bones. It comes in two natural forms: phylloquinone in vegetables, and as menaquinone when manufactured by bacteria in the body's intestines. Major food sources are leafy greens, such as spinach, broccoli and cabbage. Egg yolk, cheese, liver and pork also contain Vitamin K, but in less significant amounts.

The adult RDA for both men and women is 1 mcg for every 1 kg/2¼ lb of body weight. If you are undergoing anticoagulation therapy, however, you may be advised to reduce your Vitamin K intake, if it is considered excessive.

VITAMINS AT A GLANCE

VITAMIN	SOURCES	ROLE	RDA (M/F)
Vitamin A	Liver, oily fish, dairy produce (retinol): Carrots, green leafy vegetables, cantaloupe melon, apricots, squash (beta carotene).	Essential for good eyesight and growth. Maintains healthy skin and the lining of the respiratory and digestive tracts.	700 mcg/600 mcg; if breastfeeding, 900 mcg
Vitamin B_1	Pork, heart, offal (variety meats), wholewheat cereals, brown rice, pasta, poultry, fish, eggs, milk, yogurt, beans, some nuts.	Needed for energy release from carbohydrates, fats, alcohol. Prevents toxin build-up which otherwise could damage the heart and nervous system.	1 mg/0.8 mg
Vitamin B_2	Milk, eggs, wholegrains, yogurt, meat, poultry fish.	Energy release. Also needed as catalyst for Vitamin B_6 and niacin functioning.	1.3 mg/1.1 mg
Niacin	Pulses, potatoes, nuts, dried beans, lean meat, poultry, liver.	Metabolizes carbohydrates and fats. Needed to form neurotransmitters, maintain the digestive system and keep the skin healthy.	17 mg/13 mg
Pantothenic acid	Most vegetable and animal foods, particularly dried fruits, nuts and liver.	Energy release. Essential for fat, cholesterol and red blood cell synthesis.	3 mg–7 mg
Vitamin B_6	Soy and other dried beans, nuts, bananas, wholemeal (wholewheat) bread and cereals, chicken, fish and pork.	Releases energy from proteins. Important for immune, digestive and nervous system upkeep and for skin maintenance.	1.4 mg/1.2 mg
Vitamin B_{12}	Meat, poultry, fish, eggs and dairy products.	Vital for cell division, the making of DNA, RNA and myelin, and the transportation of folate into cells.	1.5 mcg
Folates	Leafy greens, dried beans and peas, pulses, wholemeal (whole-wheat) bread, mushrooms, avocado.	Needed for cell division, the formation of DNA and RNA and proteins in the body. Need rises while trying to conceive and in early pregnancy.	200 mcg/ (400 mcg in pregnancy)
Biotin	Present in almost all foods, particularly dried beans, grapefruit-mushrooms, egg yolk, liver.	Energy releaser. Important for synthesis of fat and cholesterol.	10 mcg–200 mcg
Vitamin C	Fruit and vegetables, particularly citrus fruit, strawberries, leafy greens, green (bell) peppers, potatoes, tomatoes.	Needed to make collagen and neurotransmitters. Aids iron absorption and is an important antioxidant.	40 mg (at least 80 mg if you smoke)
Vitamin D	Sunlight on skin, oily fish, egg yolk, fortified margarines.	Needed for absorption of calcium and phosphorus for healthy bones and teeth.	10 mcg (if confined indoors)
Vitamin E	Vegetable oils, oily fish, wheatgerm, nuts, seeds, leafy greens.	Prevents oxidation by free radicals in cell membranes and other tissues.	4 mg/3 mg
Vitamin K	Leafy greens, pork, cheese.	Promotes blood clotting and forms essential proteins.	1 mcg for every 1kg/ 2¼ lb body weight

MINERALS: ESSENTIAL FOR LIFE

On the face of it, the amount of minerals you need may seem relatively small, but your body simply cannot function properly without them. You require as many as 16 minerals in the right amounts in your daily diet, all of which are essential nutrients for life. Of these, zinc, iron and calcium are probably the most important, followed by magnesium, sodium and potassium. Some minerals are needed in tiny amounts, but they are just as vital for good health.

The body requires many different minerals in order to function at peak efficiency. Scientists have subdivided them into three categories, according to the amounts required. Minerals needed in relatively large amounts – calcium, sodium, magnesium and potassium – are known as macrominerals. Microminerals, such as iron and zinc, although just as important, are required in smaller quantities, while minerals such as iodine and selenium are known as trace elements, because, although still vital, they are only required in absolutely minuscule quantities.

GETTING ENOUGH MINERALS

Making sure that you get enough of the minerals you need may be harder than you think, although deficiency-related illnesses are relatively rare. There are two main reasons why this is sometimes the case. The minerals in food originate in the ground and enter the food chain via plants and animals. If the soil is degraded, it will be nutrient-deficient, with a knock-on effect on the food it contains. Processed foods, for their part, sometimes have minerals extracted from them as part of the manufacturing process: conversely, as in the case of breakfast cereals, some have minerals added. The alternative is to augment your intake with supplements. It is very hard to overdose on the minerals you obtain through food, since any excess is usually excreted – the risk of overdose only arises if you take too many supplements and this can be as bad for you as mineral deficiency.

You also need to make sure that you are taking in enough of the other essential nutrients in your diet, because without these, the body cannot properly absorb the minerals it needs. In order for calcium to be absorbed, Vitamin D is the necessary catalyst, and foods rich in Vitamin C help the body to absorb iron. Other food components, such as the tannin in tea and phytic acid, a constituent of brown rice and wheat bran, are less useful, because they hinder the absorption of calcium, iron and zinc.

If your diet does not contain enough of all the 'essential' minerals, the body can maintain its own balance for a short time by drawing on its mineral reserves, which are stored in the muscles, the liver, and in the case of calcium, the bones. An adequate calcium intake is particularly important: if the bones lack calcium, they become brittle, break easily, and osteoporosis may be the eventual result.

BELOW: The body needs minerals to function.

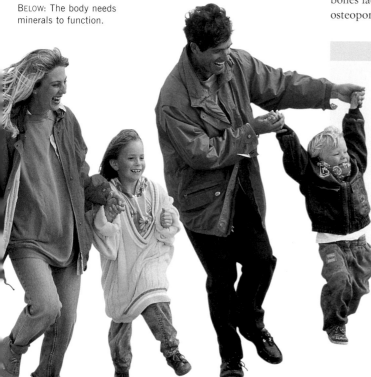

SUPPLEMENTS: PROS AND CONS

Traditional food supplements consist of vitamins and minerals sold as tablets, capsules, powders and liquids, although the term is frequently broadened to include health products containing vegetable extracts, amino acids, fish oils and herbs. If your need for particular nutrients cannot be fulfilled by diet alone, you may be tempted to make up any shortfall with supplementation. Be warned. Many of the claims made for supplements are exaggerated, while taking too much of some of them may be harmful. Too much Vitamin A, for instance, can damage the liver and bones as well as causing birth defects, while accidental iron overdosing – tablets can be mistaken for sweets easily – is one of the most frequent causes of poisoning among children.

RIGHT: Fresh food is the best source of minerals.

MINERALS AT A GLANCE

MINERAL	FOOD SOURCES	ROLE	RDA(M/F)
Calcium	Milk and other dairy products, leafy greens, sesame seeds, fish, such as sardines, which can be eaten with bones.	Builds and maintains healthy teeth and bones. Vital for cell, muscle and nervous system functions, and for blood clotting.	700 mg; if breastfeeding, 1250 mg
Chloride	Table salt and foods containing it.	Maintains fluid and electrolyte balance. Vital for gastric juice formation.	2500 mg
Magnesium	Wholegrains, fish, wheatgerm, nuts, pulses, sesame seeds, dried figs, green vegetables, milk, soy beans.	Important constituent of teeth and bones, good for healthy muscles and nervous system functions.	300 mg/270 mg
Phosphorus	All plant and animal proteins, particularly meat, fish, poultry, dairy products, nuts, seeds and wholegrains.	Vital for healthy bones and teeth, the release of energy in cells and nutrient absorption.	550 mg
Potassium	Avocado, citrus fruit, bananas, potatoes, seeds, nuts, pulses, leafy greens, wholegrains.	Essential for nerve impulse transmission. Maintains fluid and electrolyte balances, regulates blood pressure and maintains regular heart beat.	3500 mg
Sodium	Table salt, many processed foods.	Regulates water balance and essential for nerve and muscle function.	1600 mg
Chromium	Red meat, liver, egg yolk, shellfish, wholegrains, cheese, molasses.	Regulation of blood sugar and blood cholesterol levels.	25 mcg
Copper	Offal (variety meats), shellfish, nuts, seeds, cocoa, mushrooms.	Present in many enzymes. Helps in iron absorption. Needed for formation of connective tissue and bone growth.	1.2 mg
Iodine	Shellfish, seaweed and iodized table salt.	Vital for thyroid hormone secretion.	140 mcg
Iron	Lean meat, leafy greens, nuts, beans, sardines, iron-fortified cereals.	Essential part of haemoglobin and many enzymes needed for energy metabolization.	8.7 mg/14.8 mg
Manganese	Brown rice, cereals, nuts, pulses, wholemeal (whole-wheat) bread.	Triggers energy-producing enzymes. Helps to form bones and connective tissue.	1.4 mg
Molybdenum	Liver, whole grains, pulses, leafy vegetables.	Essential component of DNA- and RNA-producing enzymes. May help to combat tooth decay.	50 mcg–400 mcg
Selenium	Meat, fish, wholegrains, dairy products, avocados, lentils, Brazil nuts.	Antioxidant. Vital for normal foetal development.	55 mcg/60 mcg
Sulphur	Animal and vegetable protein.	Component of two protein-forming amino acids and at least three B vitamins.	No set RDA
Zinc	Oysters, red meat, wholegrains, sunflower seeds, dried beans, wholemeal (whole-wheat) bread.	Aids the work of many enzymes. Vital for normal growth, reproduction and effective working of the immune system.	7 mg–9.5 mg

FOOD ALLERGIES AND INTOLERANCES

Whenever a food triggers a hostile response from the body's immune system, the result is an allergy attack, which on occasion may be life-threatening. Although it is relatively simple to identify problem foods, avoiding them completely is not always that easy. Food intolerance is more complicated than allergies. It may be caused by a metabolic problem, such as the inability to digest the gluten in wheat or the lactose in milk, but more often than not, its causes are unknown.

If you are following the rules of good food combining, your chances of provoking an allergic response to food should be lessened. Nevertheless, attacks can occur. The reasons why this happens are unknown, although it is thought that heredity may play a part: if both parents suffer from food allergy, it is more than likely that their children will inherit the tendency, although the same foods may not be involved and the symptoms may differ.

Symptoms can be mild or severe. Acute symptoms include skin rashes, swelling in the mouth or throat, itchy eyes, sneezing, a runny nose, stomach pains, vomiting, diarrhoea, swelling of the joints, breathing problems, and in severe cases, anaphylactic shock. Chronic symptoms include eczema, hives, asthma, a runny nose, catarrh, and in babies, vomiting and diarrhoea into the bargain.

The offending allergen usually triggers the same symptoms every time you eat it, although their extent and severity can be influenced by other factors, such as stress, the amount of food you have eaten and how it was prepared. Identifying and avoiding the culprit food altogether is the only way to prevent such reactions, but this is not always as easy as it might appear. Sometimes, people can outgrow an allergy, but even after a particular allergen has been identified and eliminated from the diet, new allergies may surface occasionally, sometimes years later.

IDENTIFYING THE ALLERGENS

The cause of an allergic reaction may be obvious, especially if the symptoms occur immediately or shortly after a specific food has been eaten. However, in certain circumstances the symptoms may take hours or even a couple of days to appear. In these cases, health experts recommend that you try keeping a food diary listing what you eat and the symptoms each food provokes, as this may well reveal what is known as an allergic pattern. Blood tests and skin-

LEFT: Keep a food diary to help identify food allergies.

prick tests may also be advised – skin prick tests are the more reliable of the two.

If all else fails, an elimination diet may be the only answer, but you should never embark on such a diet of your own accord – you will need expert guidance from a doctor, dietician or nutritionist. Any restricted diet can put health at risk, especially since, if the elimination diet is a last resort, more than one food is likely to be involved. In this case, eliminating one food from the diet is rarely effective. All suspect foods have to be eliminated simultaneously for up to a fortnight, then reintroduced to the diet one by one at intervals of a few days, and the body's reactions to them must be observed.

COMMON INTOLERANCE TRIGGERS

As well as gluten and lactose, many other foods or food constituents are suspected of triggering intolerance. The most common are given below. In addition, genetic makeup, age and any illness generated by the intolerance all play their part in the condition.

Sulphite
A common food additive found in prawns (shrimp), dried fruit, processed potatoes, wines, beer and in some restaurant dishes. Sulphite can cause severe allergic reactions. If it triggers an intolerance in you, always check food labels for its presence, especially if you suffer from asthma.

Histamine
Found in fish. It can cause stomach and chest pain, nausea, vomiting and diarrhoea, rashes, swelling, and a fall in blood pressure.

Methylaxantine
A compound that occurs naturally in coffee, tea, chocolate and cocoa, and is also added to some colas. It can cause headaches, palpitations, vomiting and anxiety attacks.

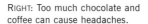
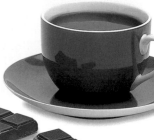
RIGHT: Too much chocolate and coffee can cause headaches.

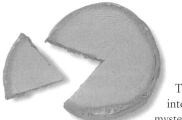

FOOD INTOLERANCE – AN ONGOING MYSTERY

The causes of food intolerance are often a mystery, although in certain instances, it is obvious that metabolic problems are involved. It is known that allergic antibodies are not responsible for intolerance. One school of thought claims that environmental pollution and an increased reliance on processed, mass-produced foods may be to blame. Other possible causes have included oral contraceptives (birth control pills), the long term use of antibiotics, steroids and other drugs, viral illness, candidiasis and stress. The symptoms are similarly far-reaching, including, a range of disorders from food cravings, diarrhoea, constipation, cystitis and irritable bowel syndrome to depression, pre-menstrual syndrome and, in children, hyperactivity.

The theories are partly backed up by science. It is known that at least 50 per cent of people with irritable bowel syndrome also suffer from food intolerance – generally gluten in wheat. Research has also indicated that three out of ten sufferers of rheumatoid arthritis can be helped to some extent by careful attention to diet. Sufferers from chronic migraine show a similar positive response; in this case, cheese (or the tyramine it contains), chocolate, citrus fruit and coffee are the classic culprits.

LACTOSE AND GLUTEN INTOLERANCE

Milk can trigger food intolerance when the body reacts adversely to the lactose it contains. People who suffer from this are deficient in lactase, an enzyme in the lining of the intestine that breaks lactose down into its constituent sugars. The consequence is that milk, and other foods containing lactose, are impossible to digest. Symptoms of the intolerance include wind, bloating, stomach cramps and diarrhoea. People with gluten intolerance suffer from an impaired ability to absorb nutrients as a result of gluten damage to the lining of the small intestine. Gluten is a protein that is found in wheat, rye, oats and barley, and appears in foods such as bread and pasta, cereals, wheat flours, cakes, biscuits (cookies), sausages and beer.

Like food allergies, intolerance tends to run in families, often making its first appearance in babyhood. In adults, the symptoms, which include diarrhoea, stomach pain, vomiting, tiredness, weight loss, breathlessness and swollen legs, can develop gradually over months or even years. If left unresolved, coeliac disease, a dietary disorder of the intestines, can result.

MIGRAINES

Migraines are among the commonest symptoms of intolerance. They can be triggered by many foods, including chocolate, citrus fruit, coffee, red wine, sherry and port, strong cheese, ingredients in meat extracts and stock (bouillon) cubes, cured meats, such as bacon and smoked ham, and pickled herring and mackerel.

FOOD COMBINING, ALLERGIES AND INTOLERANCE

People with a known food allergy may experience a rapid improvement in their condition if they concentrate on food combining. Although allergy is a disorder of the immune system, food combining removes the factors that induce the reaction. Eating different foods, mixed together, disrupts the digestion: gases and toxins are formed, and protein residues remain in the intestines. These are absorbed through the intestinal wall into the bloodstream, causing an allergic reaction.

Food combining results in perfect digestion, improving the metabolism and making allergic reactions less likely.

ELIMINATION DIET

Before starting an elimination diet, you must stop drinking alcohol and smoking and cut out tea, coffee, chocolate and processed foods for three to four weeks. If the symptoms persist, you proceed to the full elimination diet reintroducing suspect foods in a set order, trying only one new food every two days. If there is a reaction, you avoid the causative food for another month. This way, it is usually possible to establish which foods your body tolerates.

HOW THE DIGESTION WORKS

Helping the digestive system to remain healthy and do its job efficiently and effectively lies at the heart of good food combining practice. To help you achieve this the following pages focus

specifically on key aspects of the anatomy and physiology of digestion, so that you develop an even clearer insight into how correct food combining works.

The point of food combining is to be sure of easy and normal digestion of different foods eaten together. As with animals, early man ate only one kind of food per meal.

It is sometimes pointed out that cows munch other plants along with grass, or consume more than one type of grass at the same time. but the variety is still limited to gramineous or herbaceous plants. Moreover, each cow is scrupulously fastidious in its selection of food – all herbivores are equally careful – steering well clear of buttercups, for example, or any grass that has grown up through a patch of dung. By instinct, animals know what to eat, and which foods do or do not go together.

ABOVE: Food combining guarantees efficient digestion of food

DIGESTION AND DIET

Humans are now supposedly civilized. We cultivate crops to eat, and go to elaborate lengths to prepare our food. Some commentators see these activities as signs of improvement, but humans cannot change their evolutionary nature quite so easily. They are still bound by a number of physiological laws, especially those relating to the digestion. It should not be forgotten that the human digestive system has actually changed very little since prehistoric times. However delicious and appetizing manufactured food products are made to be they do not take human physiology into consideration.

At the same time, people cannot be expected to eat nothing but limited natural foods, such as fruits and nuts, although this eating pattern is so simple that it is virtually impossible to transgress food combining rules. The average person, however, and anyone who has some respect for their health, prefers a varied diet to the isolation of adhering to rules that few others follow. Eating can be a highly social activity. Food should never dominate one's lifestyle, never become more than simply a part of life.

THE DIGESTION IN ACTION

The human digestive system, the alimentary canal, is a long tract that begins at the mouth and ends at the anus. Its overall length is usually 7–8 metres/23–26 feet, but its overall surface area is a staggering 400 square metres/4300 square feet. This huge surface area is made possible by the complex structure of the stomach and intestinal wall. Just as plants obtain their nourishment from the ground, the human body absorbs its nourishment from the surface of the digestive system. The larger the surface area, the easier it is to absorb nutrients.

The process of digestion takes place on the inner surfaces of parts of the alimentary canal. The mechanism is one of decomposition: the breaking-down of many substances into their basic constituents. An apple, for example, is made up of water, protein, fat, carbohydrates, vitamins, minerals, fruit acids, flavouring, fibre and so on. Digestion releases all these substances – many of which are themselves compounds – to be used for nourishment. Of these released substances, those that are not used as building-blocks of tissue, or to assist the safe passage of food through the system, contribute to the process of metabolism by their conversion into energy.

Digestion takes place through the agency of enzymes – catalysts that promote biochemical processes. Their effect depends on the degree of acidity (the pH value) present in the environment in which they are active. If the degree of acidity changes rapidly or markedly, their activity comes to a halt.

THE PHYSIOLOGY OF DIGESTION

The digestive system does not exist in isolation, but is connected intimately with the nervous and vascular systems and regulated by the hypothalamus, a delicate, cherry-sized area of the forebrain behind the eyes.

It is incredibly elaborate and sensitive – all of the senses and the emotions can affect its functioning. The careful practice of food combining is not enough to guarantee good digestion: our disposition, the way we obtain food and what food means to us are just as important.

A person who eats a meal without anticipation or in anger, fear or exasperation, will not benefit, even from well-chosen combinations of foods. It must be understood that humans eat not only with their mouths, but with all their senses.

HOW THE DIGESTION WORKS

The digestive process starts as soon as food enters the mouth, continuing as the food passes down through the digestive system. At each stage, it is broken down into its various constituent elements, which are then converted into a form that the body can use for energy.

❶ The teeth break up food while the tongue mixes in saliva, turns the food into a bolus and pushes it towards the throat, where it is swallowed.

❷ The salivary glands release saliva into the mouth when food is present, or its presence is anticipated.

❸ The oesophagus, a muscular tube, contracts in a wave known as peristalsis to push the food bolus from the throat to the stomach.

❹ The stomach mixes the food with gastric juice; the food is churned around, turned into chyme and, little by little, moves into the duodenum.

Protein: The stomach's main function is to partially break down protein; a protein is a long chain of amino acids, which, through the action of the enzyme pepsin, is chopped into smaller sequences.

Carbohydrate: The stomach does not break down carbohydrate – the environment is too acidic to allow the necessary enzymes to do their job.

Fat: Very little fat is broken down by the gastric juice.

❺ The duodenum releases hormones into the blood when the food arrives; these stimulate the pancreas to secrete an enzyme-rich alkaline juice into the duodenum; the alkali neutralizes any stomach acid and the enzymes break down the food.

Protein: The enzymes trypsin and chymotrypsin chop this into even shorter amino-acid chains.

Carbohydrate: Amylase breaks this down into small sugar molecules.

Fat: The detergent action of bile turns fats into small globules, which are then split by the enzyme lipase.

❻ The liver secretes bile, which helps to break down fats.

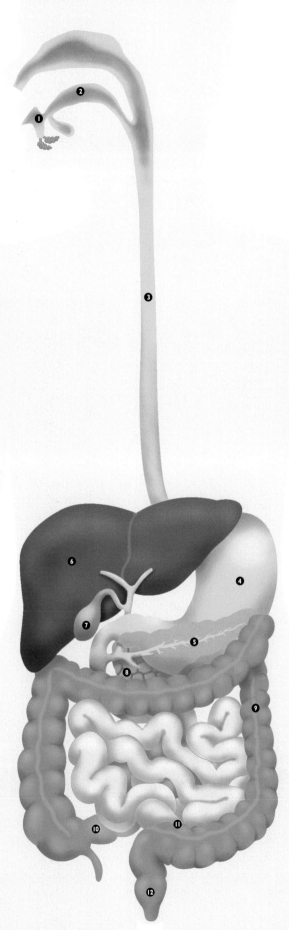

❼ The gall bladder, behind the liver, stores and concentrates bile; a hormone causes the gall bladder to contract and release bile into the intestine in response to the arrival of food in the duodenum.

❽ The pancreas secretes the hormones insulin and glucagon into the blood, additionally pumping its juice into the duodenum; these two hormones control the blood glucose level, coming into action once glucose has been absorbed by the small intestine.

❾ The small intestine, divided into the duodenum, jejunum and ileum, is where digestion and absorption occur; once digestion has broken down the food, it is absorbed into the bloodstream through the millions of tiny, finger-shaped projections called villi, which line the intestinal walls.

Protein: Proteins are absorbed from the intestine in the form of their constituent units, amino acids; cells requiring proteins for growth or repair remove the amino acids they need from the blood, and any surplus is converted into urea by the liver.

Carbohydrate: Carbohydrates are absorbed as glucose, fructose and galactose – all forms of sugar; glucose is used directly by all cells for energy, while fructose and galactose are converted into glucose by the liver; any excess carbohydrate is converted into glycogen and stored until it is needed.

Fat: Droplets of fat are absorbed by lymph vessels in the villi called lacteals; the vessels transport fat to the thoracic duct of the lymphatic system, which feeds it into the large vein above the heart; it is then stored in the body.

❿ The caecum is a pouch located at the point where the small intestine meets the colon.

⓫ Although the colon plays no part in digestion, it absorbs large quantities of water and electrolytes; residual faeces are moved into the rectum by the muscular contractions of peristalsis.

⓬ The rectum, the second part of the large intestine, is usually empty; as it fills with faeces, a reflex triggers its muscles to contract and expel the faeces through the anus.

THE MOUTH

The mouth surrounds the oral cavity – the space confined by the lips, cheeks and jaws – and is lined with epithelial cells in the form of a mucous membrane. Structures in the mouth include the teeth and gums, the soft and hard palates, and the tongue. Three pairs of salivary glands produce saliva to lubricate the mouth. Some 10,000 taste buds – four different types spread over eight major areas, predominantly on the tongue – help us to discern flavours.

The whole process of digestion starts in the mouth. There, as the teeth grind and cut food into lumps and the tongue rolls them into a pellet called a bolus, ptyalin, an enzyme contained in the saliva, starts the starch breakdown. The saliva, from salivary glands underneath the tongue, also lubricates the food, making it easier to swallow. The body produces as much as 1.5 litres/2½ pints/6¼ cups of saliva a day, although only a little is actually used, since the ptyalin stops working as soon as the bolus is swallowed.

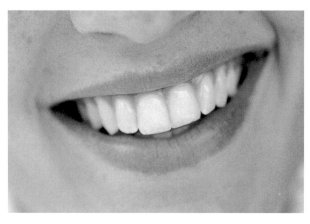

ABOVE: Digestion starts in the mouth.

WHAT THE TEETH DO

The function of the teeth is to crush food. The incisors cut and slice food into pieces, the molars grind it into pulp, and the canine teeth are used both to hold food steady as the incisors bite into it, and to reduce hard, large pieces of food into smaller, more manageable chunks. Only when eating fresh food in a natural manner – such as apples, berries and raw carrots – do we make complete use of our teeth. Most of the time, the food we eat has already been chopped into small pieces and cooked or baked in the kitchen.

In many ways the preparation of food in the kitchen has taken over the duties of the mouth. One consequence of food that is chopped smaller or softened beforehand is that we run the perennial risk of not producing enough saliva: the food may be swallowed too quickly for the saliva to come into play.

THE ROLE OF SALIVA

Saliva has not one but at least two effects on food. It is the first element of the digestive process, acting on starch and protein even before the food is swallowed. In addition, it forms a wrapping around the food, a protective and lubricating layer that facilitates swallowing and the subsequent passage down into the stomach. This wrapping, moreover, kills inimical bacteria.

The composition of saliva is not uniformly the same, but depends on the site of secretion and the speed at which it is produced. One important constituent is alpha-amylase ptyalin, an enzyme capable of breaking down starch. This effect on food before it is swallowed is known as predigestion.

Saliva is produced initially by reflex action, prompted by the stimuli of taste and smell. Then, the presence of the food in contact with the mucous membrane of the

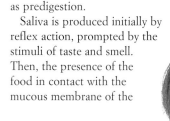

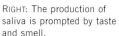

RIGHT: The production of saliva is prompted by taste and smell.

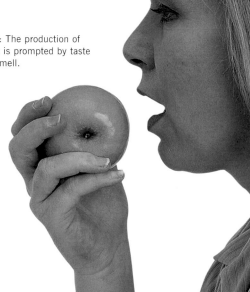

HOW WE TASTE FOOD

The surface of the tongue is covered by four kinds of papillae, which have around 10,000 taste buds lying within them. The vallate papillae, the largest of the four, contain a moat in which the food that has been dissolved in saliva comes into contact with the taste buds through tiny hairs that project from their cells into the moat. Between eight and ten vallate papillae form a V-shape at the back of the tongue: their taste buds detect the bitter content of food. When the receptors in the taste buds respond to the chemical in the food, messages about bitterness are sent, together with impulses from all the other papillae, to the brain, where the total taste of a particular food is determined. Sweetness and saltiness are tasted at the front of the tongue, and sourness at its sides.

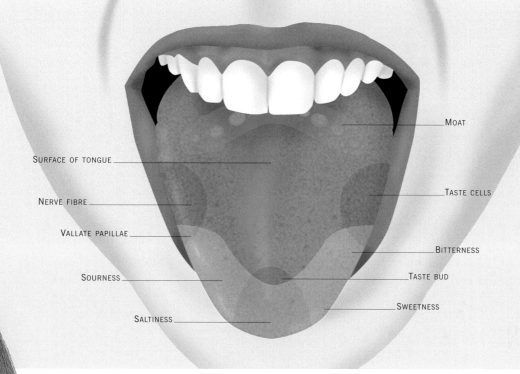

SURFACE OF TONGUE

NERVE FIBRE

VALLATE PAPILLAE

SOURNESS

SALTINESS

MOAT

TASTE CELLS

BITTERNESS

TASTE BUD

SWEETNESS

mouth and the chewing movements of the lower jaw elicit further secretion of saliva. Every day, our mouths produce about 1.5 litres/2½ pints/6¼ cups of saliva. Among other constituents, it contains calcium salts and phosphates, which, between them, regulate the degree of acidity (the pH) of the saliva. This is of great importance to the overall function of ptyalin. Researchers of former decades, like the good doctors Hay and Shelton, believed that ptyalin was active only in an alkaline environment. We now know better. The enzyme functions best in an environment that is between neutral and slightly acid, optimally between pH values of 7 and 5.5. In any case, no food is neutral or alkaline, as such.

FOOD AND SALIVA

The production of saliva is also influenced by the type of food placed in the mouth. Foods rich in starch, such as bread, potatoes or chestnuts, elicit large amounts of saliva, whereas high-protein foods generate lesser quantities. A chestnut has to be chewed for a long time, and an abundance of saliva is produced; a hazelnut or an almond simply does not have the same effect. To cut short the time spent chewing, humans took to roasting chestnuts and toasting bread. But by heating, the starch is destroyed. Without the starch, or at least the digestible starch, the chestnuts might just as well be hazelnuts or almonds, and, accordingly, a lesser amount of saliva is produced.

Food that is rich in starch should be combined only with foods that do not reduce the pH value in the mouth. Acid with starch is a bad combination: foods that are excessively acidic nullify the function of ptyalin.

THE STOMACH

The stomach – a bulbous sack in the shape of a flattened J – is the digestion's food processor, its muscles gently churning and mixing food into a porridge-like mass called chyme, which is slowly released into the small intestine. The rate at which chyme is passed through depends on its carbohydrate or protein content. The stomach also releases several enzymes, the most important of which is pepsin, secreted by the gastric glands in the stomach wall, which digests proteins.

BELOW: The food we eat mixes with gastric juices.

The human stomach is a small structure, with an outer wall made up of layers of muscle. Although the organ has more than one function, it is primarily where food descending from the mouth, chewed and bathed in saliva, is mixed with gastric juice. The acidity of gastric juice depends upon the type of food it is digesting: large amounts of high-protein food lead to a high degree of acidity (with a corresponding low pH value).

No matter what kind of food is eaten, the contents of the stomach are always bathed in acid. The acids produced by and in the stomach have three major purposes: first, to rid the food of inimical bacteria; second, to stabilize the sugars released under the influence of the salivary enzyme or eaten directly; and third, to break down protein into chains of its constituent amino acids. This last function is carried out by the enzyme pepsin, which can work only in an acidic environment.

GASTRIC JUICE AND PEPSIN

The adult stomach secretes some 3 litres/5¼ pints/13 cups of gastric juice every day. Its most important constituents are pepsin, hydrochloric acid (HCl), and mucus (mucin).

There are several varieties of pepsin – eight different types are created when parts of the molecules of the substance's precursor, pepsinogens, are split off. Pepsin has a pH value of less than 6. Hydrochloric acid has a pH value of around 1. The mixture is increased to between pH2 and pH4 by the buffer effect of chyme, the pulpy food-and-acid mixture to which the stomach contents are reduced. Pepsins work best at these acidity values.

The mucous membrane on the fundus and the corpus (see diagram opposite) contains primary cells, secondary cells and surface cells. Primary cells produce pepsinogens, surface cells produce hydrochloric acid, and secondary cells secrete the mucus that protects the stomach wall against the effects of hydrochloric acid.

In infants, gastric juice is less acidic, because milk fat undergoes an initial digestive phase through the agency of the enzyme lipase. The phase is only of minor significance in adults, although if lipase is not present, lactose intolerance can result.

HOW THE DIGESTIVE JUICES ARE PRODUCED AND REGULATED

Digestive fluids are produced as a result of any of three stimuli: the influences of the senses and the mind, local stomach mechanisms, and intestinal mechanisms. Seeing, tasting, and/or smelling food causes the secretion of gastric juice as a reflex action. Even just thinking of food can start it off. Emotions strongly influence the stimulation, or inhibition, of gastric juice secretion. Tension and aggression cause more gastric juice to be produced, and can lead, over time, to a stomach ulcer, as the acidic juice overcomes the

BELOW: Tension causes an increase in gastric juices.

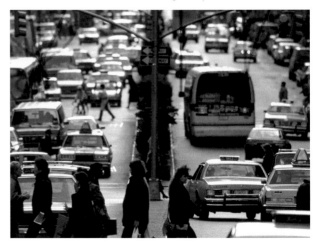

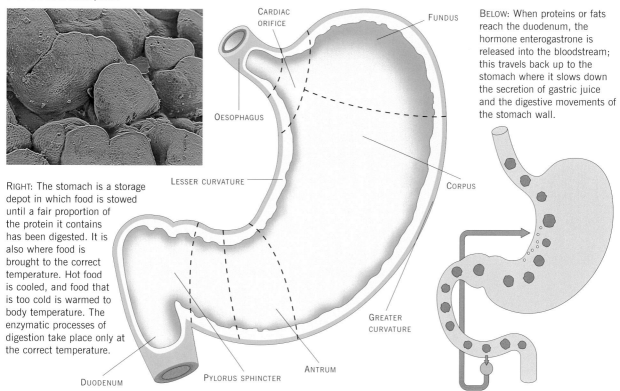

BELOW: The interior of the stomach, where all the hard work takes place.

RIGHT: The stomach is a storage depot in which food is stowed until a fair proportion of the protein it contains has been digested. It is also where food is brought to the correct temperature. Hot food is cooled, and food that is too cold is warmed to body temperature. The enzymatic processes of digestion take place only at the correct temperature.

BELOW: When proteins or fats reach the duodenum, the hormone enterogastrone is released into the bloodstream; this travels back up to the stomach where it slows down the secretion of gastric juice and the digestive movements of the stomach wall.

CARDIAC ORIFICE

FUNDUS

OESOPHAGUS

LESSER CURVATURE

CORPUS

GREATER CURVATURE

DUODENUM

PYLORUS SPHINCTER

ANTRUM

resistance of the mucous membrane and attacks the stomach wall. Fear, on the other hand, retards the production of gastric juice, the absence of which can make digestion extremely difficult.

When the chyme arrives in the lower areas of the stomach – in particular, the antrum – the hormone gastrin is released into the bloodstream. Gastrin circulates back up to the higher parts of the stomach, where it causes further secretion of gastric juice. This is part of the mechanism by which the stomach keeps track of exactly where food is and what stage of digestion it has reached, secreting gastric juice as required.

Gastrin is also released outside the stomach, in the first part of the intestine – the duodenum. In the duodenum, the hormone secretin and a specific peptide are also released into the bloodstream – substances which slow down the secretion of gastric juice, negating the action of the juice-stimulating gastrin. The contrasting actions of gastrin and secretin thus act as another regulatory mechanism.

HOW THE STOMACH RELEASES FOOD

Chyme moves slowly towards the pylorus at the base of the stomach, where a sphincter, or muscular ring, guards the entrance to the duodenum, jejunum and ileum – the constituent parts of the small intestine. Not only does the

pyloric sphincter allow only a small portion of chyme to pass through it at a time, different types of food pass through it at different speeds. The rate is controlled by enterogastrone, a hormone secreted by the stomach and small intestine when protein or fat is detected in the chyme. Its effect is to inhibit the nerves that control stomach action, and so delay the progress of food. Carbohydrates can be released from the stomach after two hours; protein takes three hours and fat as long as four hours.

The presence of fat in the duodenum, for instance, immediately causes the muscular contractions of the stomach wall to slow down and weaken. Once gastric motility is reduced, food automatically clings to the stomach wall for longer, allowing the enzymatic reaction more time – this is most advantageous for the digestion of protein. High-protein foods contain large proportions of fats, and foods low in protein contain little or not fats. This is a measure of the natural relationship between protein and fat.

Cereals, however, do not contain much in the way of fat (1.7 per cent to 7.1 per cent by volume), in spite of their relatively high protein content (7.4 per cent to 12.6 per cent). This is why combining cereals with fat makes the protein much easier to digest. Vegetables, which are difficult to digest because of their solid structure, also benefit greatly from the addition of fat in the form of salad dressing or mayonnaise.

THE STOMACH IN ACTION

When the stomach gets into gear, its first task is to bring the food it has ingested into contact with the stomach wall, where the glands that secrete gastric juice are located. It does this by initiating a process called peristalsis, which activates the

muscles in the stomach wall to mix and churn up the food and turn it into chyme. This is partly a reflex action, but mostly a response to gastrin, which encourages the secretion of gastric juice and the action of peristalsis.

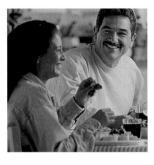

ABOVE: As a meal is eaten, the food fills the stomach in a series of layers, starting from the outside and working inwards.

As the stomach fills – this occurs in layers, each one on top of the last – the stomach walls gradually enfold the food. Real and continued contact between the food and the stomach walls is facilitated by strong muscular waves that create kneading movements. The kneading begins the moment that food touches the stomach wall, brought about partly through reflex action, but mostly through the effect of the hormone gastrin in the bloodstream.

MOVING FOOD THROUGH THE STOMACH

The muscular waves (tonic contractions) mix the stomach contents thoroughly and bathe them in gastric juice. They begin at the top of the stomach (the fundus) and travel the length of the entire organ in progressive contractions that cease only at the pyloric sphincter, the entrance to the duodenum. In fact, the antrum and the pylorus together are the main agents of kneading, the antrum forcing the food towards the muscular pylorus, the latter restricting the exit of the food and so squeezing it. This is the most important area of the stomach's function. The fundus and the corpus may be seen as simply a reservoir for food awaiting processing by the antrum and pylorus.

How quickly the stomach empties depends upon the kind of food that has been eaten, the combination of foods, how the acid-base balance is affected, and, most of all, on the overall quantity of food consumed.

PERISTALSIS AND FERMENTATION

Peristalsis in the stomach makes sure that the pulpy chyme is well mixed with gastric juice. Digested food is pressed on towards the pylorus and out into the duodenum, in order to make room for food that, as yet, has not been digested.

We shall now consider a traditional four-course lunch – an appetizer, soup or side dish, main course and a dessert. The appetizer will form the first layer in the stomach, the side-dish will lie on top of it, then the main course, and finally the dessert. Depending on the kind of food, a lot of time may be required for each of these contents, separately, to mix with the gastric juice – and, as we have seen, such mixing is essential in order to kill inimical bacteria, stabilize the sugars and break down the protein. If the mixing takes place too

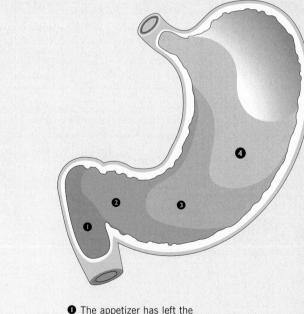

There are many misconceptions about how the stomach deals with food. Most people seem to imagine the stomach as some kind of cauldron within which food simmers in a seething stock of gastric juice. The organ, however, is a highly mobile one, and digestion relies on its inner surface only.

❶ The appetizer has left the stomach, with the other dishes following behind.

slowly, as is often the case, there is a risk of fermentation occurring in the stomach, or, less commonly, later in the digestive system. This fermentation is possible only in areas of the stomach not in contact with the gastric juice – notably in the middle. A sugary dessert or fruit on a full stomach always causes fermentation because the sugar cannot make contact with the gastric juice.

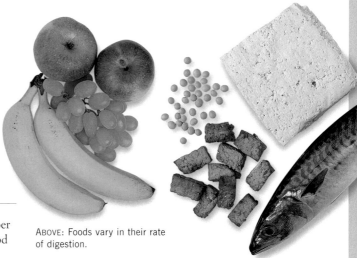

ABOVE: Foods vary in their rate of digestion.

EMPTYING THE STOMACH

How long the stomach takes to empty depends on a number of factors, the most decisive being the total quantity of food eaten. Other influences include the type of food, the composition of the menu (including whether an attempt at harmonious food combining has been made), the state of the body's acid-base balance, how well the food is eaten (and especially chewed), and the current state of the digestive system. If the meal consists largely of fruit, digestion will be quite rapid. Adding whipped cream to the fruit, however, slows digestion down. Raw vegetables and boiled food both

take longer to digest, and high-protein dishes of meat, fish, leguminous vegetables or soy products, also take a long time.

A stomach containing around 900 ml/2 pints/3¾ cups of food belonging to a traditional-style menu takes between 6 and 7 hours to digest. Particularly heavy, fatty foods may stay in the stomach for much longer, and may therefore risk fermentation and toxic degradation.

FILLING THE STOMACH

These diagrams show how the food you eat during a four-course meal arrives and progresses through the stomach.

❶ APPETIZER
❷ SOUP OR SIDE DISH
❸ MAIN COURSE
❹ DESSERT

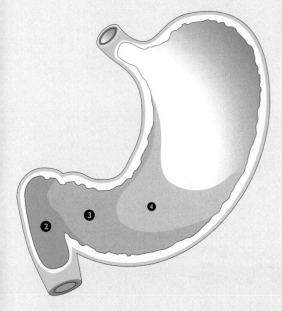

❷ The soup or side dish has left the stomach.

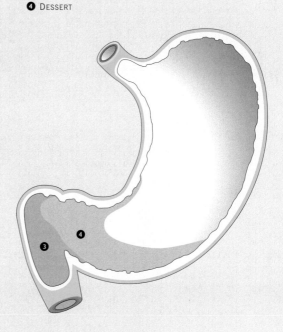

❸ The main course has left the stomach. The dessert will follow afterwards.

STOMACH PROBLEMS

What goes on in the stomach, as far as digestion is concerned, is by no means a simple business. It is all too easy to upset it, as the examples given here clearly demonstrate. The responsibility for making sure that this does not happen lies firmly in our own hands. Ignoring the digestive facts of life is a foolhardy mistake to make – if you do, stomach and digestive problems will be the inevitable result. Good eating habits, on the other hand, result in good digestion and good health.

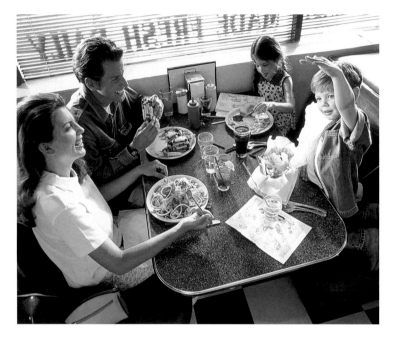

LEFT: Good eating habits will result in good digestion.

whether the food is all of one type, or a ripe old mixture. The stomach is not particularly large, and we should accustom ourselves to the idea that a moderate amount of food is enough for any meal. 'Little but often' is a well-known description of good eating habits – it is quite right, and should be brought firmly to mind whenever stomach and digestive complaints occur. It really is a pity that most people wilfully ignore this rule and insist on having three (or only two) meals a day, at set times. Actually, by eating so few times a day, we are encouraging ourselves to eat too much on each occasion. It is logical in one way, in that we need a certain quantity of food every day, but for the stomach, there is a considerable difference between whether that same quantity is better spread over two meals or five.

One commonly asked question is: does the stomach have to be empty before we start a new meal? The answer depends on what the stomach contained just before the meal. The stomach empties itself only slowly: after heavy, fatty meals, it can take 6 or even 7 hours, but after eating easily-digestible food, it may take a much shorter time.

After a night's rest, the stomach should be empty. If it is not, we feel nauseous, with bad breath and a thickly-coated tongue. An empty stomach is very receptive to the next food: the food enters in sequence and empties in the same sequence without any problem. If this is not the case, for example when a high-protein meal that has not been fully digested is joined by a meal rich in starch or sugar, a bad combination of foods forms inside the stomach – and the fireworks start.

IF THE STOMACH GETS TOO FULL

One of the most frequent causes of digestive problems involving internal fermentation and toxic degradation is undoubtedly the consumption of too much food at one time,

HOW MUCH FOOD DO WE NEED?

Several biologists have pointed out that the ideal volume for a smoothly digestible meal is somewhere in the region of 250 ml/½ pint/1¼ cups, as this represents a quantity that does not cause the exterior wall of the stomach to expand. Double that quantity and the stomach wall does expand, but still within acceptable margins. Six times the initial quantity, however, is just about the maximum a stomach can take at full expansion, and we can assume that the stomach suffers as a result. The elasticity of the stomach wall is reduced, perhaps permanently, and the abdomen begins to sag.

Ideally, any one meal should not exceed 500–600 g/1–1½lb in overall weight. A volume of 1.5 litres/2½ pints/6¼ cups is very difficult for the stomach to cope with. The risk of fermentation in the middle of the stomach is high: there is just too much material to be mixed properly with the gastric juice. Eating food that is rich in water, however, greatly reduces the volume once it reaches the stomach, because water leaves the stomach faster. This is why the maintenance of the acid-base balance is so important to a good diet.

A DISTENDED STOMACH

If you eat too much mixed foods at one meal, the stomach becomes heavily laden and begins to bulge. There are three common shapes into which the stomach distends: in this book, they are described as the hooked stomach, the long stomach and the moose-horn stomach.

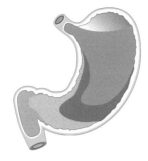

ABOVE: When the stomach is overfilled it becomes distended.

The hooked stomach occurs quite frequently, although it is perhaps the least similar to the original stomach shape. Much of the outer wall is vertical, so that about half of the stomach is almost cylindrical, before curving into a rather badly-kinked hook. The long stomach is found more in women than in men: the stomach arches downwards for a surprising distance, to the fourth lumbar vertebra or even lower. The food accumulates in a lump at the bottom – as it does in the hooked stomach – making fermentation likely to occur in the fundus and corpus. The moose-horn stomach is caused by the distended coils of the small intestine pressing up against the stomach from beneath. The distension is because of the sheer quantity of food being forced through the coils.

AIR IN THE STOMACH AND ACID INDIGESTION

It is all too easy for an air bubble to form in the fundus, the uppermost part of the stomach. These bubbles are caused by swallowing air while eating, and especially while eating too rapidly. This is why babies have to be burped. Eating too much too fast creates a large air bubble in the stomach. As the stomach starts muscular peristalsis to knead the food, while the pylorus is still closed, an unpleasantly tense sensation is felt. If the lower oesophagal segment allows the air to escape upward, it causes belching. Nervous tension encourages this process. Acid indigestion can also occur if gastric juice is brought up out of the stomach and into the lower oesophagus. Fermentation or toxic degradation in the stomach can make the situation even worse, as gases accumulate within the stomach and pressurize it.

DRINKING DURING MEALS

Drinking during meals has little or no effect on the digestion of solid food for the simple reason that liquids are filtered off much faster. When we eat soup, for instance, the water of the soup flows straight down special folds in the shorter, curved, inner wall of the stomach, and on to the pylorus: liquids always take the most direct path consistent with gravity. Once

the liquid has quickly drained away, the rest of the food is left in the form of a usefully pliable mass. Nor does drinking dilute the gastric juice, as is sometimes suggested. Gastric juice is produced from the stomach wall whenever necessary, and in whatever quantity is needed. Indeed, people who have a peptic ulcer suffer from overproduction of gastric juice. Wouldn't it be just a little too easy to cure this problem simply by drinking a glass of water to dilute the gastric juice in their stomachs? The nutritional biologists J. F. de Wijn and W. T. J. M. Hekkens have no truck with any such notion: 'It is a figment of the imagination', they say, 'to suppose that drinking during a meal might be harmful because it causes the gastric juice to be diluted'.

During meals that largely consist of cereals and bread, however, it is not advisable to take a drink while there is still food in the mouth, for drinking makes chewing impossible. For similar reasons, dipping bread or biscuits (cookies) in liquids is not to be recommended. The bread becomes so soft that it cannot be chewed properly, and the possibility of predigestion in the mouth is lost.

There is one golden rule in relation to drinking: drink when thirsty. But what kind of drink we choose may affect the digestion. Still spring water has no effect at all on digestion. Soft drinks (sodas), cola, beer and wine are altogether different. Cola, for example, has a very high degree of acidity,

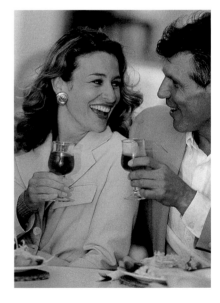

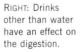

RIGHT: Drinks other than water have an effect on the digestion.

with a pH level of 1.9, and, as a consequence, disrupts the digestion of starch by making the saliva more acid. It also interferes with the digestion of high-protein foods by inhibiting the gastric juice. Remember the old schoolroom precept – acid inhibits acid. Real health fanatics eat their soup at the end of the meal, or long before or after they have eaten, which does not make much difference, nutritionally.

THE DUODENUM

The duodenum is the central part of the alimentary canal, where the major part of the digestive process takes place. It triggers the release of the hormones and enzymes that make subsequent absorption of the nutrients possible. This is not its only role, however. It also sparks off the release of secretin, which stimulates the manufacture of an alkali-rich secretion by the pancreas, and this in turn neutralizes the acids that are still present. Achieving this acid-base balance is essential to the principles of successful food combining.

The duodenum may be described as the heart of the digestion, because this is where the main digestion of protein, starch and fat takes place. In relation to what happens in the duodenum, the digestion of a proportion of starch in the mouth and protein in the stomach may both be considered no more than part of the process of predigestion. Similarly, the later and much more limited processes in the small and large intestines may be described as post-digestion. As this suggests, the digestive process is, over all, highly complex.

NEUTRALIZING THE ACIDS

The fact that the duodenum brings the acid-based food contents received from the stomach into acid-alkali neutrality has considerable relevance to food combining. Pancreatic juice ducted into the duodenum contains water and alkaline sodium bicarbonate, a substance that has a considerable capacity for combining with acids. The environment of the stomach, as we have seen, is strongly acidic, but the duodenum and intestines – thanks to the influence of pancreatic and intestinal juice – are alkaline, or only very slightly acidic (pH6.5 to pH8), allowing the local enzymes to function properly. The pylorus does not open to allow food to leave the stomach and enter the duodenum until the correct pH value has been attained in the duodenum.

The neutralizing process actually begins at the very end of the stomach, and takes place over a total linear distance of only about 10 cm/4 inches. The pylorus releases only a very small amount of food into the duodenum at a time, which is one of the reasons why the stomach empties so slowly. This is an advantage, however, as it allows digestion to take place in the duodenum at a comparatively slow, steady and therefore thorough pace.

RIGHT: The main digestion process of protein, starch and fat takes place in the duodenum.

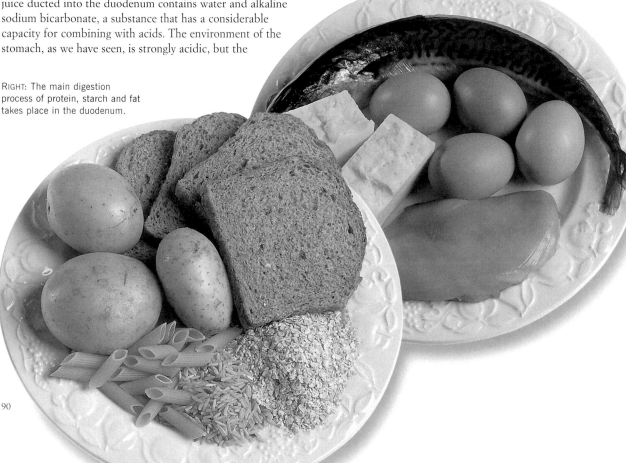

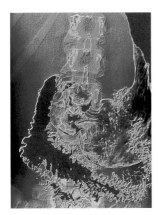

ABOVE: The role of the duodenum in digestion is vital.

THE IMPORTANCE OF GLUCOSE

1. A high level of glucose in the blood results from eating a meal that is rich in carbohydrates, or from the excessive release of glucose from its store in the liver; a low blood glucose level is the result of excessive insulin, eating a diet low in carbohydrates, or simply not eating.

2. The pancreatic cells in the islets of Langerhans monitor the level of glucose in the blood; if the level becomes excessive, they secrete the powerful hormone insulin.

3. Insulin lowers the level of blood glucose; it affects every tissue in the body, enabling glucose to enter the tissue cells; in liver and muscle cells, insulin causes glucose to be stored as glycogen, or used as fuel for energy. The hormone also prevents the conversion of protein into glucose and encourages the absorption of protein from the intestines.

4. Glucagon is released by the cells in the islets of Langerhans when the blood glucose level is too low. The glucagon frees glucose from the liver to normalize the blood sugar level.

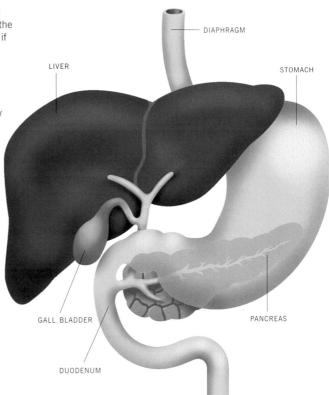

DIAPHRAGM

LIVER

STOMACH

GALL BLADDER

PANCREAS

DUODENUM

THE ORDER OF DIGESTION

Each food contains protein, carbohydrate and fat. But the pancreas cannot secrete three different enzymes simultaneously, one to cope with each, because there is only one duct linking the pancreas to the duodenum. So the pancreas effectively chooses the order in which the food constituents are to be digested, depending on the proportions of those constituents in the food. After a high-protein meal, the first enzyme to be secreted is protease; following a meal rich in starch, the enzyme amylase comes first; after a meal rich in fats, the first enzyme is pancreatic lipase.

The enzyme secretion of the pancreas can be disrupted by inappropriate combinations of food. Disruption may occur if several different foods are consumed at once, and enter the duodenum in the form of chyme of a mixed composition, containing as much protein as starch, or worse, protein or starch that hasn't touched by earlier digestive processes.

THE ROLE OF BILE

Bile enters the duodenum from the gall bladder. It contains no digestive enzymes, but serves instead as an emulsifier, altering the structure of the fat in food with the help of pancreatic lipase, which attacks triglycerides (fats composed of one molecule of glucose and three molecules of fatty acids) and splits them into their constituent parts. The duodenum stimulates the gall bladder to secrete bile by releasing the hormone cholecystokinin, and stimulates enzyme secretion from the pancreas through the release of pancreozymine.

Bile is also secreted in some quantity by the liver, and flows with bile from the gall bladder into the duodenum. The presence of fats, peptides and egg yolk in the stomach and duodenum thus effectively causes the production of bile.

THE ROLE OF THE PANCREAS

As well as the production of enzymes which are secreted into the duodenum for the digestion of food; the pancreas also produces four main hormones. In response to food entering the duodenum, it releases secretin and cholecystokinin into the bloodstream. Specialized cells, known as the islets of Langerhans, secrete insulin and glucagon when the blood sugar level changes. These hormones play crucial, complementary roles in the mobilization and distribution of glucose; maintaining and regulating the necessary glucose levels in the bloodstream. Without this the body is subject to erratic fluctuations in blood sugar, with consequent ill health.

THE INTESTINES

It is in the small intestine, which is divided into the jejunum and the ileum, that the process of absorption gets under way. Sugars, amino acids and tiny globules of fat cross the intestinal wall to enter the body's transport system. In the large intestine, which also consists of more than one constituent part, further reabsorption of water and valuable mineral salts takes place, wastes are compacted into faeces for excretion, and some vitamins, notably Vitamin B_{12}, are synthesized.

To all intents and purposes, digestion is completed in the small intestine. The constituents into which the food has been broken down during digestion, such as vitamins and minerals, now travel through the intestinal wall and are absorbed or transported via the bloodstream.

The small intestine is known for its forceful peristaltic waves, which not only press the food onwards on its continuous path, but bring it into good contact with the intestinal wall, thereby completing the various digestive processes. Let us now review the digestive process as it has been presented so far, noting in particular a number of significant physiological aspects.

STARCH, PROTEIN AND FAT

Through the agency of the salivary enzyme ptyalin, starch undergoes predigestion in the mouth. In the stomach, the sugars already released are stabilized by gastric juice to prevent fermentation. No further digestion of starch takes place in the stomach. In the duodenum, however, the complex sugars that constitute starch undergo further breakdown by pancreatic amylase to become disaccharides. These receive the final digestive treatment in the small intestine. Glands in the mucous membranes of the intestinal wall produce various enzymes: maltase, which breaks down maltose into glucose; saccharase, which breaks down saccharose (cane or beet sugar) into fructose; and lactase, which breaks down lactose (milk sugar) into galactose.

The digestion of protein begins in the stomach, where hydrochloric acid activates pepsinogens to form all or most of eight different pepsins – the first stage of protein breakdown. In the duodenum, pancreatic juice converts trypsinogen and chymotrysinogen to trypsin and chymotrypsin; breaking down the protein into dipeptides. In the small intestine the dipeptides are finally broken down into individual amino acids under the influence of the enzyme dipeptidase. Various reabsorption systems then transport the amino acids from the intestine into the bloodstream.

Fat is always the last nutrient to undergo digestion. Babies predigest some milk fat in the stomach, but, in adults, fat digestion takes place in the duodenum, where it is effected by bile and pancreatic lipase. In the small intestine, fatty acids and monoglycerides are absorbed by the mucous membrane of the jejunum, and biliary salts are absorbed in the ileum.

THE LARGE INTESTINE

The large intestine consists of the caecum, from which the appendix dangles, the ascending colon, the transverse colon, the descending colon and the rectum, which ends at the anus. It has various functions, specifically the reabsorption of water and mineral salts, the compaction and excretion of faeces, the synthesis of certain vitamins (notably Vitamin B_{12}), and the final sorting out of digestive difficulties. The human organism should work extremely efficiently – nothing need be wasted. The role of the large intestine mainly concerns controlled fermentation, in which the caecum plays a prominent part. The small intestine injects small quantities of chyme into the caecum via the ileo-caecal valve. There, in the initial 'chamber' of the large intestine, a fermentation process takes place under the influence of the bacillus *Escherichia coli*. This is where the intestinal flora chiefly reside.

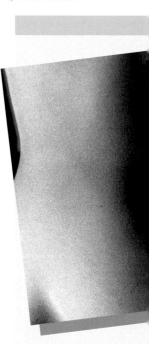

IMPROVING THE PROCESS

One goal of food combining is to improve the working of the large intestine. The natural process of fermentation is becoming rare in industrialized countries because of the persistent consumption of the wrong foods. In most people, the large intestine has degenerated into a receptacle for wastes and the results of fermentation and toxic degradation from earlier in the sequence of digestion. The effects are constipation, intestinal disease and disorders, distension of the intestinal walls through gas and stretching, and a lot of discomfort.

ABOVE: A flat stomach, indic of good digestion.

WHAT THE VILLI DO

The inner surface of the wall of the small intestine is folded to make a greater surface area available for the absorption of nutrients from food. On the folds of the wall are millions of tiny projections known as villi and microvilli. Each villus contains a network of arteries and veins – which are part of the portal circulation linking the intestines and the liver – and a branch of the lymph system called a lacteal. The portal blood vessel and lacteals absorb carbohydrates, proteins and fats in food. The small intestine itself is around 3 metres/ 10 feet long, but the folds of the intestinal wall, the villi and the microvilli increase the surface area available for absorption to as much as 40 square metres/430 square feet – the size of a large room.

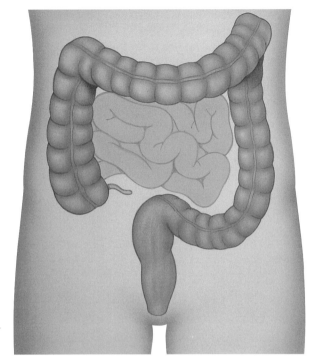

RIGHT: The intestines – where nutrients are absorbed from food.

HOW INTESTINAL GASES ARE FORMED

Gas and wind in the intestines are produced by the fermentation and degradation or breakdown of food matter; toxic residues can also be involved. Over-eating, eating food that is too concentrated to maintain a proper acid-base balance, and eating without paying attention to harmonious food combining, causes digestive problems. The complex digestive system, with its many enzymatic and hormonal processes, is simply unable to digest the food in an optimal fashion. As a consequence, indigested residues are left behind – mostly starch, sugar and protein residues. Starch and sugar start to ferment, but protein residues begin degradation.

There are a number of different fermentation processes, mostly named after the result of the process (alcoholic, lactic, butyric, acetic, propionic and so forth). The intestine forms a perfect site for fermentation processes: the temperature is ideal, the appropriate bacteria are present, and there is a comparatively alkaline environment (a high pH value). In natural circumstances, the process should not take place there, but in the caecum, after which any food residue that remains in the chyme can be digested at the right time and place. This important process is often disrupted by fermentation and degradation at an earlier stage, causing very unpleasant effects.

Residues of protein stimulate the growth of certain bacteria, unbalancing the equilibrium of the intestinal flora, but also converting the residues into gases, some of which can be extremely poisonous.

In addition to nitrogen and oxygen, they may contain hydrogen and methane, although the overall smell is determined mostly by the proportional presence of amines and hydrogen sulphide. Some of the intestinal gases may be taken up by the bloodstream and eventually exhaled by the lungs as bad breath. The bacteria do not convert food residues only into gases, however. They can also produce toxic substances: 14 potentially serious toxins have been detected in human intestines and faeces.

In addition to flatulence, gases in the intestines may cause inflation, in which the contents of the abdomen distend outwards and upwards, pushing against the stomach and exerting pressure on the diaphragm. This pressure can then be relayed by the diaphragm to the heart and lungs. In this way, intestinal gas may be responsible for heart palpitations and shortness of breath.

When no pathological cause can be found, intestinal gases are caused by bad digestion. In the stomach, they are produced mainly by the fermentation of sugars in the middle of the organ, or by a disruption in the breakdown of protein. The pressure of the diaphragm on the heart and lungs caused by gas in the stomach is even stronger than the pressure caused by intestinal gas.

Latent fermentation and degradation processes can cause acute symptoms after a meal. This is because a full stomach transmits impulses to the intestine, increasing peristalsis. This causes a heavy sensation in the abdomen and in some cases a sudden urge to defecate.

METABOLISM

Inside each one of the millions of cells that make up the human body, a complex but vital bodily process – metabolism – creates building blocks for new tissue and repair materials for existing tissue. Most importantly of all, metabolism is the means by which food is converted into the body's energy supply. This is essential even when we are at rest. Without fuel, the body cannot function and if the necessary raw ingredients cannot be processed, the tissues and, eventually, the entire body will die.

During the process of digestion, food is broken down and sorted into its three main constituents – carbohydrates, proteins and fats. Although each of these is made up of a different group of chemicals, they share basic similarities – in particular, they all contain carbon, oxygen and hydrogen. After digestion, each group of chemicals enters the bloodstream in a different form.

All carbohydrates pass through the intestinal wall and enter the circulation through the villi lining the intestinal wall and the blood vessels known as the portal veins. They do this in the form of simple sugars, of which glucose is the most common. Proteins are more complex, chemically, each being composed of different combinations of the 20 amino acids. Like carbohydrates, proteins enter the circulation through the portal blood vessels in their simplified, amino acid form. Fats, however, enter the circulation slightly differently. They pass into the lymphatic system through the lymph vessels in the villi, and on into the main veins of the body. They also differ from carbohydrates and proteins because they are not broken down completely before they enter the blood. Instead, they are suspended in the blood as tiny, milky globules. After a meal high in fats, the blood can become clouded by millions of these globules.

THE BLOOD: A NUTRIENT SOUP

The blood can be thought of as a kind of chemical soup, in which all the basic ingredients needed for the release of energy are transported around the body in different forms. The main oxygen supply is breathed into the lungs and then carried in the red blood cells. More oxygen, plus carbon and hydrogen, from glucose are added, from fat which has now broken down into glycerol and fatty acids, and from protein, as amino acids, which have now gained added nitrogen.

The portal veins transport the glucose and amino acids in the blood to the key organ in these processes – the liver. Here, the overall blood level of glucose is assessed – this is important, because too much glucose can have harmful health effects – and any surplus is metabolized into glycogen, a form of glucose that can be stored in the liver and the muscles until needed. Controlled amounts of glucose and a mass of amino acids then join the main circulatory systems, transporting to the body's cells all the basic components of food.

WHAT HAPPENS IN THE CELLS

Each part of the body is made up of microscopically small cells – the smallest independent units of life. Blood, with its rich cargo of glucose, amino acids and fats flows to and around each one of them. It also carries oxygen, the other main requirement for the release of energy. The process by which energy is released is known as cellular respiration.

Inside each cell, carbon, hydrogen and oxygen react together to produce energy, heat, carbon dioxide and water. The energy enables the cell to maintain itself and fulfil its functions, while the heat produced keeps the body temperature at a constant level. The waste products pass back into the blood and are eventually excreted from the body – carbon dioxide in exhaled air and water in urine and faeces. Because the oxygen, carbon and hydrogen in the blood is used up by the process, their levels must be constantly replenished through eating, drinking and breathing.

The food chemicals pass through the cell walls into another chemical soup called cytoplasm and are further simplified into a chemical known as acetyl coenzyme A, which can be stored until it is needed, or used by the enzymes in the

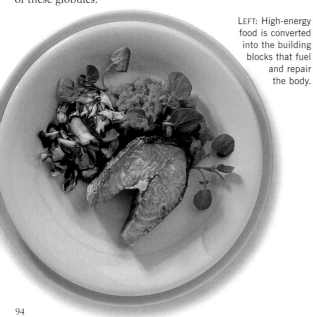

LEFT: High-energy food is converted into the building blocks that fuel and repair the body.

HOW A CELL PRODUCES ENERGY

Every cell in the body needs energy to carry out its functions and to generate sufficient heat to keep the body at the optimum temperature for chemical reactions to take place within them. The fuel for this comes from the broken-down products of food – glucose, fat and, in certain instances, amino acids. The final conversion is performed by the mitochondria, which initiate a process known as the Krebs cycle, in which the carbon and hydrogen atoms are stripped from acetyl coenzyme A, resulting in the release of heat, carbon dioxide and energy. The hydrogen combines with the oxygen to form water, while the carbon dioxide is transported by the blood to the lungs, where it is exhaled through the respiratory system.

GLUCOSE The carbon and hydrogen atoms which make up glucose are used by the cells of the body to produce heat and energy; any surplus glucose is stored in the muscles and liver as glycogen or converted by the liver into fat and stored in the adipose tissues. When the demand for energy increases, these reserves are mobilized so that more fuel can be supplied to the cells.

PROTEIN Proteins are composed of varying combinations of around 20 amino acids; because amino acids are vital for the growth and repair of tissues, they are used as fuel only as a last resort.

FAT Fat is stored in the adipose tissue, which lies beneath the skin and in the abdomen; when there is not enough glucose available to meet the body's needs, fat is transported to the liver, where it is broken down into glycerol and fatty acids to make up the shortfall.

A membrane of protein and fat surrounding each cell controls chemical movements in and out of the cell; some hormones work by making the membrane more permeable, making it easier for glucose to access the cell.

The Golgi apparatus is a series of flattened sacs and vesicles which store and release protein.

The mitochondria are the site of cellular respiration; they produce all the energy needed for the cell to fulfil its role in the body.

The cell's nucleus contains 23 pairs of chromosomes; the genes on each chromosome organize and control the chemical reactions of the cell.

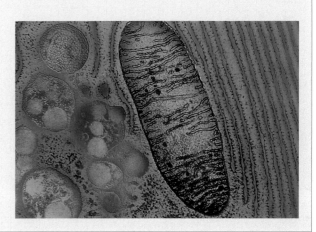

RIGHT: Magnification of a mitochondrion.

The liver

❶ The bile manufactured and secreted by the liver is carried to the gall bladder and passed into the duodenum; the salts contained in bile are essential for the breakdown of fats and Vitamin K absorption.

❷ The hepatic artery supplies the liver with oxygenated blood which contains fat globules; the liver converts the globules into glycerol and fatty acids.

❸ The portal vein supplies the liver with blood that is rich in nutrients. Proteins, in the form of amino acids, and carbohydrates, such as glucose, are delivered to the organ for storage, breakdown or redistribution.

❹ Glucose, amino acids and fats leave the liver, passing through the hepatic vein to enter the inferior vena cava; they move on from here to the heart, which pumps them around the entire body. On the journey around the body, the glucose and amino acids are used as fuel and for the creation and repair of tissues, while the fats are stored.

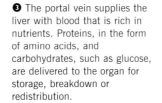

LEFT: The liver and its function.

mitochondria (the cell's energy factories).The speed at which this works is controlled by the brain through the endocrine system. When extra energy is needed, the glands are stimulated to produce hormones, which act on the cells in the areas of the body in which the energy is required.

GROWTH, MAINTENANCE AND STORAGE

Not all the food products circulating in the blood are used in the release of energy, however. Glucose, obtained from carbohydrate, is the main energy source. Amino acids are used in this way only in an emergency, because their main and most important task is to build and repair tissues. Fats that are not required for energy production are stored in special cells in the body: excess glucose is turned into fat and stored in the same way. If the body's energy needs cannot be met by the food products in the blood, stored fat is broken down and released to supplement the available supplies. If you are overweight, this means that you can lose weight by reducing your intake of food. The rate at which energy is required for body maintenance varies from individual to individual, which is why some people can eat large amounts of food without getting fat, while others find that they put on weight very easily.

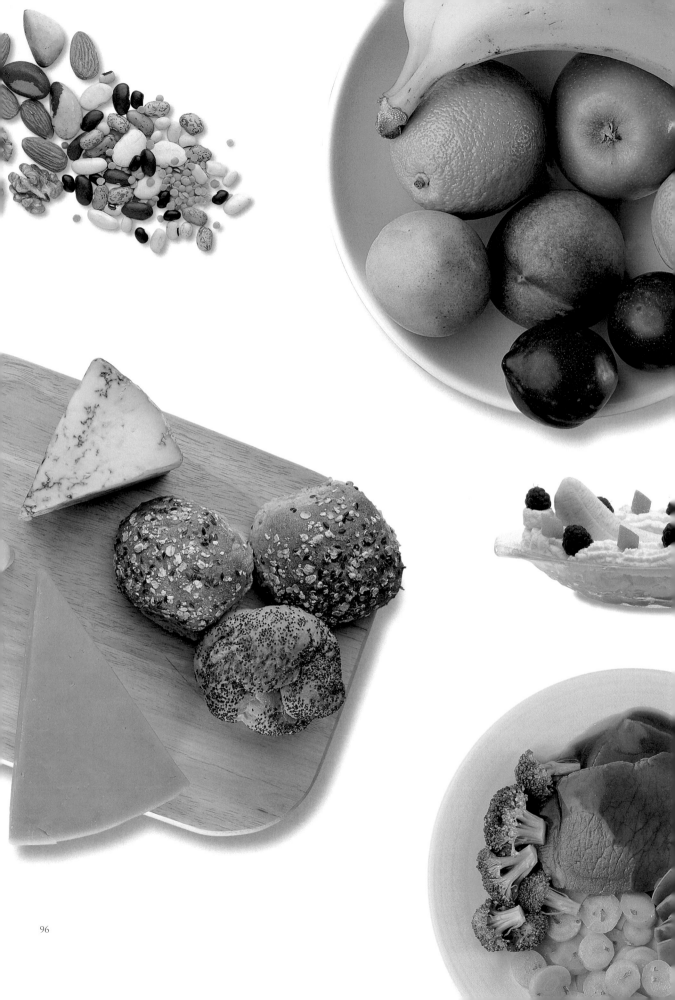

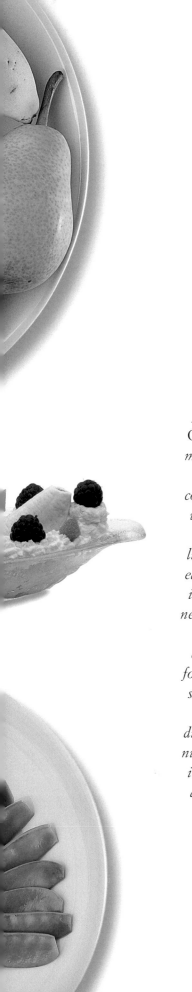

CHAPTER 3

FOOD COMBINING: GOOD AND BAD COMBINATIONS

*D*r *Herbert M. Shelton was undoubtedly correct when he wrote in his* Food Combining Made Easy *in 1951 that 'one of the most common causes of poor digestion, prevalent all over the country, is the consumption of combinations of foods that are incompatible'. He went on to say – again correctly – that 'the fact that just about everybody chooses to forget the limited capabilities of the digestive enzymes and eats pretty well anything at any time is responsible in large measure for the indigestion from which nearly everyone suffers more or less continuously'. Food combining can put all this right. Food combiners believe that certain combinations of food can be digested far more easily and with less stress on the system than other combinations. If you follow food combining principles, your digestion will improve, your body will absorb the nutrients it needs efficiently and your vitality will increase. All you need to do is to sort out which are good combinations and which are bad – it's really as straightforward as that.*

Which Foods with Which?

Establishing which nutrients go well together is the key to food combining. Knowing what proportions of nutrients are in each potential combination will help you to prepare meals that consist of good combinations of food. To achieve effective digestion, you also need to consider how to maintain the body's acid-base balance, how much food you eat and the speed at which you eat.

As we know, the five key nutrients from a food combining standpoint are protein, fat, sugar, starch and acids. Other substances – roughage (dietary fibre), vitamins, minerals, water, aromatic substances and so on – are also conducive to good digestion and essential for overall health and wellbeing. However, these substances have no influence, good or bad, on food combining, although the body's acid-base balance may feel the benefit of metallic trace elements in the diet and benefit from drinking water.

Some nutrients in combination react against each other, either preventing each other from imparting their full benefit, or generally disrupting the smooth function of the digestive processes. Foods that contain large proportions of such incompatible nutrients should not be eaten in combination at all: these are not appropriate to food combining. Nutrients that go together well, on the other hand, should be combined freely.

POSSIBLE COMBINATIONS

By now, you should be familiar with the pentagon that shows the good and bad combinations of food types (see pages 44–45). There are six bad combinations and four good combinations on the pentagon. In practice, however, there are many more. (Mathematically, the five nutrients can be combined in pairs in more than 3,100 different ways.) Here, I will stick to the original ten, plus one or two others that can be mentioned separately.

Opponents of food combining may point out that every type of food tends to have at least four nutrients in it, and not uncommonly five. They are right, up to a point. Every type of food does contain protein, fat and acid. It usually contains either starch or sugar as well, and indeed may

contain both. So, even if we eat only one type of food, without variation, the digestive system does have four or five nutrients to contend with. But crucially not at the same time: they are digested in a specific sequence.

CHANGING NUTRIENT PROPORTIONS

In combining foods, we affect the overall proportions of nutrients within the meal. If we know what the proportions are, it is possible to put together meals that combine well. Many combinations hardly change the proportions of nutrients within individual foods at all, allowing digestion to take place smoothly and efficiently, even though several different foods are being eaten together. Food combining consists of a set of dietary rules that allow you to eat several different foods in one meal, or even in one dish, with unimpaired digestion. It is a healthier, more natural way of eating that everyone can benefit from and enjoy.

DOMINANT NUTRIENTS

Nutrients occur in certain proportions in foods, and there is nearly always a dominant nutrient. The proportions of nutrients are thus of great significance and central to the overall composition of every food. In food combining, the objective should be to retain the ratio of those proportions. In many foods, protein and starch are both present, as in potatoes. However the ratio of one to the other is so favourable (the starch is the dominant nutrient and far outweighs the amount of protein) that the combination does not interfere with the digestion. But if we were to eat meat with the potatoes, the overall proportions would be completely different, the effects unfavourable and the combination bad.

Eating a single food would guarantee excellent digestion, and foods that are suited in evolutionary terms to human digestion, such as fruit, always have favourable proportions of nutrients. However, in many agricultural products – cereals, milk products, soy and leguminous vegetables – the protein-starch ratio is unfavourable. And in manufactured products – biscuits (cookies), soft drinks (sodas), desserts, chocolate, and processed meats – the ratio is arbitrary. To eat a random selection of different foods is to confront the digestive process with several dominant nutrients and, if this happens, digestion becomes difficult, or occasionally, even impossible.

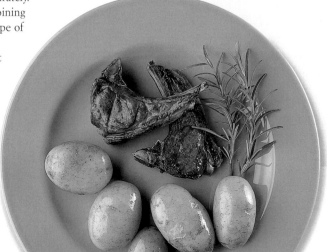

CHICKEN FACTS

Chicken is one of the healthiest foods of animal origin that you can eat. It is an excellent source of protein, rich in B vitamins, and contains some trace minerals, notably zinc. Most of its fat content is polyunsaturated – the polyunsaturates are the so-called 'good' fats that do not raise blood cholesterol levels – and much of this can be eliminated simply by removing the skin either before or after cooking. The table here compares the relative calorie, fat and protein levels in a typical single serving of roast chicken, with skin and without it. It also highlights the health benefits of the vitamins and minerals that chicken contains.

	CALORIES	FAT	PROTEIN	VITAMINS	MINERALS
Meat and skin	216	14g	23g	Rich in B vitamins, especially niacin. A single serving provides up to 85 per cent of the recommended daily niacin intake. Contains only traces of vitamin B12.	White meat is rich in potassium and phosphorus; dark meat also contains them, but to a lesser extent. However, there is double the iron and zinc in dark meat compared with white.
Skin removed	148	5g	25g		

COMBINING CHICKEN WITH RICE

An example of a popular meal that combines incompatible foods is chicken with rice. The chicken and cooking butter is dominated by protein, supported by fat – protein-fat is a natural combination. The rice is dominated by starch. When the three are combined protein and starch vie for dominance, turning the combination into a bad one (see below).

- **250 G/8 OZ CHICKEN AND 15 G/½OZ BUTTER**
  PROTEIN 52 G   FAT 29 G   STARCH 0 G

- **55 G/2OZ POLISHED RICE**
  PROTEIN 3.5 G   FAT 0.3 G   STARCH 39 G

- **300 G/10 OZ CHICKEN WITH RICE**
  PROTEIN 55.5 G   FAT 29.3 G   STARCH 39 G

RICE BENEFITS

On its own, rice is easily digestible. In health terms, it is a good source of complex carbohydrate which is digested and absorbed slowly, releasing glucose into the bloodstream steadily, rather than in a massive spurt; making blood-sugar levels easier to stabilize and control. Rice is also gluten-free, and ideal for people with gluten intolerance and coeliac disease.

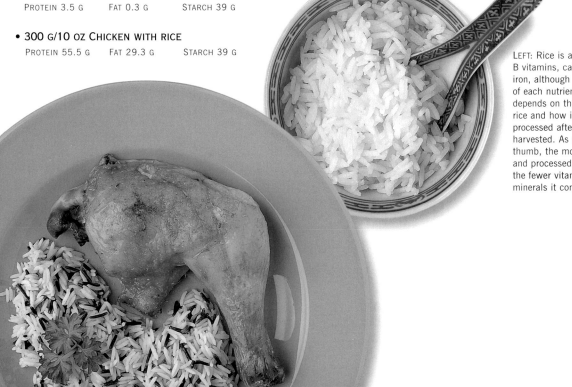

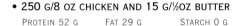

LEFT: Rice is a source of B vitamins, calcium and iron, although how much of each nutrient it contains depends on the variety of rice and how it is processed after it has been harvested. As a rule of thumb, the more refined and processed the rice, the fewer vitamins and minerals it contains.

HEALTHY DIGESTION

If you are new to food combining, its success will vary, at first, depending on how healthy your digestive system is. Existing digestive problems will need to have the the strain taken off the system to encourage it to work more efficiently. As it becomes easier to digest food, you will find that your body is able to absorb more nutrients because it is functioning efficiently.

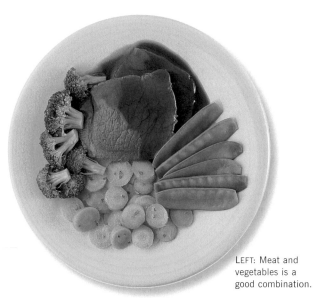

LEFT: Meat and vegetables is a good combination.

The health and condition of the digestive system has an important role to play in the success or otherwise of food combining. People who for one reason or another have weak digestive systems cannot help but suffer digestive problems whenever they eat several types of food at the same time. Good combinations of food cause only minor problems, but difficult or truly bad combinations may have serious consequences. Such people should benefit from a diet of rather bland dishes or, better still, from a diet of the same food all the time.

Bad combinations have proportions of nutrients which make them unsuitable for everyone to eat. People whose

Sensible eating the food combining way can help your body to heal. But if you have severe or persistent symptoms, such as pain, cramps, vomiting or diarrhoea, consult a doctor.

digestive systems are particularly strong and vigorous may be able to tolerate them for some time, but only at the expense of expending considerable amounts of energy digesting them.

SENSIBLE EATING HABITS

It has been pointed out already that food combining is not an end in itself, but is one of several elements of a healthy dietary regime. It is possible to eat a good combination of foods and yet still disrupt the body's acid-base balance. For example, meat with vegetables is a good combination, but a lot of meat eaten with only a few vegetables distorts the acid-base balance. Digestion becomes difficult and too many acids are formed during metabolism. Something else that can spoil digestion, even with a good combination of foods, is over-eating. If you eat too much food, no matter whether it is all of the same type, your digestion will suffer.

As well as food combining, then, it is important to take into account the acid-base balance, to restrict the amount of food eaten in any one meal, to eat as slowly as possible – especially when eating fruit – and to concentrate on what is being eaten. At the same time, the aim should be to avoid thinking too much during a meal and, above all, to enjoy the food in the excellent combination in which it has been prepared. If all these parameters are observed, food combining will turn out to be the blessing it ought to be.

IS BRAN GOOD FOR YOU?

The origins of the so-called 'bran revolution' go back to the early 1970s, when Dennis Burkitt, a British doctor, first put forward his theory that a lack of fibre in the diet and the constipation that resulted was a likely cause of diverticulitis and could even lead to bowel cancer. At about the same time, Commander T.L. Cleave, a naval surgeon, similarly suggested that the low-fibre diet served to seamen in the Royal Navy caused constipation, which in turn could result in haemorrhoids and varicose veins. The bran bandwagon took off from here.

Unfortunately, it has now been shown that excessive consumption of bran can cause more problems that it solves. Eating too much bran can result in flatulence and abdominal bloating, while the phytic acid bran contains can restrict the body's ability to absorb the iron it needs, with anaemia as a possible result. In one research project, more than half of people with irritable bowel syndrome taking part in the study said their symptoms got worse, not better, after they had eaten bran.

DIGESTIVE DISORDERS

COELIAC DISEASE
A dietary disease of the intestines, coeliac disease is caused by a reaction to gluten, a protein that is a major constituent of wheat, barley and other cereals. It can strike at any age and the only remedy, once it has been diagnosed, is to eliminate all foods that are not gluten-free from the diet.

Eat
Fresh fruit and vegetables, salads, beans, nuts, pulses, poultry, cheese, potatoes, rice.

Avoid
Breakfast cereals, bread, cake, biscuits (cookies), processed meats, beers in which barley is a major ingredient, wheat flour and all foods that contain cereal.

DIARRHOEA
You need to adapt your diet to include foods rich in soluble fibre, at the same time making sure that you are getting enough protein, vitamins and minerals, particular dietary iron to help offset the loss of blood.

Eat
Fruit, leafy greens, oily fish, lentils, parsley and watercress. Liver is recommended by doctors for its high vitamin A content, but you should avoid it if you are pregnant.

Avoid
Nuts, seeds, bran, sweetcorn (corn), any other foods that aggravate the symptoms.

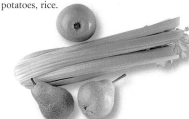

DIVERTICULAR DISEASE
This condition arises when, as a result of pressure building up in the bowel, areas of the colon wall balloon outwards to form miniature sacs, which can become infected and inflamed. You should cut down on refined foods and eat more vegetables, wholegrain cereals and plenty of other fibre-rich foods. You should also increase the amount of water you drink to at least 1.7 litres/3 pints/7½ cups a day.

Eat
Wholemeal (whole-wheat) bread, porridge, pulses, lentils, fresh and dried fruit, brown rice and other wholegrain cereals.

Avoid
Refined carbohydrates.

TRAPPED WIND (GAS)
Wind (gas) that is not expelled can cause uncomfortable bloating. It is not a serious condition in itself, but it can be a symptom of a more chronic complaint, such as constipation, an ulcer, irritable bowel syndrome or Crohn's disease, an inflammatory disorder that can affect any part of the gastrointestinal tract. Avoiding heavy meals, eating slowly and cutting back on fizzy drinks (sodas) all help to minimize the effects of flatulence. Another helpful step is to add digestion-aiding herbs and spices to your food.

Eat
Live yogurt, herbs such as sage and thyme, caraway and fennel seeds; and drink peppermint and fennel teas.

Avoid
Peas, beans, lentils and other pulses, artichokes, Brussels sprouts, and cabbage. If you are eating food that is high in fibre, cut back on the amount you eat.

GASTROENTERITIS (STOMACH UPSET)
An inflammation of the stomach lining and of the intestines, gastroenteritis results in bouts of diarrhoea, vomiting, painful stomach cramps, and mild fever. An attack can last for up to three days. A diet of plain boiled rice, bananas, apples and dry toast, which should be made with white bread, can help to settle the stomach. You should drink plenty of water to replace lost fluid, as otherwise dehydration can result.

Eat
Bananas, apples, plain boiled rice, dry white toast. Drink plenty of water. Camomile tea may help to relieve symptoms, as may ginger or cinnamon tea, sweetened with a little honey.

Avoid
All foods (especially dairy) products) except for those listed opposite for the first 48 hours of an attack. After that, you can eat potatoes, cooked vegetables, particularly carrots, and egg.

IRRITABLE BOWEL SYNDROME (IBS)
Irritable bowel syndrome is not caused by what you eat – it is a condition brought on by stress, although a high intake of sorbitol, a sugar substitute, and lactose (a sugar in milk) can sometimes trigger the condition. A change in diet can help to mitigate its effects, which include bloating, general discomfort and alternating bouts of constipation and diarrhoea. You should eat regular, moderate-sized meals, including plenty of food rich in soluble fibre, and make sure that you are drinking sufficient water not to become dehydrated. The minimum amount recommended is 1.7 litres/3 pints/7½ cups a day.

Eat
Apples, pears, dates, oats, barley, rye, plenty of vegetables and live natural yogurt.

Avoid
Wheat bran, pulses and any other foods to which you are allergic. Bran used to be recommended but should be avoided. It is now thought that it is an irritant.

BAD COMBINATIONS: PROTEIN AND STARCH

Eating protein and starch together is little short of dietary suicide as far as successful food combining is concerned. Indeed, it is one of the classic bad food combinations. The simple fact is that protein-rich and starchy foods should never be combined.

Such a combination distorts the vital acid-base balance, making digestion far more difficult as a result. If two types of protein are involved, matters become even more problematical. You should never mix foods like these that fight each other.

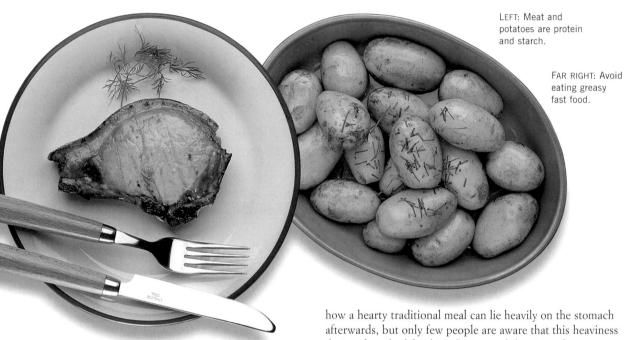

LEFT: Meat and potatoes are protein and starch.

FAR RIGHT: Avoid eating greasy fast food.

Protein and starch is one of the most common bad combinations. Particularly popular examples include bread and cheese, meat and potatoes, chicken and rice, peanut butter (or other nut-based spread) sandwiches, and so on. Meat, meat products, fish, cheese, cereals and potatoes are the dietary mainstays in industrialized countries. They have an ancient tradition as such and represent the heart of the modern food economy.

It may be said that most of these foods are not suitable for human consumption – but it is not realistic to think that we can do without them. Many nutritionists have pressed for a reduction in the amount of meat we eat in order to cut down on the consumption of animal protein. Furthermore, there is a growing trend towards eating more low-protein foods, resulting in an increased interest in fruit and vegetables. Yet particularly for those who stick to the traditional diet of meat, fish, cheese, bread and so forth, there is a considerable advantage in trying to combine foods better. Everyone knows

how a hearty traditional meal can lie heavily on the stomach afterwards, but only few people are aware that this heaviness derives from bad food combining and that it can be prevented easily by not eating high-protein and starch-rich foods at the same time.

WHERE HAY AND SHELTON WENT WRONG

The protein-starch combination was particularly favoured by the old school of nutritionists, including Dr Hay, Dr Shelton and others. Indeed, Dr Hay based his entire theory upon this very combination, wrong as it is, and it was later also adopted by Dr Shelton. Why they should have done so – and so misguidedly – demands an explanation.

According to their theories, starch is digested in the mouth by the salivary enzyme ptyalin, an enzyme that required an alkaline environment in order to function. This is not the case: ptyalin actually requires a mildly acidic environment. But because protein is digested in the stomach by the enzyme peptin in a highly acidic environment, it was thought that the digestion of starch was impossible there, and starch was

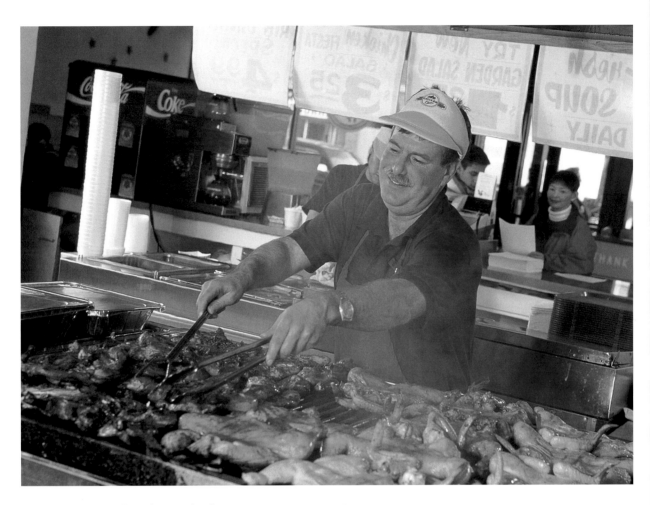

therefore digested only in the mouth. This is not quite accurate: the digestion of starch in the mouth is indeed halted by gastric juice once the starch arrives in the stomach, but resumes again when the starch reaches the duodenum.

It was also thought that starch in the stomach begins to ferment because the alkaline-requiring ptyalin was destroyed. But fermentation cannot actually occur in an acidic environment. The gastric acids do not cause the released sugars to ferment, as Hay and Shelton thought. On the contrary, gastric juice stabilizes the sugars so they cannot ferment – completely the opposite effect. No doubt, some will now say that a bloated feeling in the stomach is quite common. It certainly is – but the feeling is not caused by the juxtaposition of sugars and gastric juice, as the theorists of the old school imagined.

As we know, the stomach is filled layer by layer from the outside in. If we over-eat, part of the food remains in the middle of the upper area of the stomach for too long, not coming into contact with the inner stomach wall, and so is not mixed with gastric juice. When this happens, the sugars start to ferment, and gas accumulates.

HOW DIFFERENT FOODS ARE DIGESTED

From this, you will see why it is totally understandable that the theory of food combining never used to be accepted by classical dieticians: the principle, as stated by its proponents in those days, was incorrect. However, food combining, as outlined in this book, conforms in every detail with modern physiological science.

No foods have a pH value of seven or higher: neutral and alkaline foods do not exist. If they did, they would not last for long, since all foods need to contain some acids, which are needed to destroy bacteria. The storage life of food thus depends totally on its acid content. (Note that the acids described here are free acids, not the bound or conjugate ones that determine the acid-base balance.)

When we eat starchy food, predigestion takes place in

RIGHT: Courgettes
(zucchini) are mildly
acidic vegetables.

103

PROTEIN MYTH

Not so long ago, sports nutritionists recommended athletes eat extra protein to boost physical energy as part of their preparation for sports events and competitions. Modern nutritionists have stood this advice totally on its head. Too much protein, they say, makes the body produce too much acid. To counteract this, the body's calcium and sodium reserves can become drained. Losing calcium in this way can have serious consequences since it can lead to weakened bones. Current advice is to rely on complex carbohydrates for 67 per cent of the extra calories you need. Good sources of these include potatoes, rice, bread and pasta. Some 20–30 per cent of additional calories should come from fats and only 10–15 per cent from protein.

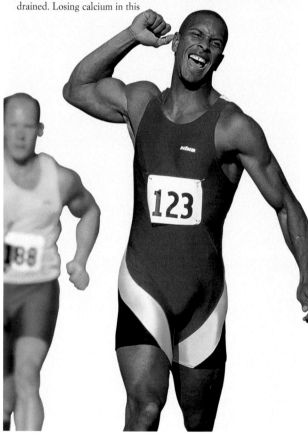

the mouth. As we chew, the starch is partly converted first into disaccharides and, if we chew long enough, into monosaccharides. If we are eating just starchy foods, the sugar that is released is stabilized by the gastric juice in the stomach. All foods contain protein, if sometimes only in a tiny quantity. This protein is partly digested in the stomach.

The secretion of gastric juice depends upon a number of factors. At the maximum level, secretion of hydrochloric acid gives the gastric juice a pH value of around one, which is extremely acidic. The type of food that is being digested reduces this acidity to a pH value of anything between two and four as a buffer effect: pepsins function at their best at this degree of acidity.

According to the proponents of the old school of thought, gastric juice becomes neutral if starchy foods, such as potatoes or bread, are eaten, in which case ptyalin can then continue its digestive activity on starch. But this is not what actually happens. If we were to eat only cauliflower or courgettes (zucchini), which are mildly acidic vegetables with a pH value of about 5.9, the pH value of the gastric acid would still remain at around four, and the available protein would still be broken down.

BREAD AND CHEESE: A CLASSIC EXAMPLE

Let us look at bread and cheese; first, at how they are digested separately and then at how they are digested when eaten together. It is then easy to understand why they should never be eaten together.

When we eat bread or bread and butter, the saliva in the mouth partly breaks down the starch to sugars. When the food reaches the stomach, the gastric juice secreted is of a type that is geared to cope with such starch-rich material. The protein in the bread (about seven per cent) is partly broken down by pepsins in the acidic environment. Those sugars that have already been released during chewing are stabilized in the stomach, so preventing them from fermenting.

Gradually, the stomach contents are passed on to the duodenum, where the starch, protein and fat are digested one after the other.

When we eat cheese by itself, the well-chewed cheese proceeds to the stomach, where the gastric juice secreted is of a type that is geared to cope with high-protein food – cheese contains around 25–35 per cent protein – and so remains quite acidic.

So what happens when we eat bread with cheese? The digestive process is pretty much the same as with bread alone: the digestion of starch and protein happens virtually simultaneously and, as we have seen, can do so without difficulty, because there are effectively two separate digestive processes in operation, one in the mouth and the other in the stomach. All the same, experience tells us that this combination is not a good one.

By eating bread with cheese, we are putting together two dominant nutrients – starch and protein. Because neither bread nor cheese can satisfy the stomach, it is all too easy to eat too much of both of them. But too much of these foods in the stomach makes for fermentation, because of the excess starch. The presence of two dominant nutrients in the stomach causes digestion to become difficult: the process takes place slowly and incompletely. The quantity also adds to the digestive difficulty.

As the material proceeds to the duodenum, small intestine and large intestine, digestion becomes even more troubled. The pancreas, in particular, has a difficult task, with large quantities of protein, starch and fat all present. Digestion is necessarily incomplete. Part of the protein degrades; part of the starch ferments. The intestine provides an environment suited to fermentation and the process continues apace. The result is an intestine bloated with gases, caused specifically by the bad combination of protein and starch.

It is worth repeating once more the golden rule that high-protein foods and starchy foods should not be combined. The protein-starch combination distorts the acid-base balance and makes digestion difficult. If two types of protein are involved, digestion becomes even more problematical.

TOO MUCH PROTEIN?

Nutritionists and health experts of all persuasions agree that eating too much protein can be bad for you. The body cannot store the excess, so it is converted into glucose, a process that puts unwanted strain on both the liver and the kidneys. It may also increase the excretion of calcium and other important minerals that the body needs for good health. Official food guidelines state that, to be sure of a balanced diet, you should eat complex carbohydrates six times daily, fruit and vegetables five times, milk and yogurt twice, and protein twice daily. Your daily intake of fats and oils should be between 15 g/½ oz and 25 g/1oz as a minimum and maximum amount.

Food combiners certainly do not quarrel with these guiding principles. In addition they insist that it is important to eat such a diet in the right combinations to maintain digestive good health and full nutrient absorption. They agree with the official view that, at least in the industrialized world, people on the whole are eating far more protein – especially animal protein – than they need. The normal recommended daily levels are no more than 55 g/2 oz of protein for men and 45 g/1½ oz for women, although, of course, there are exceptions. If you are pregnant, for instance, the advice is to increase your protein intake by half as much again.

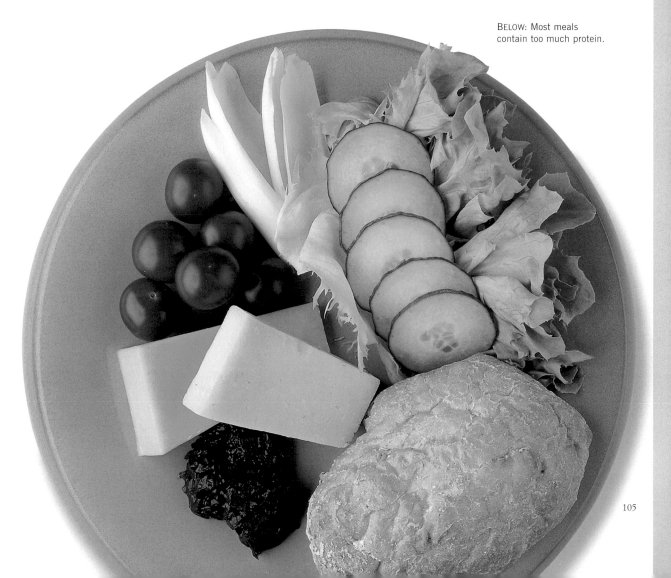

BELOW: Most meals contain too much protein.

BAD COMBINATIONS: STARCH AND SUGAR

In food combining terms, eating starch and sugar together is almost as bad a combination as protein and starch. Eating too much sweet food should be discouraged in any event. Too many sugary treats and sugar-rich drinks, such as beer, can result in a paunch and then obesity. The latter is now the commonest nutritional disorder in the Western world. If you are obese, you need to lose weight. Food combining can help by changing what you eat and, far more importantly, the way you eat it.

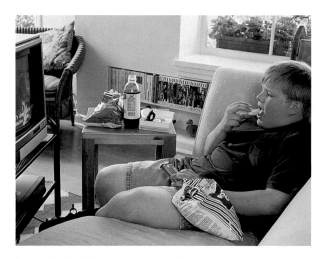

ABOVE: Obesity is the commonest nutritional disorder in the West.

The combination of starch and sugar is almost as common as that of protein and starch. Fillings in sandwiches are generally sweet, except when sliced meat or cheese is used instead, and bread with jam (jelly), chocolate, sweet spreads, syrup, honey and bananas is widely eaten and can cause fermentation. A sweet tooth is common in Europe: sugar consumption varies between 35 kg/7 lb and 5 5kg/120 lb per person per year. Pastry, which is a combination of starch, sugar and fat, honey-cakes, raisin bread, custard tarts, doughnuts and other such delicacies are all upsetting to the digestion.

These much loved sweet foods are also the direct cause of the obesity evident in a large proportion of the populations of industrialized countries. Weak abdominal muscles are often said to be responsible for a paunch, but this is to ignore the fact that the weakness of the muscles is not so much the cause as the result. A 'beer belly' is caused by the fermentation of the sugars the beer contains, and not by the quantity of liquid consumed.

WHY THE COMBINATION IS BAD

How can starch and sugar represent such a bad combination if, as we have seen, one of the main effects of gastric juice is to stabilize sugars, so preventing fermentation? The answer is the relative proportions of the nutrients. To combine starch and sugar is to juxtapose two dominant nutrients that are digested in totally different ways: we are mixing two different digestive processes.

When we eat a food rich in sugar, for example a spoonful of honey, a ripe banana, or a lump of sugar, digestion takes place quite fast: the breaking down of disaccharides in the mouth to become monosaccharides happens smoothly and effortlessly. In the stomach, the sugar is stabilized by the gastric juice, proceeding intact to the duodenum and onwards, so that absorption can occur in the small intestine.

But as we have seen, the digestion of a food rich in starch takes place slowly, mainly because of the presence also of protein and fat. If we eat starch and sugar in one meal, or even in one dish, we run the risk that a part of the sugar will end up in the fermentation zone of the stomach, in the middle, away from the gastric juice. There, it will begin to ferment. Slow and incomplete digestion leads to the presence of undigested disaccharides and starch residues in the chyme within the intestines, where further fermentation takes place, with intestinal bloating as the inevitable result.

Imagine a jam (jelly) sandwich passing through the digestive system. If it is by itself, things may not be too difficult. But, if there is more than one sandwich, there is the risk of fermentation. The stomach is confronted with too large a quantity of sugar to be mixed with gastric juice for the sugars to be stabilized effectively. As we know, fruit, a sweet dessert, or any other type of sweet food should not be eaten on a full stomach. Whatever is last to be eaten settles itself in the middle of the stomach, far from the stomach wall, in the fermentation zone.

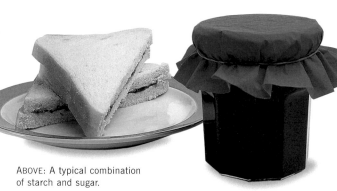

ABOVE: A typical combination of starch and sugar.

SAFE ALCOHOL LIMITS

Drinking too much alcohol of any kind can be bad for you in both the short and long term, especially if you are a regular drinker. It takes the liver, on average, an hour to break down each unit of alcohol you drink: a high alcoholic consumption will slow the rate of absorption down further, irritate the stomach and, eventually, damage the liver severely. The chart here shows you how much alcohol a variety of popular drinks contains, expressed as percentages and as alcoholic units. The upper limit, according to health experts, is 28 units a week for men and 21 units a week for women. Women should drink less than men because they tend to have smaller livers and more body fat, which means that they metabolize alcohol more slowly. If you are trying to conceive or are pregnant, you should give up alcohol completely until at least the thirteenth week of pregnancy. You can then have the occasional drink, but no more. Remember, too, that the units should be spread

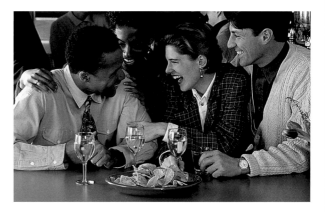

ABOVE: Too much alcohol irritates the stomach.

evenly through the week and certainly do not concentrate them in one or two binges. Men should not drink more than four units per day and women no more than three.

DRINK	ALCOHOLIC VOLUME	UNITS	MAXIMUM WEEKLY CONSUMPTION (MEN/WOMEN)
Spirits (single measure)	40%	1	28/21
Wine (small glass)	8%–14%	1–2	14–28/10–21
Standard beer or lager (large can)	3.5%	1.5	18/14
Strong beer and lager (large can)	7%	3	9/7

BELOW: Drinking more than the recommended alcohol intake can result in a paunch, then obesity.

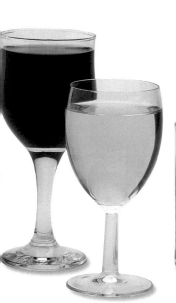
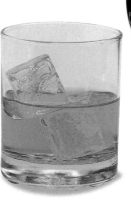
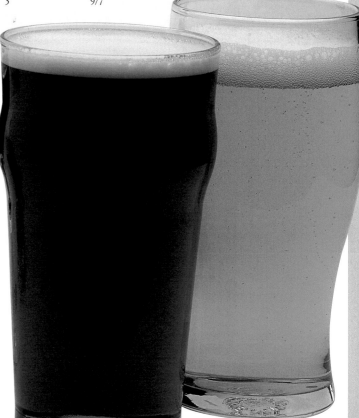

BAD COMBINATIONS: STARCH AND ACID

These two together create problems as the examples that follow show. If there is too much acid present, the starch cannot undergo its essential predigestion in the mouth, as ptyalin, the enzyme responsible for the predigestion, cannot act in an over-acidic environment. If this happens, fermentation of undigested starch, wind (gas) and uncomfortable bloating are the likely results.

The predigestion of starch occurs in the mouth as a result of the presence of the salivary enzyme ptyalin, which works in an environment that is mildly acidic with a pH of 5.5–7. If we eat food with a degree of acidity higher than 5.5, the saliva becomes too acidic and the ptyalin has no effect. Exactly the same thing happens if we mix acidic beverages with a meal, for they, too, are mixed with saliva in the mouth.

If the starch is not predigested, digestion has to start in the duodenum, under the auspices of the pancreas. It is a heavy burden for the pancreas, and there is a risk that part of the starch will not be broken down and that sugar residues will undergo fermentation in the intestines, causing intestinal bloating and flatulence. It is always in our own interests to try to make sure that starch is properly predigested – particularly if we have weak digestive systems.

The old school of food combining was under the misapprehension that sugar started to ferment in the stomach if ptyalin was eliminated. But in a combination of starch and acid, there is no possibility of fermentation in the stomach: any problem that does occur with fermentation crops up in the intestines, as stated above. It is there that the insufficiently digested starch begins to ferment, causing distension of the intestines, bloating and flatulence.

COMMON ACID-STARCH COMBINATIONS

It is all too easy to eat starch and acid together, for very few people know enough to be aware that the combination prevents predigestion and may cause digestive problems. Sourdough bread, for example, much enjoyed around the world, is a starch-acid combination. The sourdough, in fact, makes the saliva so acid as to render the predigestion of the starch the bread contains impossible. In consequence, sourdough bread is in itself difficult to digest. Worse still, if we eat it with honey or jam (jelly), we are presenting our digestive systems with a starch-acid-sugar combination; and if

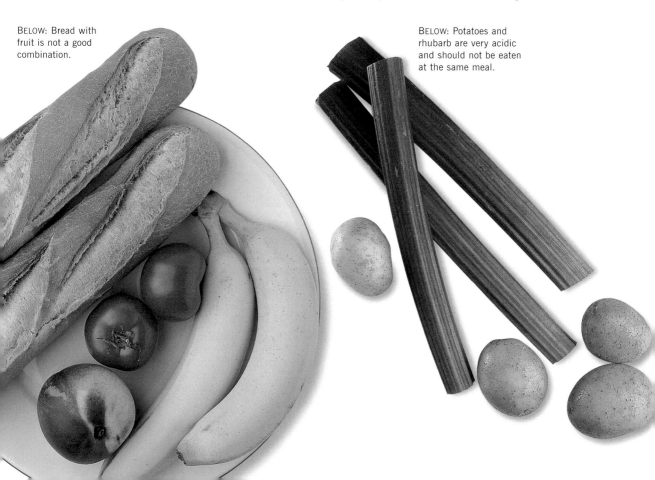

BELOW: Bread with fruit is not a good combination.

BELOW: Potatoes and rhubarb are very acidic and should not be eaten at the same meal.

we eat it with cheese, cold meat or nut spread, it is a starch-acid-protein combination. Eating food like this is contrary to the principles of food combining.

Similarly, bread together with fruit is a bad combination in general, for fruit contains acids. Certainly, some fruits are more acidic than others: the more acidic a fruit is, the more difficult it is to combine with starch. But even sweet fruit, such as bananas with a pH value of 3.8, can have a high degree of acidity.

COMBINATIONS TO AVOID

The combination of bread or potatoes with particularly acidic fruit and vegetables, such as tomatoes and rhubarb, should be avoided. Combinations of starchy foods with vegetables that contain lactic acid, or with yogurt, buttermilk, sour cream and such like should also not be eaten. In all of these cases, the saliva becomes too acidic for the ptyalin to fulfil its digestive function.

While on this subject, we should mention sauces that include yogurt, vinegar, cider (apple) vinegar or lemon juice. These, as well as manufactured sauces and gravies, ketchup, curry sauces, garlic and mustard dressings are invariably highly acidic because of the preservatives they contain. Commercial sauces of this kind have a pH value of between 2.9 and 3.6. Because we generally pile on a lot of sauce, these otherwise delicious dressings interfere with the digestion if

BELOW: Cola drinks and wine increase acidity in the saliva.

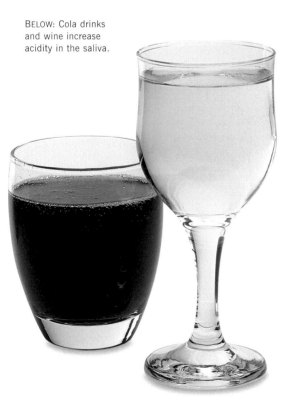

DRESSINGS ALERT

Edible oil has a pH value of about 4.5, which means that dressings made of oil or mayonnaise to which a little lemon juice or vinegar has been added have an even higher degree of acidity. Even if we use these dressings sparingly, the combination makes for difficult digestion, while to go overboard and use them in quantity is simply inviting serious digestive trouble. Commercially produced mayonnaise and other salad dressings should never be used in combination with starchy foods.

Not all vinegars are what they seem. White malt vinegar is simply brown malt vinegar which has been filtered through charcoal to remove the colour: the vinegar provided in many cheap restaurants and cafés is, in reality, non-brewed condiment (NBC). It is made from synthetic acetic acid, artificial colouring, vinegar flavourings, salt and sugar.

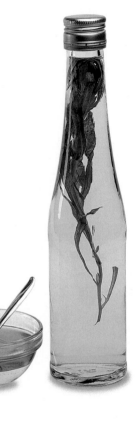

BELOW: Manufactured dressings and vinegars are highly acidic.

they are eaten with potatoes or pasta. They are safe to eat, however, with vegetable meals.

Sauerkraut and vegetables containing lactic acid may be combined with other vegetables, but should not be put together with potatoes, rice, buckwheat, bread, or other farinaceous food. Chips with vinegar is another bad combination, and sweet-sour gherkins (dill pickles) or cocktail onions should not be combined with starchy foods because of their vinegar content.

Many drinks are highly acidic, too. Cola, for instance, is especially acidic, with a pH value of 1.9. Many soft drinks (sodas), coffee and all alcoholic drinks, including wines, beers, lagers and spirits, greatly increase the degree of acidity of the saliva.

BAD COMBINATIONS: PROTEIN AND ACID

Combining food rich in protein with highly acidic foods is a bad idea. The high level of acidity in the stomach that such a combination causes virtually guarantees that pepsin, the enzyme that is secreted to break down the protein, and the gastric juices that are involved in its digestion cannot do their jobs properly, if at all. Waking up feeling drugged, with a furry tongue, a sour taste in the mouth and bad breath are all clear signs that the acids are starting to take over.

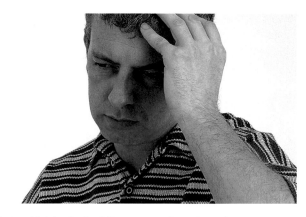

ABOVE: High levels of acidity causes unpleasant symptoms.

The digestion of protein begins in the stomach under the influence of the enzyme pepsin, which comes in eight forms. Pepsin works well in the environment of the stomach – it operates in an acidic environment of pH value 2–4. The process continues in the duodenum in a more alkaline setting involving the enzymes trypsin and chymotrypsin. Many people think that eating foods that have a high acid content assists the acidic gastric juice in the stomach. According to Shelton, however, the presence of acids from such food actually stops the secretion of gastric juice, so preventing protein from being digested.

STOPPING THE DIGESTION WORKING

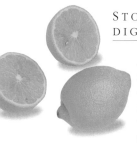

ABOVE: Lemons are an acidic fruit.

As we have seen earlier, acid inhibits acid, with the obstruction of digestion in the stomach as a result. This is only logical, because the degree of acidity in the stomach may be altered by the kind of food present. The maximum degree of acidity in the stomach may be as high as pH 1.0, but the food that arrives there can certainly change that. If the food is highly acidic, the degree of acidity remains high – perhaps too high for the pepsin to function. Moreover, with such a degree of acidity present, the secretion of gastric juice may also be inhibited. Not enough may be produced and protein may remain undigested as a result. Whichever approach is taken, eating highly acidic food with protein does the digestive system absolutely no favours at all. (Mildly acidic foods, however, have no such adverse effects on the workings of the stomach and the secretion of gastric juice.)

With a combination of protein and acid, the digestion of protein is disrupted: its breakdown remains incomplete. Protein residues may stay in the stomach for too long and begin to degrade, which can lead to an unpleasant taste back up in the mouth. The incomplete digestion then further obstructs protein breakdown in the duodenum and protein residues continue degrading in the intestine.

Because high-protein foods contain fat, a combination of protein and acid is less harmful than a starch and acid

RIGHT: The digestive system is complex, and needs maintaining correctly.

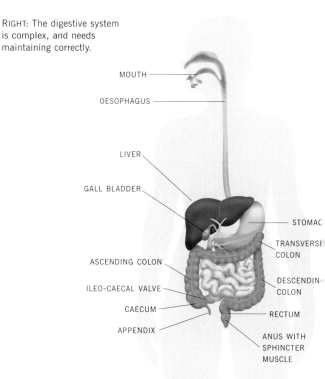

MOUTH

OESOPHAGUS

LIVER

GALL BLADDER

STOMAC

TRANSVERSE COLON

ASCENDING COLON

DESCENDIN COLON

ILEO-CAECAL VALVE

CAECUM

RECTUM

APPENDIX

ANUS WITH SPHINCTER MUSCLE

combination. The salivary enzyme functions better in a mildly acidic environment and is more susceptible to acids. The enzymes of the stomach require a more acidic environment (pH 2–4), and consequently can be influenced only by strong acids. Exactly how much acid is present is also significant. Acid and fat form a good combination of foods, because emulsification occurs, in which a part of the fat is actually absorbed by the acid.

EXAMPLES AND EXCEPTIONS

In general, high-protein foods should not be eaten together with vegetables that contain lactic or other acids, sauerkraut, proprietary sauces and gravies, mustard or any kind of fruit. Many people sprinkle cooked fish with a little lemon juice or garnish it with a couple of slices of lemon. They do this with the intention of improving their digestion of the fat. In actual fact, the small quantity of lemon juice involved has absolutely no effect on gastric function. Pickled herrings and the vinegar on them, on the other hand, actively obstruct gastric function.

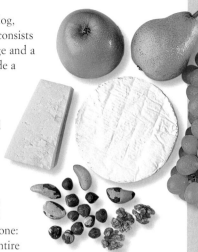

ABOVE: Cheese and nuts balance each other out as a fat and acid.

The original form of hot dog, from north-west Europe, consists of a hot frankfurter sausage and a helping of sauerkraut inside a split roll. Sauerkraut and frankfurter is an example of a bad protein-acid combination. Another bad acid-protein combination is adding mustard to cheese (as in toasted Welsh rarebit).

These last two examples show how to extend a bad combination into a worse one: starch-protein-acid. The entire fast-food culture is based on bad food combining. In addition to the combination of protein and starch, a lot of other acidic material is added to food, particularly ketchup, mayonnaise and vinegary dressings. These extra items all hinder the digestion of both starch and protein.

But there are one or two exceptions: high-protein foods like cheese and nuts can be eaten in combination with fruit and vegetables (which are acidic). How, you ask, can there be exceptions? Is this not a contradiction of the principles of food combining? This is where the proportions of the nutrients in the foods come into play. Cheese and nuts have a very high proportion of fats in them, often even higher than protein. So, in this situation, what is effectively happening is that it is not so much a combination of protein and acid as one of fat and acid which is involved. The latter is a good combination, provided that the proportions of just a little cheese or a few nuts eaten with a much larger amount of fruit and vegetables, is maintained.

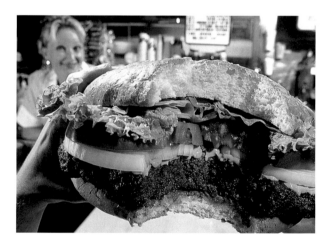

ABOVE: The fast food culture is based on bad food combining.

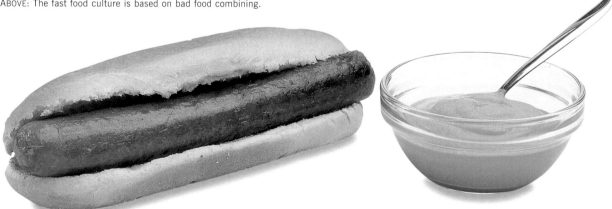

ABOVE: A hot dog with mustard is a bad starch-protein-acid combination.

BAD COMBINATIONS: FAT AND SUGAR

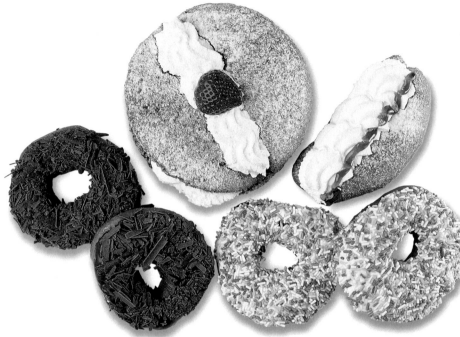

LEFT: Cakes and pastries
are a bad combination.

In Nature, high-sugar foods do not contain much fat and vice versa. We should learn from this and avoid the fat-sugar combination, which means cutting down and finding alternatives for quite a few tasty treats, such as chocolate, ice cream, nougat, cakes and marzipan. In digestive terms, these foods are a bad combination and, in any case, excessive eating of sweets (candies) is bad for health. Not only do high-fat, sugary foods cause tooth decay, but they contain so-called 'empty calories', rather than sustaining, healthy nutrients.

A combination of fat and sugar is unfavourable to digestion. Foods rich in fat almost always have a low content of sugar (carbohydrate). Conversely, foods rich in sugar – such as high-sugar fruits – are low in fat; honey, for example, is actually fat-free. Food combining says we should learn this lesson from Nature and plan our own diets accordingly.

Wherever there is sugar in a food, there is generally also a lot of water. Some nutritionists like to say 'Sugar swims in water', by which they mean that sugar is easy to digest if eaten in foods that contain plenty of water. The effect of this is that sugar in naturally occurring foods is always present only in low concentration. Fruits that are comparatively rich in sugar contain a very high proportion of water. Bananas, for example, which are rich in sugar, are no less than 76 per cent water by volume.

Water and fats are opposites. Again, this highlights the fact that fat and sugar do not belong together.

ENCOURAGING UNHELPFUL FERMENTATION

In the average Western diet, the fat-sugar combination is very common. Chocolate, sweetened whipped cream, ice cream, cakes and biscuits (cookies) are all examples of fat-sugar combinations, while nut spreads are almost always sweetened with honey or sugar in order to create a sweet sandwich filling. These foods do not help the digestion in any way.

If we eat sugar together with high-fat food, the sugar is mixed with the fat. On its own, sugar is easy to digest. It is broken down into monosaccharides and absorbed into the bloodstream fairly rapidly. It proceeds to the stomach, where it is bathed in and stabilized by gastric juice; then it is conveyed to the duodenum before travelling on to be absorbed in the small intestine. The presence of fat, however, slows this process down. Fat inhibits the kneading movement of the stomach wall. Sugar that is completely surrounded by fat cannot make contact with the gastric juice, is not stabilized and all too quickly begins to ferment.

According to Dr Shelton, sweet nuts and fruit comprise a particularly reprehensible combination, despite their

CHOCOHOLIC ALTERNATIVES

Chocolate itself is high in fat – its fat content is around 30 per cent by weight. It contains variable amounts of sugar, but quite enough to make it a problematic food combination at best and a bad one at worst. Although some food combiners recommend carob chocolate as a healthier alternative, you should note that this is far from being a low-fat food. Because coconut or hydrogenated vegetable oil is used to make it, carob is often just as high in fat as conventional chocolate, while the carob pods themselves are rich in natural sugars, such as sucrose, glucose and fructose. Other possible alternatives to chocolate include fruit bars, cereal bars, dried figs and other dried fruit, natural liquorice and sesame seeds.

RIGHT: Cereal bars are a healthier alternative to chocolate.

delightful aroma together. Sweet fruits, of course, are rich in sugar. He points out that the combination of fat and sugar is a bad one, and states that avocado and sweet fruits are better not eaten together, presumably for the same reason.

QUANTITIES AND PROPORTIONS

Foods that contain a high proportion of fat should not be sweetened, so you should not sweeten cream for example. A much-loved combination of foods is fruit with whipped cream, which, at first sight, would appear to be a fat-sugar combination. But that is not quite the case. In fact, it is more of a fat-acid-sugar combination. And it all depends on the overall quantity, the constituent proportions and the specific type of fruit. Fruits that have an acidic content obviously have a lower sugar content than sweet fruits. Whipped cream, for its part, may contain 10–30 per cent fat and we may use just a little or a lot of it.

Some people cannot eat bananas with whipped cream. People who have weak digestive systems may also experience problems after eating sweet fruits with whipped cream. The combination is a difficult one for anybody. Acidic fruits with whipped cream, however, should not cause such difficulties.

THE FAT-SUGAR RATIO

This table demonstrates that in general high-fat foods are low in sugar, although there are exceptions like cashew nuts.

FOOD	FAT	SUGAR	RATIO
Brazil nuts	67%	2.3%	29:1
Avocados	23.5%	0.9%	26:1
Green olives	13.3%	1.5%	9:1
Black olives	35.8%	4.9%	7:1
Sunflower seeds	49%	8.3%	5.9:1
Hazelnuts	61%	10.6%	5.8:1
Almonds	54%	9.3%	5.8:1
Linseed	35%	6%	5.8:1
Cashew nuts	42.2%	30.5%	1.4:1

❗ ALLERGY ALERT

Nuts are one of the commonest food allergens, the main culprits being peanuts, walnuts, cashews and pecans. Peanut allergy is the most dangerous, since, in extreme cases, it can cause death as a result of anaphylactic shock, in which the respiratory and circulatory systems both stop functioning. If you are allergic to peanuts, you must avoid them and all foods and food products that might contain them, such as nut-flavoured breads, biscuits (cookies), ice cream and cooking oils. Even the smallest trace can cause a severe allergic reaction. Other symptoms of nut allergy include swellings, rashes, eczema, intestinal and breathing problems and, if you are asthmatic, asthma attacks.

Bad Combinations: Protein And Sugar

There are few foods rich in protein that naturally contain very much sugar. To maintain digestion, we should take our lead from Nature and avoid combining these two nutrients. For example, food combining authorities always advise avoiding ending a meal with a sweet dessert if, say, the previous main course has been packed full of protein-rich food.

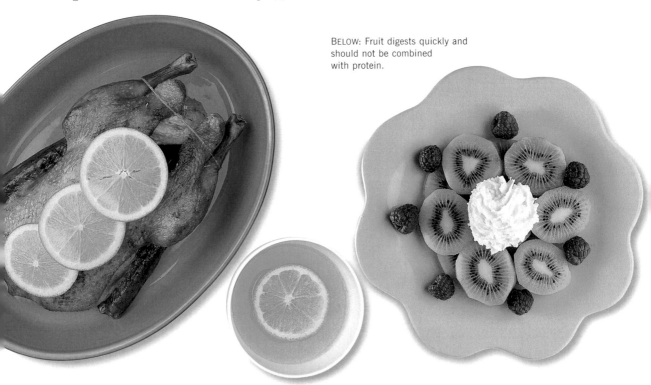

BELOW: Fruit digests quickly and should not be combined with protein.

High-protein food seldom contains much in the way of simple carbohydrates (sugar). Among meats, only meat deriving from internal organs (non-muscular tissue) contains carbohydrate in the form of glycogen, and then the quantity is minimal. In vegetable foods, such as nuts and seeds, the proportion of carbohydrates is similarly very small, although there are exceptions, for example cashew nuts, lupin seeds, pine nuts, sesame seeds, and, of course, leguminous vegetables.

HIGH IN PROTEIN, HIGH IN FAT

High-protein food, on the other hand, always contains a lot of fat. In this sense, the fat-sugar combination and the protein-sugar combination overlap to an extent. If we add sugar to a high-fat food, we are most likely to arrive at a bad protein-sugar combination as well. Avocado is an exception to this because it actually contains very little protein – 1.9 per cent by volume. For all that, avocado is described as a high-protein fruit/vegetable because its protein content is higher than that of other fruit and vegetables, although in comparison with high-protein foods, its protein content is very low.

What can make things worse are misguided combinations. A sweet dessert at the end of a high-protein meal, for instance, is always a mistake. It is a classic example of a bad food combination. Some recipes pair meat and fish with fruit (for example duck with orange) a combination that does not aid digestion. High-protein foods remain in the stomach for a relatively long time and are difficult to digest: sugar is not digested fast enough in a well-filled stomach, which may very well lead to unwanted fermentation, with consequent flatulence, bloating and other unpleasant signs of digestive discomfort.

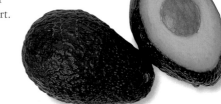

RIGHT: Avocados contain a little protein.

114

ICE CREAM AND FOOD COMBINING

Along with sweet desserts, ice cream is best avoided if the previous courses in a meal have been centred around protein-rich foods. Not only are most brands of ice cream rich in fat, but they also have a high sugar content into the bargain. The protein content of ice cream is around the same as that of milk. Much of the fat in ice cream is saturated, although the percentage varies from a low of around six per cent to a high of 15 per cent. Anything containing less than five per cent fat cannot be called ice cream: instead, it must be labelled as a 'frozen dessert'. The table here shows the nutrient breakdown of a 100 g/3½ oz average serving of a number of popular varieties.

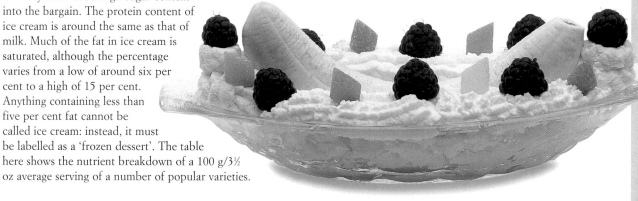

Dairy ice cream, by law, must only contain milk fat: if other non-milk or vegetable fats are substituted, this must be specified on the product's label. Remember, too, that the extremes of very cold foods can upset the digestion just as much as very hot ones: If you eat them, do so sparingly.

TYPE	PROTEIN	SUGAR	FAT	CALCIUM	CALORIES
Dairy	3.6 g	24.4 g	9.8 g	130 mg	194
Dairy, flavoured	3.5 g	24.7 g	8.0 g	110 mg	179
Non-dairy	3.2 g	23.1 g	8.7 g	120 g	178
Non-dairy, flavoured	3.1 g	23.2 g	7.4 g	120g	166

ABOVE AND BELOW: Ice cream should be avoided after a protein meal and eaten only sparingly because it has a high fat and sugar content.

SUGAR SUBSTITUTES

Nutritionists agree that people should try to cut down on the sugar in their diet, but opinions differ as to whether artificial sweeteners are an acceptable substitute. Some people report adverse side-effects, such as headaches, from taking them, while leading food combining authorities and some nutritional therapists believe that they may throw the levels of glucose in the blood out of kilter and actually serve to increase, rather than reduce,

sugar cravings. Instead, while you are weaning yourself away from sugar, you could try fruit sugar (fructose) powder. This is nearly twice as sweet as conventional sugar, so you need only half the quantity you would have taken normally. Otherwise, try honey or frugo-oligosaccharide (fructolite), cutting back on quantities by degrees.

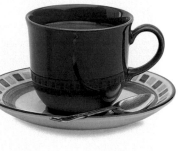

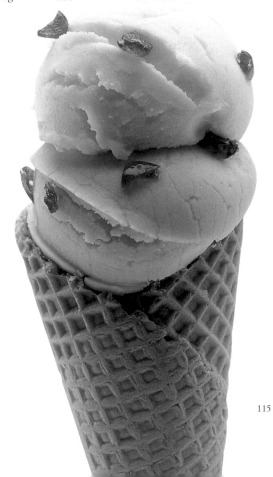

OTHER BAD COMBINATIONS

There are other bad combinations that are more complicated and require special attention. The most important of them are dealt with below, while others, such as protein-fat-starch and protein-fat-sugar, just need a passing mention. The first is effectively the same as a combination of protein, fat and starch: if the amount of fat added is large, problems may result. The second is essentially the same as the combination of protein and sugar plus fat and sugar, for protein is always accompanied by fat.

LEFT: A combination of meat and dairy fats should be avoided.

COMBINING FAT AND FAT

In dietary science, it is usual to distinguish between animal fat and vegetable fat. For convenience, we make the further distinction between animal fats (meat and fish), milk fats (milk, butter, whipped cream, full-fat cheese), egg yolk and vegetable fats. Fats themselves are composed of saturated, unsaturated and polyunsaturated fatty acids. Their digestion is relatively simple: there should be no digestive problems at all if the gallbladder and the liver are working well.

Fats are found in almost all foods, but can occur in different proportions. We should try to avoid mixing different kinds of fat at the same time. To fry meat in margarine, for example, is to mix animal and vegetable fats. Some say that grilling meat in its own fat improves the digestion.

To date, there is no scientific evidence that eating different types of fat is unfavourable to the digestive system. At the same time, we do know that no extra fat should be added to a food that is already rich in fat, for a disproportionate amount of fat in food does cause digestive problems. The digestive system is simply not capable of processing a lot of fat all at one time, for reasons of capacity rather than anything else. The other disadvantages of a diet that contains too much fat are well known.

COMBINING PROTEIN, FAT AND FAT

The combination of protein and fat is a natural one. All high-protein foods contain fat. The protein remains the dominant nutrient because of its crucial influence on the digestion. But to add fat to a high-protein food is to end up with a protein-fat-fat combination. In particular, the addition of single and concentrated fats, such as edible oil, margarine and animal fats (beef dripping and lard) to high-protein foods can obstruct digestion.

As we have seen, fat slows down the function of the stomach, which can be a good thing when digesting protein. But, if there is too much fat, stomach movement may be over-restricted. Adding fat to a food that already contains fat, for example frying meat in margarine, may make the overall quantity of fats altogether indigestible. The decisive factors in relation to this combination are exactly how much fat is being added, and how strong and healthy the digestive system is.

COMBINING FAT, ACID AND STARCH

This combination requires particular attention because it is a frequent subject of misunderstanding. Fat and acid is a good combination, as is fat and starch. But what happens if both combinations are used together, when what is eaten is effectively a fat-acid-starch combination? The proportion of acid is the crucial factor. If the quantity of acid is minimal (for example a few drops of lemon juice or wine vinegar in mayonnaise or in an oil-based salad dressing) it can be ignored. Lashings of acidic sauce on top of starch-rich food, on the other hand, is asking for real trouble. Ready made commercial sauces tend to be extremely acidic and thus go very badly with starchy meals. The acid makes the degree of acidity in the food even higher, altogether eliminating the effect of the enzyme ptyalin in the mouth.

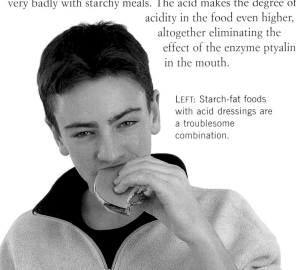

LEFT: Starch-fat foods with acid dressings are a troublesome combination.

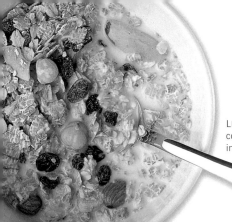

LEFT: Muesli (granola) contains many incompatible foods.

COMBINING PROTEIN, FAT, STARCH AND ACID

This is a dreadful combination, of course, but is one that is consumed every day in industrialized countries in such traditional dishes as meat with potatoes and acidic gravy, or chicken curry with rice. Four out of five nutrients are competing for dominance. Cakes or pastries, for example, may contain four dominants – protein, fat, sugar and starch. In a cake decorated with whipped cream, there may even be five dominants – protein, fat, starch, sugar and fat again (the whipped cream).

Without doubt, the worst example of a bad combination of foods in one single dish must be muesli (granola). Swiss pioneer of the natural-health movement Dr Max Bircher-Benner popularized muesli (granola) as the ideal healthy start to the day. Although some food-combiners go along with his views, it is, in my opinion, an extremely bad food combination that should be avoided, despite the fibre it contains. No other dish contains so many combinatory incompatibles. Its ingredients are nuts, oat flakes, raisins, honey, milk and fruit: nutritionally, this means that you are eating a combination of protein (nuts) + protein (milk) + starch (oat flakes) + sugar (honey and raisins) + fat (nuts) + acids (in the fruit). We might more graphically express it in symbols – $P + P + St + Su + F + A$. No fewer than six dominant nutrients are being eaten in equal proportions.

RIGHT: There is a vast choice of fresh and dried fruit that can form the basis of a healthy, cleansing, nutrient-rich breakfast. Do not mix melon with other fruit, but otherwise mix and match from apples, apricots (fresh and the dried Hunza variety), bananas, blackberries, cherries, figs, grapefruit, grapes, guavas, kiwi fruit, mangos, oranges, nectarines, peaches, pears, pineapples, pomegranates, strawberries, raspberries and more.

WHAT MAKES THE BEST BREAKFAST?

As we have seen above, muesli (granola) is a nutritional solecism. It would be much better for everybody to eat just fruit instead. If you cannot face the thought of solid food first thing in the morning, you should eat a few pieces of fruit as soon as you can manage it. In fact, the food combining authorities all agree that fruit, provided that it is eaten on its own, is probably the healthiest breakfast you can eat. The argument is that the natural rhythm of the human digestive system makes fruit the easiest foodstuff for the body to digest first thing in the morning. It certainly helps to keep the bowels moving and the colon healthy. Because it is high in water and low in calories, it also aids in the removal of unhealthy toxins. Breakfast cereals, on the other hand, present problems. Conventional nutritionists say that they are a good high-fibre, low-fat start to the day. They contain both insoluble and soluble fibre, the former aiding bowel movement, while the latter helps to reduce cholesterol levels in the blood. Most commercial varieties also have added vitamins and minerals – notably B vitamins and iron – to boost their health-giving qualities. However, they may also contain salt and hidden sugars, while, because the majority of them are rich in starchy carbohydrates, they should not be mixed freely with milk, which is a protein food. Many nutritionists recommend starting the day with a bowl of porridge, especially if you are a diabetic, because of the slow-release energy the complex carbohydrates in porridge provides. The trick here is to accompany the porridge with just a little milk, diluted half-and-half with water. It should never be eaten with sugar or syrup.

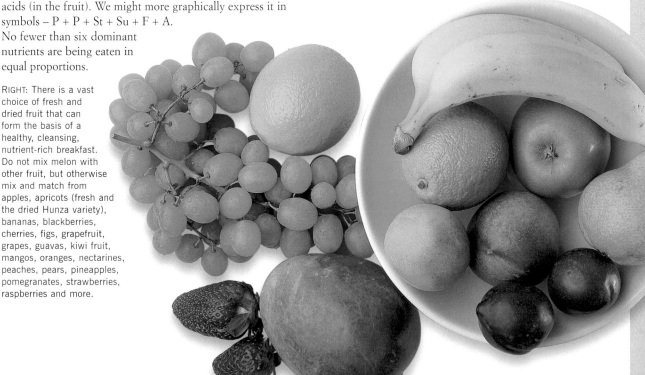

GOOD COMBINATIONS: PROTEIN AND FAT, STARCH AND FAT

Looking at the long list of bad food combinations, we may well wonder what combinations of food are actually good. In fact, there are four good combinations – protein and fat, sugar and acid, fat and acid, and fat and starch – but in practice only the last three are taken into account when putting a meal together. The protein-fat combination is found naturally in high-protein foods, but is not useful to take into account, while, though a good one, the starch-starch combination is rarely used.

The best way to forget bad combinations of food is to start applying these good ones. Limited as they are, they are enough to allow for a great variety of different dishes. Although the following pages present information in terms of combination of nutrients, we should be aware that from a practical standpoint, although the number of nutrient combinations may be small, dozens of foods may be combined. The many delicious recipes on pages 190–329 illustrate this very point.

COMBINING PROTEIN AND FAT

Protein and fat are a natural combination of nutrients in high protein food. They belong together and occur in virtually all foods, although often in very small quantities. The great advantage of fat in nutritional terms is that it slows down the

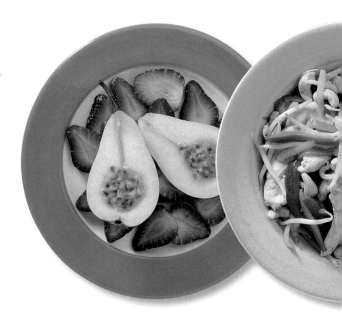

ABOVE: A sensible three-course meal combines protein and fat, and starch and fat.

function of the stomach so that the accompanying protein has more digestive time and effort devoted to it.

However, the protein-fat combination is found only in diets that consist solely of one type of food, or as part of another combination (as, for example, a combination of protein, fat and starch). Remember, too, that, across the whole field of nutrition, it is widely considered that, in the industrialized world at any rate, too much high-protein food is being eaten for good health. This advice applies particularly to high-protein food of animal origin. Current thinking is that we should be eating more starchy foods because of the slow-release carbohydrates they contain.

COMBINING STARCH AND FAT

Foods that are rich in starch – other than potato – contain quite a lot of protein (7–12 per cent by volume), although the protein-starch ratio in cereals and potatoes is actually the same. And they are low in fat.

The way in which starch is digested is extremely complex. Initially, predigestion takes place in the mouth, thanks to the enzyme ptyalin. This enzyme, however, is much affected by the presence of acids and fats (from a chemical point of view, fats consist of fatty acids). In addition, fats contain antioxidants

BELOW: Meat contains protein and fat.

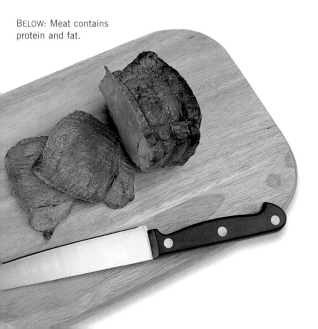

Here are some menus to try, which include some of the recipes to be found at the back of this book.

LIGHT LUNCHES

Minestrone (page 218)
Mexican Stuffed Tomatoes (page 202)

Artichoke Bisque (page 218)
Steamed Vegetables (page 250)

FRUITY IDEAS

Stuffed Apricots (page 320)
Summer Fruits in Berry Sauce (page 322)

Cinnamon Apples (page 315)
Stuffed Pineapple (page 314)

THREE-COURSE MEALS

Fennel au Gratin (page 202)
Raw Tomato Soup (page 211)
Oven-Baked Aubergine (Eggplant) and
Tomatoes (page 256)

Pumpkin Soup (page 218)
Stuffed Cabbage Rolls with
Spiced Rice (page 255)

that prevent them from becoming rancid. So fats can inhibit or even nullify the reaction of the salivary enzyme. However, on the other hand, the presence of fat improves digestion in the stomach by lengthening the digestive process. This is because the presence of fat slows down the peristaltic motion of the stomach wall so that starchy foods stay in the stomach longer, permitting the enhanced digestion of their protein.

Combining starchy and fatty foods is favourable to digestion, provided that the overall degree of acidity is not too high. Fat generally has a pH value of 4.5, which would be high enough technically to render the saliva rather acid were it not for the fact that the added fat – like butter in a sandwich or on spaghetti – is in sufficiently small quantities that the overall dish contains very little fat in relation to the large quantity of starch. The starch-fat meal has a lower degree of acidity as a result. Starchy foods, moreover, have a high water content usually. The water dilutes the acid and a higher, more alkaline pH value is the result.

The ratio of starch and fat is critical to predigestion, because the permitted level of acidity is exceeded easily. If that is something of a disadvantage, it is more than made up for by the favourable influence fat has in the stomach on the digestion of protein in starchy foods. The combination is undoubtedly a good one overall.

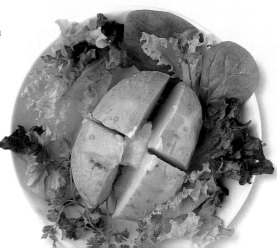

GOOD COMBINATIONS: FAT AND ACID, SUGAR AND ACID

Although fat and acid is a good combination, you should remember that concentrated fat is hard to digest. Although the acid in the combination makes this possible, this means that the combination does not sit well with high-protein

foods or starch-rich foodstuffs. Sugar and acid is a relatively new food combination. Traditionally, it was a combination that was frowned on by old-style food combiners, but recent scientific research has shown it to be perfectly acceptable.

COMBINING FAT AND ACID

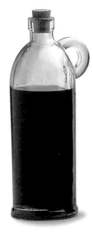

This passes for a good combination, although there are conditions. Fat that is used in a concentrated form (for example, beef dripping, coconut oil, table oil, or fats used in deep- or shallow-frying) is difficult to digest. So these should be used only in restricted quantities. Eating a small amount of fat is not harmful because sugar can be converted to fat so there is never any shortage of fat in the body.

Acid has a useful effect on fat, which, through its agency, becomes emulsified and virtually dissolved. In this way it becomes easier to digest. A small quantity of lemon juice, wine vinegar, vinaigrette (which usually contains wine vinegar) or ordinary vinegar can make fat lighter to digest and, indeed, mayonnaise or an oil-based dressing may be almost indigestible without the addition of some such acid. The fat may otherwise remain in the stomach for too long, particularly in people whose digestive systems are not in good health, resulting in an unpleasant sensation. If this happens to you, drinking a glass of lukewarm water mixed with a little lemon juice should bring immediate relief.

Dressings and mayonnaise combine rather well with vegetable meals. Because of their high acid content, however, they should not be put together with high-protein foods and especially not with foods that are rich in starch. An ideal constituent for a vegetable meal is avocado sprinkled or mixed with lemon juice or vinaigrette.

Nuts or cheese eaten together with acidic fruit represents a good fat-acid combination. Fruit is low in protein, so the proportions of fat and acid are not influenced by it and the acid in the fruit duly emulsifies the fat in the cheese or nuts. Nuts or cheese can also be eaten together with such acid fruits as tomatoes and rhubarb, or with vegetables that contain lactic acid. However, as the acid limit for good digestion can be easily exceeded, making the digestion of

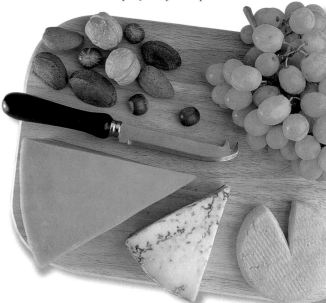

LEFT: A small amount of vinegar makes fat easier to digest.

ABOVE: Nuts, cheese and acidic fruit are a good fat–acid combination.

protein difficult, it is usually better to minimize the proportion of vegetables.

In general, fat and acid are a good combination, as long as acid is not added to the fat in a quantity that makes for more than merely a light emulsifying process. If this happens,the level of acid becomes so high that the food can no longer be combined with starch-rich foods or even high-protein foods (see the protein-acid and starch-acid combinations).

COMBINING SUGAR AND ACID

Nobody has ever really considered this combination before. It used to be thought that sugar fermented in the stomach because the salivary enzyme ptyalin, which helps digest sugar and starch, was destroyed by gastric juice there. Modern knowledge of the physiology of digestion and the practical experience of thousands of patients have proved something

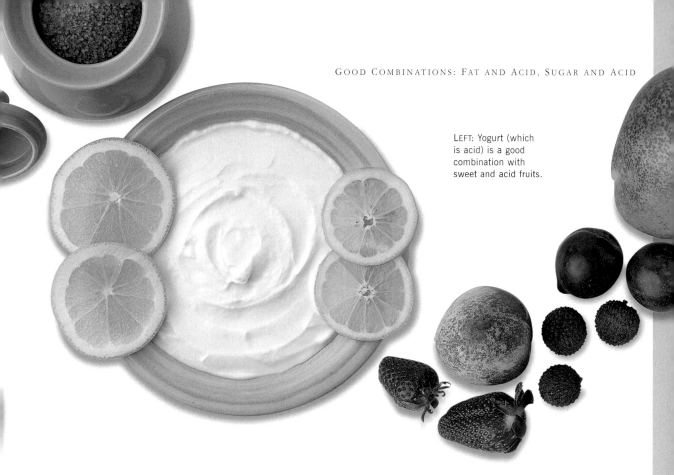

LEFT: Yogurt (which is acid) is a good combination with sweet and acid fruits.

entirely different. The digestion of sugar that begins in the mouth is temporarily halted in the stomach, where the sugars are stabilized. But the gastric juice does not only stabilize the sugars, it also has protective and bactericidal properties. Any fermentation that does occur is not as a result of the destruction of ptyalin, but is owing to the presence of unstabilized sugars that have not made contact with the gastric acid, which prevent the ptyalin from continuing its reaction. The upper part of the stomach (the fundus and corpus) acts as a storage chamber. In a well-filled stomach, the food in the middle of this chamber does not touch the walls to come into contact with gastric acid, and in the warm, damp conditions of the stomach starts to ferment.

This contention is completely contrary to the ideas propounded by the doctors Hay and Shelton. Nonetheless, it is striking that Dr Shelton considers yogurt, which is acid, a good combination with sugary honey, as he does yogurt with sweet fruit, sugar and other sweet foods. On the other hand, he comes down strongly against combining sweet and acidic fruits – a point of view that is not consistent with his favouring the yogurt and honey combination, for that combination is identical in terms of the nutritional elements. So, contrary to Dr Shelton's assertion, the combination of sweet and acid fruits is good.

Fruit represents a natural sugar-acid combination and such harmonious combinations do not have much effect on digestion. There is nothing in modern science to contradict this. We can eat lightly acidic, semi-acidic and acidic fruits together without any digestive problems. If any combination does turn out to be more difficult than others, it is a problem of the individual digestive system and not a problem linked to the combination of foods.

MAKING YOUR OWN YOGURT

A useful source of calcium and phosphorous, essential ingredients for strong bones and healthy teeth, yogurt is also packed with vitamin B_2, which the body needs in order to release energy from food, and vitamin B_{12}, which helps to keep the nervous system in peak condition. It is generally made by heating pasteurized milk to which yogurt or yogurt culture is then added. The yogurt bacteria remain 'live' when they enter the body and medical experts believe that live yogurt is a probiotic, meaning that it encourages the proliferation of 'friendly' bacteria in the gut (see page 49). As well as aiding the digestion, yogurt may also help to prevent bad breath, constipation and diarrhoea.

1 Bring 1 litre/1¾ pints/4 cups of skimmed (skim) or full-cream (whole) milk to the boil. Allow to cool to 41°C/106°F. (You will need a cooking thermometer to measure the temperature accurately.)
2 Add two tablespoons of the milk to the yogurt starter (from health food stores), or use two tablespoons of plain live yogurt.
3 Mix thoroughly with the remaining milk and store in a large covered bowl. Leave in a warm place for 12 hours, or until the mixture sets.
4 Transfer to plastic yogurt containers and store in the refrigerator. You should not keep the yogurt for longer than 7–10 days, so it does not pay to make too much at once.

GOOD COMBINATIONS: STARCH AND STARCH

How many forms of starch you can put together in a single meal is a matter of debate among food combining authorities. Traditionally, the consensus was against it – not because the combination was believed necessarily to be a bad one in itself, but because it was thought that it could be a green light to overindulge and overeat, with inevitable consequences. However, provided that this risk is kept firmly in mind – and that the body's acid-base balance does not become disrupted – there is nothing at all wrong with this type of combination.

There is, for example, a clear difference between potato starch and cereal starch. Modern research has confirmed Dr Shelton's view that eating different types of starch together does not cause digestive problems. In one type of bread there are five different types of grain, for instance, so five different types of grain starch are mixed, yet it does not cause digestive problems. Mixing grain starch and soy flour is slightly more problematical, however: it leads to an increased proportion of protein, and this may cause digestive difficulty.

OVEREATING AND THE ACID-BASE BALANCE

Dr Shelton's warning about overeating is apposite enough, but the danger of overeating naturally exists even when only one form of starch is being consumed. Starch is slow to break down into its constituent sugars. So how full we feel when eating starch is dependent not so much on the rise in blood-sugar level, but on the physical pressure of food against the stomach wall. We therefore go on eating until our stomach feels full – we do not stop after eating only one sandwich or one pancake.

Too much starch, in addition, disrupts the body's acid-base balance, which thus can cause digestive difficulties. It is remarkable that Dr Shelton said nothing at all about this aspect of the combination, whereas Dr Hay made it the basis for his argument in favour of keeping starch and protein separated. In effect, Dr Shelton probably took it into account anyway, if perhaps subconsciously. He recounts that for more than 50 years previously, nutritionists had been used to helping themselves to a liberal serving of vegetable salad together with a meal rich in starch, the salad always piled high on the plate and consisting of fresh, raw vegetables. This would have prevented them from eating too much starch.

ABOVE: Different forms of starch can be combined.

It has been asked whether it is healthy to eat two kinds of starch during one meal. Dr Shelton, discussing the matter, stated that nutritionists recommend only one form of starch per meal, not that there is anything particularly indigestible about such nutrients, but because eating two or more starch-rich foods during one meal almost inevitably means overeating. He therefore suggested that everybody – especially those who were ill – should restrict themselves to one form of starch per meal.

Starch is of vegetable origin and belongs to the group of substances known as polysaccharides. The composition of starch can vary, so that one form is different from another.

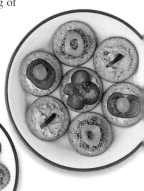

RIGHT: Buffet snacks are starch based.

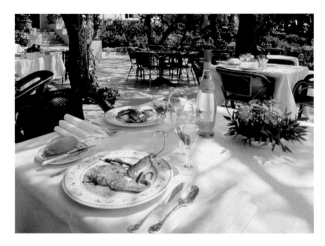

ABOVE: The Mediterranean diet is considered to be very healthy.

The combination of starch and starch is a good one. Like Dr Shelton, I recommend a diet low in starch for people who are ill, as well as for healthy people.

It must be admitted, though, that starch-starch combinations are comparatively rare in any case. There is nothing unwholesome about them, but people seldom eat sandwiches with potatoes, for instance. It is doubtful whether anyone has ever considered baking a cake with potato flour. One frequently found form of starch-starch combination however is the potato croquette, in which a mashed potato roll is covered in breadcrumbs and deep-fried, but this is really a starch-starch-fat combination.

Buffet snacks are often based on farinaceous ingredients. Such dishes included potato salad, potato croquettes, mini pizzas, different kinds of sandwiches and savoury biscuits (crackers) with different toppings. It is not wrong to have several of these attractive little treats on our plate.

PASTA AND THE MEDITERRANEAN DIET

Contrary to what some people still believe, pasta and other starchy foods are not fattening, even though they may be filling. Breads and cereals contain no more calories per gram than lean meat – and they are far lower in fat into the bargain. According to the health experts, carbohydrates, of the kind starch-packed pasta contains, should provide around half of the daily energy intake. The carbohydrates in pasta are classed as complex as opposed to sugars, which are simple ones. Complex carbohydrates are broken down slowly and turned into glycogen, which the body stores and then converts into glucose to fuel its energy needs. Pasta itself consists of a paste or dough made with flour and water. It is a main component of the Mediterranean diet, which nutritionists believe is one of the healthiest in the world and can significantly reduce the risk of heart disease. Other important elements of the diet include rice, bread, potatoes, and cereals, such as couscous, accompanied by liberal quantities of fresh vegetables, olive oil and red wine. It has been calculated that, on average, the Mediterranean diet includes five servings of vegetables and fruit a day.

AVOIDING HEART DISEASE

The Japanese staple food is rice, which is starch-rich and consequently carbohydrate-high. This, combined with the fact that they eat far less fat than people do in the West, means that they enjoy one of the lowest levels of heart disease in the world. To avoid heart disease, the doctors advise increasing consumption of starchy carbohydrate and decreasing the fat. An average Japanese meal consists of steamed rice, miso soup, made from soy bean paste, and small dishes of fish and varieties of shellfish, vegetables, noodles, chicken and meat.

RIGHT: Foods rich in starch and fibre, such as wholemeal (whole-wheat) bread and rolls, rye, crispbread and Granary (multigrain) bread, may help to keep unhealthy blood cholesterol levels in check. Raised blood cholesterol levels are now considered to be the main enemy of heart health. Other foods in a heart-friendly diet include fruit, such as oranges, pears and bananas, and vegetables, such as sweetcorn (corn), mangetouts (snow peas), garlic, onions and various types of beans.

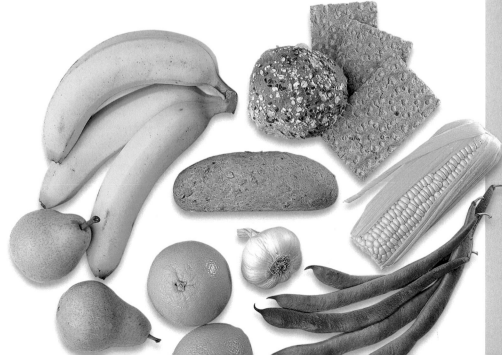

PROBLEMATIC FOOD COMBINATIONS

With food, just as in life, nothing is quite as simple, straightforward and clear-cut as it might seem on the surface. Nowhere is this more true than in what might well be described as the 'grey areas' of food combining. So much here depends on the exact proportions of the nutrients involved, as well as on individual digestive tolerance, which can vary greatly from person to person. What can never be achieved, however, is the transformation of a completely bad food combination into a good, healthy one.

After reading this far, it may well seem that there are a few good combinations of foods and a lot of bad ones. But nothing on the subject of food can ever be quite so clear-cut. Every type of food has a different composition. By combining foods, the proportions of nutrients in them are changed for the better or worse. The idea of a limit of tolerance (the level at which a food simply becomes indigestible) has been mentioned once or twice. Yet it is not easy to define that limit in relation to specific combinations, although, of course, some foods should never be combined. There are, however, combinations that people can tolerate if they have a strong enough digestive system.

INFLUENCING THE COMBINATION

The protein-starch combination is a bad one. An example is the ubiquitous cheese sandwich. But there is a great difference between a sandwich with a thick slice of cheese and the same sandwich with a thin slice. There is a similar difference between a sandwich with a lot of butter or margarine spread over the bread and the same sandwich with only a little. A cheese sandwich is easier to digest if salad is added, rather than pickle. Whether we eat one sandwich or a whole plate of them also makes a considerable difference. So many factors have a crucial influence on digestion.

It should be made clear from the outset, however, that a bad combination can never be transformed into a good one. All that can be done with a bad combination is to try to improve it by restoring the acid-base balance somehow – perhaps by adding salad – or by limiting the quantity consumed.

RIGHT: Starchy vegetables.

IMPROVING THE COMBINATION

So, provided that our digestive systems are functioning reasonably well, we can improve on the combinations in this book that are described as difficult or problematical. Those people whose digestive systems are in poor health should restrict themselves to the good combinations of food because they cannot tolerate the slightest deviation. Do not be too quick to believe, however, that you are one of the exceptions who can digest everything and anything. Acid indigestion, a stomach bloated with food and wind (gas), flatulence, diarrhoea or constipation are all clear symptoms of digestive difficulty even when you are not ill.

It is not possible to describe basic problematical combinations in the way that we did with the bad and the good combinations. Rather, here we deal with a number of different types of food that are difficult, but not impossible to digest when used as the sole constituent of a diet, or which can cause problems when combined with other foods. It should also be noted that the list is by no means exhaustive.

COMBINING PROTEIN WITH FOODS LOW IN STARCH

Protein and starch form a bad combination. There are foods that contain only minimal amounts of starch, but even this tiny quantity can cause serious problems in those who have a weak digestive system (although it does not cause problems in

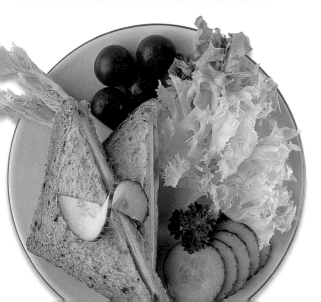

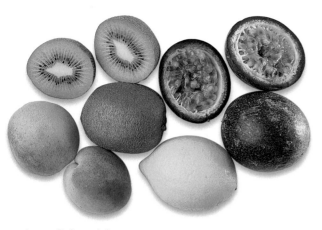

ABOVE: Fruits contain
sugar and acid.

healthy systems). What we are talking about here are
vegetables that have a starch content of around and slightly
more than four per cent such as Jerusalem artichokes: a
content of less than four per cent is negligible.

COMBINING PROTEIN WITH MILDLY ACIDIC OR SEMI-ACIDIC FRUIT

As we have seen, protein with acidic fruit is a bad
combination, unless the fat present is dominant. This is the
case, for instance, with a combination of nuts or cheese with
acidic fruit. For people with a sensitive digestive system, even
the acid in a mildly acidic fruit may cause problems:
moreover, this combination very much depends on individual
digestive reaction.

COMBINING FRUIT AND VEGETABLES

Fruit and vegetables are almost nutritional opposites. Fruits
are acidic, vegetables are usually not. Fruits contain a lot of
sugar, most vegetables contain only a trace. Eating fruit and
vegetables together can cause digestive problems. As far as

BELOW: Fruit and
vegetables should
be eaten separately.

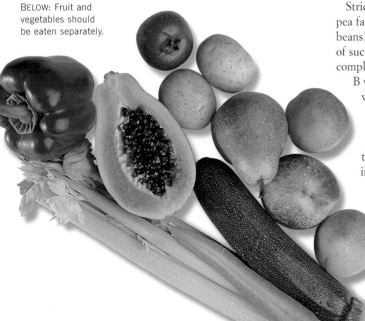

possible, they should be eaten separately – and vegetable
juice counts as vegetables in this connection. Nonetheless, as
has been stated earlier, this combination is not a bad one, just
a difficult one.

MILK

Milk is not easily combined with other foods. It is a drink
that pretty well has to be taken and used on its own. With
fruit or vegetables, milk forms a problematical combination.

LEGUMINOUS VEGETABLES

Legumes are always difficult to digest. However, their
digestion can be improved by combining them with other
types of vegetables, which has the effect of restoring the acid-
base balance. Even in the most favourable
circumstances, though, every dish that contains
leguminous vegetables remains a difficult
combination. The same applies to
soy products, with the
exception of tofu
(bean curd).

RIGHT: Combining peas and
beans with other vegetables
improves their digestion.

Strictly speaking, legumes are defined as any member of the
pea family of vegetables: they include chickpeas (garbanzo
beans), runner (string) beans, soy beans and lentils. The seeds
of such plants are known as pulses. Legumes are high in fibre,
complex carbohydrates, minerals, such as calcium, and the
B vitamins. They also contain some protein, although,
with the exception of soy beans, not in significant
amounts, and are extremely low in fat. They can be a
difficult food owing to their tendency to cause
flatulence, particularly if you are not used to eating
them. If this is the case, take care how quickly you
introduce them into your diet. It is worth noting that soy
beans are a common food allergen, while pulses in
general should be avoided by gout sufferers
because the purines they contain can further
inflame affected joints.

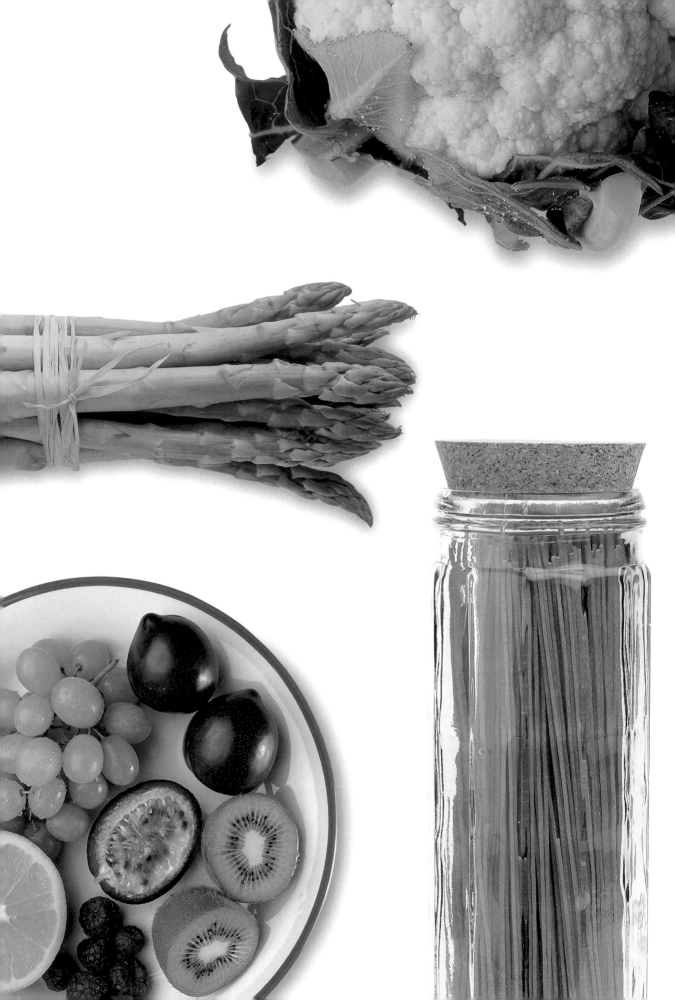

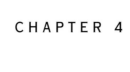

CHAPTER 4

HOW TO COMBINE FOOD CORRECTLY

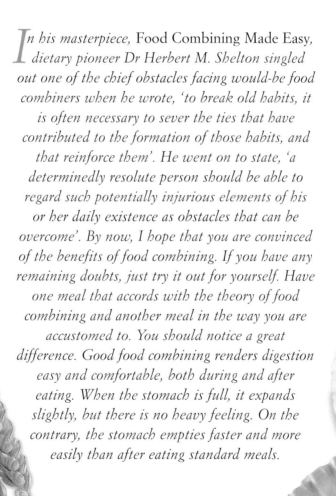

*I*n his masterpiece, Food Combining Made Easy, *dietary pioneer Dr Herbert M. Shelton singled out one of the chief obstacles facing would-be food combiners when he wrote, 'to break old habits, it is often necessary to sever the ties that have contributed to the formation of those habits, and that reinforce them'. He went on to state, 'a determinedly resolute person should be able to regard such potentially injurious elements of his or her daily existence as obstacles that can be overcome'. By now, I hope that you are convinced of the benefits of food combining. If you have any remaining doubts, just try it out for yourself. Have one meal that accords with the theory of food combining and another meal in the way you are accustomed to. You should notice a great difference. Good food combining renders digestion easy and comfortable, both during and after eating. When the stomach is full, it expands slightly, but there is no heavy feeling. On the contrary, the stomach empties faster and more easily than after eating standard meals.*

MOVING FROM THEORY TO PRACTICE

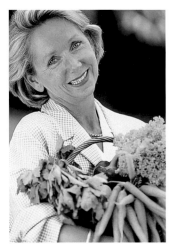

ABOVE: Many people enjoy the advantages of food combining and the benefits of improved health.

The advantages of good food combining should be clear by now, but the obvious question that arises is how best to put this wonderful theory into daily practice. It may look a little complicated at first, but learning how to combine foods correctly is not difficult at all. The starting point is, as ever, the familiar pentagon diagram on which the five main nutrient groups (fats, carbohydrates or starch, proteins, sugars and acids – see pages 130–1) are shown with their good and bad combinations displayed. Remember, it is the dominant nutrient in any two particular foods that determines whether or not they may be combined healthily.

Thousands of people already enjoy the advantages of food combining, and it has helped many of them to fight off disease and regain good health. Its principles – eating good combinations of nutritious food – are scientifically sound and correspond to present-day knowledge of the physiology of digestion. Mastering these principles involves having a fair understanding of the five food groups around which the food combining system is built and on which it relies.

If I were to ask you which group jelly (flavored gelatine), jam (jelly), honey and syrup belonged to, you would know the answer immediately: sugar. If I were to ask you to list several high-protein foods, you would be able to do so easily, I'm sure. However, other groupings might be slightly more difficult to identify straightaway. Is fruit grouped with sugary or with acidic foods? The answer is, of course, that fruit contains both sugar and acids. When thinking about how to combine different types of fruit with other foods, you have to take account of both the sugar and the acid content.

EASY COMBINERS

In addition to foods that belong within the five nutrient groupings, there are some foods that have very little effect on food combining. Dr Hay pointed out that non-leguminous vegetables have something of a neutral character, for example. With the exception of the tomato (if that is a vegetable at all) and pulses, vegetables can be combined with both protein and starch. I have tended to avoid using the word 'neutral', in this sense of 'inert', for fear that it might be taken to mean a neutral position between acidity and alkalinity. A neutral food implies that it would have a pH value of seven – and such foods do not exist.

Fresh milk and eggs, however, come close to having a neutral value and so also do most vegetables, which contain a lot of water but not much carbohydrate, acid or fat, and very little protein. The protein content of vegetables is actually higher than that of fruit, but it is very low in comparison to the protein content of high-protein foods. If you add vegetables to other foods, the overall proportions of nutrients barely change, which is why vegetables may be combined with just about anything – although there are exceptions, such as combining vegetables with sugar. If vegetables are combined with sugar, the sugar content, which is always very low in vegetables, is proportionally increased by enough to alter the nutrient ratio. So sugar or honey should never be eaten with raw vegetables. Acids go well with vegetables. But because fruit contains acids and sugar, fruit together with vegetables is a problematical combination for the digestion.

MILK – A 'COMPLETE' FOOD

Milk is a whole food in liquid form – one of Nature's most nourishing foods. It contains high-quality protein and is a good source of the essential B vitamins, notably thiamin, riboflavin and niacin, as well as minerals such as phosphorus and zinc. Above all, it is an excellent source of calcium, which is vital for the growth and maintenance of strong healthy bones and good teeth. The daily adult calcium requirement is around 700 mg, which is the amount contained in 600 ml/1 pint/2½ cups of

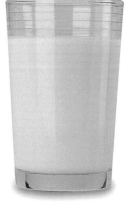

RIGHT: Milk is liquid nourishment.

MUSHROOM MAGIC

Mushrooms and other forms of edible fungi, such as truffles, are delicious, they combine well with many other foods and have very little effect at all on overall nutrient proportions since they contain remarkably little acid (their pH value is 6.4), hardly any fat or carbohydrates, and relatively little protein (2.7 per cent by volume). Truffles contain slightly more protein (5 per cent). The water content of mushrooms is extremely high (94 per cent), and they provide only 15 calories per 100 g/3½ oz. They are also a useful source of potassium and valuable trace elements.

Although in theory there can be no bad combination involving mushrooms, they are not usually eaten with nuts, seeds, fruit, yogurt or milk – with the exception of a milk- or yogurt-based sauce.

Some people have been concerned about the hydrazines and nitrosamines mushrooms and other edible fungi have been shown to contain, which may possibly be carcinogenic. However, you would have to eat very large amounts of mushrooms indeed to be remotely at risk. In terms of nutritional value, there is very little difference between wild mushrooms and those that have been cultivated commercially, although the former usually have an earthier flavour. If you are gathering mushrooms for yourself from the wild, take a field guide with you and be absolutely sure to identify them correctly since some of the most toxic varieties of mushrooms look just like edible ones. If you are in any doubt whatsoever, do not eat them.

Cep
Porcini to the Italians, ceps look somewhat like glossy buns when they are fresh. When dried, they have a concentrated meaty flavour.
Chanterelle
Trumpet-shaped mushrooms that are firm in texture and golden in colour. They have a peppery aroma.
Morel
A mushroom with a cap like a honeycomb and a rich earthy flavour.
Oyster
A mushroom with a somewhat chewy texture.
Shiitake
A richly flavoured tree fungus, usually sold dry, which Chinese herbalists recommend as a guarantee of a long, healthy life.
Truffles
A gourmet fungi that grows underground, usually in the roots of beech or oak trees. It is sniffed out by trained pigs or dogs. Périgord (black) and Italian (white) truffles are especially prized by connoisseurs. Until recently, truffles defied all attempts at cultivation, but in late autumn (fall) 1999 it was announced that a food scientist had succeeded in growing them, at least experimentally, by grafting them on to other plants.

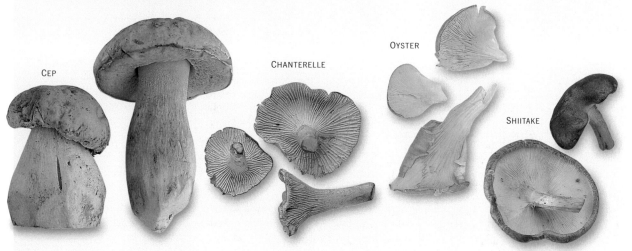

CEP CHANTERELLE OYSTER SHIITAKE

milk, but this requirement varies according to age and circumstance. Growing teenagers, for instance, need between 800 mg and 1000 mg of calcium a day, while breastfeeding mothers need around 1250 mg daily.

Milk readily increases in acidity, so improving digestion, but can be combined well only with acidic foods. Milk with fat, milk with fruit, or milk with vegetables should be regarded as problematical combinations. Food combiners argue that whole cow's milk is not the best type of milk to include in the diet. They advocate using goat's milk or skimmed (skim) or semi-skimmed (low-fat) cow's milk – this is milk from which all or most of the fat has been removed, leaving the nutrients intact – as healthier alternatives.

TYPE	CALORIES PER 100 ML (3½ FL OZ)	FAT CONTENT
Whole milk	66	3.9%
Semi-skimmed (low-fat) milk	46	1.6%
Skimmed (skim) milk	33	0.1%
Single (light) cream	198	19.1%
Whipping cream	373	39.3%
Goat's milk	30	2.5%

FOOD COMBINATIONS & NUTRITIONAL GUIDELINES

To simplify food combining principles, here is a diagram of food combinations, grouped according to the five nutrients. Non-leguminous vegetables, mushrooms and milk are grouped separately (see pages 126–7) because these fairly common foods do not fall into any of the other categories. For further reference, here is also a version of the original food combining pentagon, plus an explanation of the food pyramid favoured by conventional nutritionists.

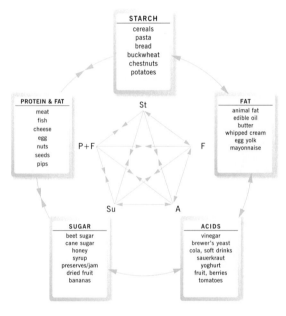

LEFT: This handy pentagon will show you which groups different foods are in.

Using the first diagram given here, everyone can participate in food combining and avoid bad combinations of food successfully. However, it is simply not possible to classify every individual food: the diagram would become far too complex. All that is necessary, after all, is a rough-and-ready working knowledge of the subject, and particularly of foods in their groups. If you wonder what buckwheat can be combined with, for example, look under its generic group, 'cereals'. Or if you want to know what a beefburger may be combined with, check under 'meat'.

The food combining pentagon is another way of looking at the same thing. It shows there is a total of ten possible combinations, four of which are good and six of which are bad. You can see at a glance, for instance, that, while starch and fat is potentially a good combination, a combination of starch, protein and fat is definitely one to be avoided.

RIGHT: This food combining chart goes into more detail, and shows you which foods combine well with others.

✔	good combination
•	good but not usual
✗	difficult combination
—	bad combination

PROTEIN	meat–fish–poultry
	cheese – cottage
	nuts – seeds – pips
FAT	oil – fat – egg yolk
	butter – whipped cream
	avocado – olive
SUGAR	sugar – honey
	fruit rich in sugar
STARCH	cereals – bread – pasta
	potato
	vegetables rich in starch
ACIDS	fruit – berries
	vinegar – mustard
	tomato
	yoghurt – butter milk
	vegetables (lactic acid)
	vegetables
	milk
	mushrooms

Legend: ✓ = combines well · – = acceptable/neutral · X = combines poorly · • = (marginal) · ▦ = shaded cell (diagonal)

	mushrooms	milk	vegetables	vegetables (latic acid)	yoghurt – butter milk	tomato	vinegar/mustard	fruits – berries	vegetables rich in starch	potato	cereals – bread – pasta	fruit rich in sugar	sugar – honey	avocado – olive	butter – whipped cream	oil – fat – egg yolk	nuts – seeds – pips	cheese – cottage cheese	meat – fish – poultry
				ACIDS					STARCH			SUGAR		FAT			PROTEIN		
1	✓	–	✓	–	–	✓	–	–	X	–	–	–	–	–	–	–	–	–	▦
2	✓	–	✓	–	X	✓	–	✓	X	–	–	–	–	–	–	–	–	▦	–
3	•	–	✓	✓	X	✓	–	✓	X	–	–	–	–	–	–	–	▦	–	–
4	✓	X	✓	✓	✓	✓	✓	✓	✓	✓	✓	X	–	–	–	▦	–	–	–
5	✓	–	✓	✓	✓	✓	✓	✓	✓	✓	✓	X	–	–	▦	–	–	–	–
6	✓	–	✓	✓	✓	✓	✓	✓	✓	✓	✓	–	–	▦	–	–	–	–	–
7	–	–	–	–	✓	•	•	✓	X	–	–	X	▦	–	–	–	–	–	–
8	–	–	–	–	✓	•	X	✓	X	–	–	▦	X	–	X	X	–	–	–
9	✓	–	✓	–	–	✓	–	–	X	–	▦	–	–	✓	✓	✓	✓	–	–
10	✓	–	✓	–	–	✓	–	–	X	▦	–	–	–	✓	✓	✓	✓	–	–
11	✓	–	✓	✓	✓	X	X	X	▦	✓	✓	X	X	✓	✓	✓	X	X	X
12	–	X	X	X	✓	X	✓	▦	X	–	–	✓	✓	✓	✓	✓	✓	✓	–
13	✓	X	✓	–	–	✓	▦	✓	X	–	–	X	•	✓	✓	✓	–	–	–
14	✓	X	✓	✓	✓	▦	✓	X	X	–	–	•	✓	✓	✓	✓	✓	✓	✓
15	•	✓	✓	✓	▦	✓	–	✓	✓	–	–	✓	✓	✓	✓	✓	X	X	–
16	✓	X	✓	▦	✓	✓	X	X	✓	–	–	–	–	✓	✓	✓	✓	–	–
17	✓	X	▦	✓	✓	✓	✓	X	✓	✓	✓	–	–	✓	✓	✓	✓	✓	✓
18	✓	▦	X	X	–	X	X	X	–	–	–	–	–	X	X	–	–	–	–
19	▦	•	✓	✓	•	✓	✓	–	✓	✓	✓	–	–	✓	✓	✓	•	✓	✓

The Food Pyramid

You can use your knowledge of food combining to improve and refine the guidelines set out in the classic food pyramid favoured by orthodox nutritionists. Like food combiners, nutritionists classify food in groups, which they then arrange into a multi-tiered pyramid (see right). Working downwards from the top, the groups within the tiers consist of sugary and fatty foods; meat, poultry, fish and other sources of protein, such as nuts, pulses and eggs; milk and dairy products; vegetables; fruit; potatoes, breads and cereals, such as wheat and rice. Nutritionists argue that if you increase your intake of foods rich in complex carbohydrates (the foods at the base of the pyramid) and cut right back on the ones containing saturated fats and sugar (the foods at the top of the pyramid), you will be laying the foundations for a healthier lifestyle, reducing the risk of developing heart disease and other diet-related illnesses and conditions.

No food combiner would disagree with this in principle. It is basic nutritional common sense. Where there may be disagreement, however, is over how best to combine the various foodstuffs contained in the pyramid to produce a healthy balanced diet. The nutritionists who devised the pyramid argue, for instance, that the position of any food within it is determined by its main ingredients. Take a quiche as a seemingly straightforward example. Because its main ingredient is egg, it falls, say orthodox nutritionists, into the category of a protein food. But this disregards the fact that the quiche's pastry, which is a mixture of flour and fat, makes it come into both the fat and carbohydrate groups as well. Food combiners believe you have to take all such facts into account before you can decide what really goes best with what in nutritional terms. Remember, too, when planning meals that a varied diet is important: no food can provide all the 13 vitamins, 16 minerals, adequate protein, carbohydrates and fats that we need each day (for nutritional requirements, see pages 70–1).

All modern nutritionists agree that vegetables should be the backbone of most diets. They are vital providers of vitamins, minerals, carbohydrates and the all-important dietary fibre.

There is disagreement, however, over when and how to eat fruit, which is an equally important dietary constituent. As far as the digestion is concerned, the food combining way is best: treating fruit as something separate – best eaten on its own, rather than as as a single component of a complex meal.

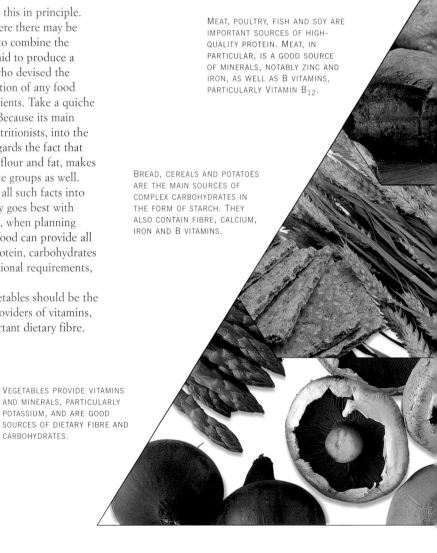

SUGARY AND FATTY FOODS CAN STILL FORM PART OF A HEALTHY, BALANCED DIET, PROVIDED THAT THEY ARE EATEN IN STRICT MODERATION.

MEAT, POULTRY, FISH AND SOY ARE IMPORTANT SOURCES OF HIGH-QUALITY PROTEIN. MEAT, IN PARTICULAR, IS A GOOD SOURCE OF MINERALS, NOTABLY ZINC AND IRON, AS WELL AS B VITAMINS, PARTICULARLY VITAMIN B_{12}.

BREAD, CEREALS AND POTATOES ARE THE MAIN SOURCES OF COMPLEX CARBOHYDRATES IN THE FORM OF STARCH. THEY ALSO CONTAIN FIBRE, CALCIUM, IRON AND B VITAMINS.

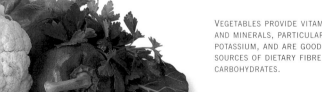

VEGETABLES PROVIDE VITAMINS AND MINERALS, PARTICULARLY POTASSIUM, AND ARE GOOD SOURCES OF DIETARY FIBRE AND CARBOHYDRATES.

HEALTHY EATING GUIDELINES

Most people who change their diet so that what they are eating is in tune with modern health guidelines find that, as a result, they are increasing their intake of complex carbohydrates, while at the same time cutting back on fats, especially saturated ones. The amount of sugar drops dramatically into the bargain. In practical terms, this means eating more vegetables, fruit, bread, potatoes, rice and pasta and fewer sugary, fatty foods. The main guidelines are:

• Eating little but often is best. Eat smaller amounts of food at regular intervals spaced through the day, rather than skipping meals in favour of a big blow-out in the evening.
• Eat a wide variety of foods.
• Maintain a healthy weight (see page 176).
• Eat plenty of starch- and fibre-rich foods and cut back on ones that are rich in fat and sugar.
• Make sure that what you eat contains plenty of vitamins and minerals.

• If you drink, keep your alcohol intake within sensible, moderate limits (see page 107).
• Cut back on the amount of salt you use in cooking and avoid adding salt to food at the table.
• Bear in mind the overall balance of what you eat during the day: remember that snacks and meals both count towards it.
• Enjoy what you eat.

MILK AND DAIRY PRODUCTS CONTAIN CALCIUM – A VITAL CONSTITUENT OF STRONG BONES AND HEALTHY TEETH – PROTEIN, MAGNESIUM, VITAMIN B_2 (RIBOFLAVIN), VITAMIN B_{12} AND VITAMIN A.

Left: The food pyramid was devised by health authorities as part of a plan to provide easy-to-follow guidelines for healthy eating. The most sophisticated food pyramid is the American version, which has six bands of food arranged in four tiers.

FRUIT PROVIDES THE BODY WITH VITAMIN C, CAROTENES, FOLATE, FIBRE AND SUGAR.

FRUIT

Fruit lies almost by definition at the heart of any successful food combining plan, although, until fairly recently, the nutritional benefits of fruit in particular tended to be overlooked by traditional food combining experts. Food combining guru Dr Herbert M. Shelton, for one, recognized just how incorrect this was when he wrote in his pioneering work Food Combining Made Easy *that fruits 'are exquisite collections of pure, rich, watery food constituents'.*

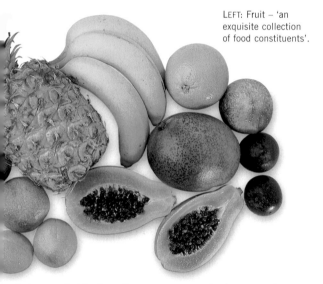

LEFT: Fruit – 'an exquisite collection of food constituents'.

It is remarkable that whereas many people shower praise upon fruits, berries and nuts, traditional cuisine tends to look down on fruit. As fruits have a low calorific value and contain little protein and fat they are therefore regarded as inferior to other foods. Contemporary cookery books cite fruits as good sources of vitamins and minerals, but then go on to warn of the dangers of eating too much of them, suggesting that one or two a day is more than sufficient. Throughout my career I have been trying to have fruit accepted as the sustaining nourishment it is, while my colleagues in traditional dietetics have been reluctant to see it as any such thing.

FRUIT PROBLEMS: FACT OR FICTION?

In alimentary medicine, fruit is very often cast as the villain. Digestive problems, wind (gas) caused by fermentation and other stomach and intestinal disorders are frequently blamed on fruit. It is at the top of the list of forbidden foods. Many

of these problems may well have something to do with how it is eaten. It is cooked, or eaten in the form of a sauce, a jelly (flavored gelatine) or a jam (jelly). Pieces of fruit are virtually always treated as a dessert. It is often eaten when unripe. And it is frequently combined with other foods unsuited to it. All these factors can give rise to digestive problems.

Fruit is difficult to combine with other foods. This is particularly true of berries and the type of fruit and vegetables known as gourds (which include melons). The nutrients in food that are decisive in food combining are sugar and acids. Fruit is a natural sugar-acid combination and therefore combines badly: its acids do not combine with starch or protein, while its sugars do not combine with starch, protein or fat. So five combinations are immediately ruled out.

Fruits, including berries and melons, cannot be combined with bread, cereal dishes, pasta, meat or fish. Avocado and olives, which are both extremely rich in fat, may be combined with starch, but not with fruits that are rich in sugar. A jam (jelly) sandwich – a sugar-starch combination – is a bad combination. A banana sandwich, which is another popular confection, is also extremely inadvisable because of its inherent sugar–starch and starch-acid combinations. Remember that tastes can be deceptive. A banana is as acidic as a tomato despite its sweet taste. (Its high sugar content masks any acidic taste.) A tomato contains only three per cent sugar, which is why the acids in it are clearly discernible to the taste buds.

HOW BEST TO EAT FRUIT

As far as possible, eat fruit as a separate dish or meal and do not combine it with other foods. Eaten as a meal in itself or as a casual snack, fruit can be digested smoothly and easily. If you still experience digestive difficulties, the cause could well be something different – irregular working hours for example. (In snatched breaks between shifts, people often tend to eat too much and too fast.)

I have often been surprised by the large quantities of fruit that some people seem to eat at a sitting. They may think they know all about fruit-eating, but they really understand little about fruit diets. Fruit should be eaten slowly and in small amounts. The fruit should be allowed to melt in the mouth, so that the sugars can be released and absorbed into the bloodstream. Sugar in the bloodstream affects the saturation centre in the hypothalamus of the brain: the appetite is satisfied relatively quickly, and the person does not feel obliged to eat more than a small quantity. This is the road to perfect digestion. If you eat too fast, you swallow large lumps of fruit that the stomach cannot break down properly, leading to undigested residues fermenting in the intestines.

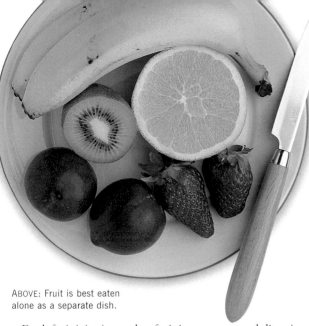

ABOVE: Fruit is best eaten alone as a separate dish.

Fresh fruit juice is equal to fruit in every way and digestion is a lot easier because it has been reduced to liquid even before reaching the mouth. Fruit juice, in fact, can be compared with breastfeeding. The idea that fruit juice contains no dietary fibre is inaccurate, for the juice is merely the liquid form of the whole food.

QUANTITIES OF FRUIT

Is it possible to eat too much fruit? It certainly is. A person who does so has to eliminate excessive quantities of potassium through the kidneys, which means an annoying frequency and urgency in urination and burdensome pressure on the kidneys and the bladder. Years of experience with cancer patients on a strict fruit diet (the Dries cancer diet) have taught me that cancer patients can get by with relatively little fruit per day as soon as they switch over to a fruit-only diet. The daily intake is not more than 1.5 kg/3 lb, and blood tests show that there are no nutritional deficiencies. For people in normal health, the amount of fruit per meal should not exceed 500–600 g/1–1 lb 4 oz. This puts no pressure on the stomach. To live only on fruit requires several meals a day, and in most cases fruits such as nuts are necessary in order to be sure the body is receiving its full complement of nutrients.

COMBINING FRUIT WITH FRUIT

In his work, Dr Shelton distinguished between sweet, semi-acidic and acidic fruits. I am not aware of what he based this division upon, but it may well have been the tastes of the each fruit. Unhappily, his classification does not work and all his contentions about food combining in relation to fruits therefore have to be ignored. It is just not the case, for instance, that, as Dr Shelton mistakenly contends, sweet fruit (fruit with few acids and plenty of sugar) may not be combined with acidic fruit (fruit with plenty of acid and comparatively little sugar).

Sugar and acid are a good combination, as I have already said. All fruit contains sugar and acid in some proportion or

other, so putting combinations of fruit together does not change anything. Mixing sweet fruit with acidic fruit means that what is digested might as well be semi-acidic fruit. Of course, the effect is not always averaged out quite so evenly, but any difference is so small that it does not influence the digestion one way or the other.

Shelton also stated that, from his experience of providing meals to the unwell, he had discovered that it was best to serve sweet and acidic fruit as separate meals. This is not true and in any case his grouping of specific fruits into sweet, semi-acidic and acidic is 80 per cent inaccurate. He considers pineapple to be an acidic fruit, for instance, when it is in fact a sweet fruit. There is no scientific reason why sweet and acidic fruits should not be combined. The stabilization of sugars in the sweet fruit is totally accounted for by the acids in the acidic fruit. Many people whom I know to have been familiar with the principles of food combining for years have told me that never once have they tried to avoid combining all types of fruit and that they have never had any problems with digestion because of it. They are quite used to eating all kinds of fruit together.

I gave a banana mixed with lemon juice to some people whom I knew had a digestive problem. The reaction was unanimous: never had they eaten a banana that digested so comfortably. Shelton was right in saying that there are ill people who cannot tolerate certain combinations of foods, but that applies also to some healthy people and is a reflection of the individual's reaction to certain foods, rather than having anything to do with the combination involved.

People whose digestive systems are weak benefit from eating only one kind of fruit at any one time, despite the possibilities of food combining. Eating solely one type of food makes for the most relaxed digestion and, technically, nothing is better than such a diet. Ordinarily healthy people should not experience any problems in mixing the types of fruit they eat, except in relation to the particular fruits they personally do not tolerate well.

RIGHT: Lemon eases the digestion of bananas.

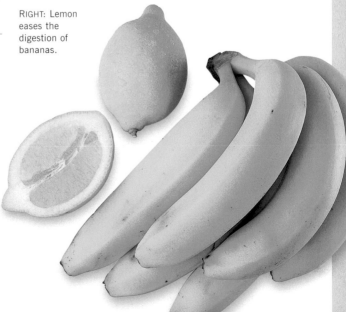

To sum up, fruit may be combined with fruit without qualms. It is not necessary to take the acid or sugar content into account at all. The sole exception to the rule is rhubarb, which contains so much oxalic acid that it is better avoided. Its leaves are particularly toxic and should never be eaten.

FRUIT AND OTHER FOODS

Fruit, especially sweet fruit, goes well with acidic foods, such as yogurt, buttermilk, sour cream and even sauerkraut. Acidic fruits may be combined with fatty foods, such as full-fat curd (farmer's) cheese, hard and semi-hard cheeses, nuts and seeds. Fruit served with unsweetened whipped cream is also a good combination because the acid is then the dominant nutrient. (Fruit can be surprisingly acid: even a 'sweet' banana has a pH value of 3.8, which makes it as acidic as a tomato). However people with sensitive digestive systems may experience difficulties if they eat large quantities of sweet fruit together with whipped cream, which is rich in fat.

Finally, fruit and sweetened whipped cream combined with foods rich in starch, such as cakes or pastries, is a bad combination for anyone.

MELONS

Melons belong to a family of fruit and vegetables known as gourds that come from climbing plants. Only the honeydew melon and the Spanish yellow melon have any genuine sugar content. The others contain mere traces. Unlike other fruits, therefore, they are mildly acidic and in food combining terms should be considered a separate group of foods.

Apart from the honeydew and the yellow melon, melons are almost 94 per cent water, with 1 per cent protein, 0.2 per cent fat and 5.3 per cent carbohydrate. (In terms of energy, melon supplies only 25 calories per 100 g/3½ oz.) Dr Shelton advises people to eat melon on its own. The honeydew and the yellow melon contain sugar, however, and so can be combined with other fruits.

The vegetable gourds – pumpkins, courgettes (zucchini), cucumbers, gherkins (cornichons) and aubergines (eggplant) are all classic examples – may be successfully combined with other non-leguminous vegetables. This is because they are similar in composition to them.

Type	Nutritional value	Effects on health
TREE FRUITS		
Apple **Loquat** **Medlar** **Pear** **Quince**	Contain Vitamin A and Vitamin C and are rich in minerals such as magnesium and calcium. As well as Vitamin C, pears are a useful source of fibre and potassium Loquats do not contain Vitamin C, but do contain beta-carotene.	Contain fructose, a natural simple sugar which is slow to metabolize and so helps to control blood sugar levels. Apples help to lower cholesterol and have antiviral properties. Pears are among the least allergenic of foods.

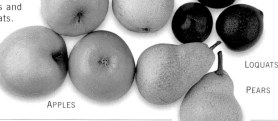

RIGHT: Apples, pears and loquats.

LOQUATS

PEARS

APPLES

Type	Nutritional value	Effects on health
SOFT FRUITS		
Bilberry **Blackberry** **Blackcurrant** **Blueberry** **Cranberry** **Gooseberry** **Huckleberry** **Loganberry** **Raspberry** **Redcurrant** **Strawberry** **Whitecurrant**	High in Vitamin C, especially blackcurrants, which, weight for weight, contain four times as much as an orange. Blackberries are rich in fibre and folate, while gooseberries are a useful fibre source. As well as Vitamin C, raspberries contain Vitamin E, folate and fibre. Strawberries have the highest Vitamin C content of any soft fruit, but they start to lose it quickly after harvesting.	All berries have antioxidant properties that may help to protect the body against cancer and other degenerative diseases. They also contain salicylates, a natural substance similar to aspirin which can cause an allergic reaction. Naturopaths believe that raspberry juice helps to cleanse and detoxify the digestive system and use it to treat complaints like diarrhoea and cystitis.

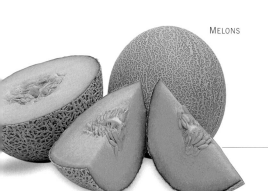

MELONS

BLACKBERRIES

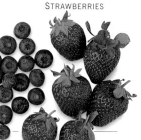

STRAWBERRIES

RASPBERRIES

BLUEBERRIES

FRUIT AT A GLANCE

Type	Nutritional value	Effects on health

STONE (PITTED) FRUITS

Apricot
Cherry
Damson
Greengage
Nectarine
Peach
Plum

Apricots, particularly dried ones, are high in beta-carotene, iron and potassium. Cherries, too, are good potassium sources, while greengages and damsons contain calcium and magnesium. Plums are highly acidic, and best eaten only in moderate quantities. These fruits all contain useful amounts of Vitamin C.

Eating cherries regularly will help to reduce uric acid levels in the blood, so helping to protect against the possibility of contracting gout. Peaches are easily digestible and are a gentle laxative.

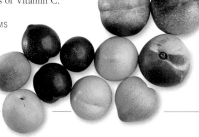

NECTARINES

PLUMS

PEACHES

RIGHT: Peaches, plums and nectarines.

CITRUS FRUITS

Clementine
Grapefruit
Kumquat
Mandarin
Orange
Pomelo
Satsuma
Tangerine
Ugli fruit

Grapefruit and oranges are particularly high in Vitamin C. Oranges also contain thiamin and folate. Citrus fruits are good sources of calcium and beta-carotene.

Pith and membranes are rich in pectin which may help to lower blood cholesterol levels, and bioflavonoids, which have powerful anti-oxidant properties. For this reason, it is better to eat the fruit rather than drink the juice and, at the least, not to discard the pulp when juicing.

ORANGES AND
GRAPEFRUIT

Type	Nutritional value	Effects on health

MELON

Cantaloupe
Charentais
Galia
Honeydew
Watermelon

Some varieties, particularly cantaloupe, are good sources of Vitamin C and beta-carotene.

High water content may stimulate the kidneys to work more efficiently. Food combiners say that, because it can ferment in the stomach, melon is best eaten on its own, although the honeydew and yellow varieties can be combined with other fruits.

HONEYDEW

CHARENTAIS

TROPICAL AND SEMI-TROPICAL FRUITS

Banana
Date
Fig
Grape
Kiwi fruit
Lychee
Mango
Papaya
Passion fruit
Persimmon
Pomegranate
Pineapple

Bananas are high in potassium, as are dates (when dried) and natural sugars. Fresh dates are a useful source of Vitamin C. Mango is quite high in sugar, and is a rich beta-carotene and Vitamin C source, the ripe flesh being particularly easy to digest. A standard serving of pineapple will supply a quarter of the body's daily Vitamin C needs.

Black grapes are a rich source of antioxidants. Pineapple contains bromelain, an enzyme that helps the body to break down protein. Ripe bananas are extremely digestible and aid recovery from diarrhoea and constipation.

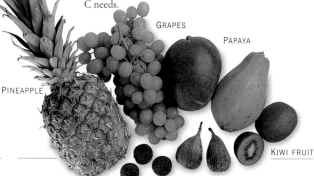

GRAPES

PAPAYA

PINEAPPLE

KIWI FRUIT

PASSION FRUIT

FIGS

137

VEGETABLES

*The composition of vegetables is completely
different from that of fruit, which is why
vegetables and fruit should never be eaten
together. They are a difficult or problematic
combination. The major difference between the
two lies in the relative proportions of protein,
carbohydrates and acids. Fruits are fairly rich in
sugar and acid, but are low in protein. Vegetables*
*are low in sugar and contain
little by way of acids, but
they are slightly richer in
protein: the lower their
sugar content, the
more fruit acids
they contain.
Acids and sugars
have a reciprocal
relationship.*

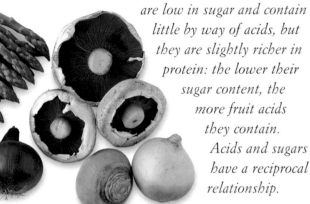

With the exception of the tomato (if it may be considered a
vegetable), vegetables do not contain much acid – their pH
value is around 5.2 to 6.6, which makes them only mildly
acidic. This is why they may be combined readily with protein
and starch. (Dr Hay regarded vegetables as neutral in relation
to protein and starch.) Their actual structure is generally
harder and more solid than that of fruit, which is one reason
why they are more difficult to digest. The problem may be
solved by adding low-fat mayonnaise or an oil-based dressing
to vegetables, which makes them remain longer in the
stomach so that digestion is given extra time to take place.
Raw vegetables with no dressing are problematical for the
digestion. Humans are not natural herbivores and you should
make sure that vegetables receive a minium of preparation.

In terms of food combining, there is no difference
between raw and cooked vegetables. If, however, you boil
vegetables, they lose much of their Vitamin C content, which
leaches away in the cooking water. The vitamin is also
sensitive to heat. Cooking, however, can make it easier for the
body to access a vegetable's nutrient stores in certain
instances. Carrots, for example, are always better cooked
rather than eaten raw, since the cooking process softens the
vegetable's tough cell membranes, making it easier for the
body to absorb the valuable beta-carotene they contain.

Type	Nutritional value	Effects on health
CABBAGE FAMILY		
Broccoli **Brussels** **sprouts** **Cabbage** **(red, green,** **white)** **Cauliflower** **Chinese leaves** **(cabbage)** **Kale** **Kohlrabi** **Mustard** **and cress** **Radish** **Turnip** **Swede** **(rutabaga)** **Watercress**	Broccoli contains folate, iron and potassium, is an excellent source of Vitamin C and a useful one of beta-carotene. Cabbage is rich in Vitamins C, K and E and a good source of potassium. Kale contains folate, iron and calcium, while kohlrabi is a useful source of soluble and insoluble dietary fibre. Swede (rutabaga) is a useful vitamin source and may help to protect against cancer. Watercress is a rich source of Vitamin C, beta-carotene and iron.	All members of the cabbage family are cruciferous plants, containing valuable phyto-chemicals, including indoles, which are thought to lessen the risk of contracting breast cancer, and isothio-cyanites, which may help to fight cancer of the colon and of the rectum. Eating too much swede (rutabaga) may cause an iodine deficiency, which can affect the thyroid gland.

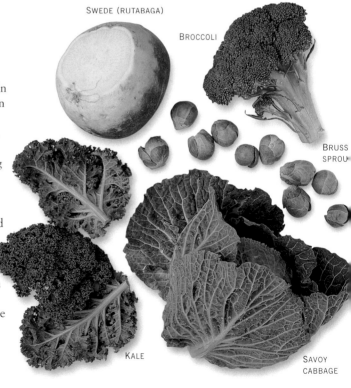

SWEDE (RUTABAGA)

BROCCOLI

BRUSS
SPROU

KALE

SAVOY
CABBAGE

VEGETABLES AT A GLANCE

Type	Nutritional value	Effects on health

BEET FAMILY

Beetroot (beet)
Spinach
Swiss chard

Beetroot (beet) is potassium-rich, a good source of folate and contains Vitamin C. The edible leafy tops contain beta-carotene, calcium and iron. Spinach is an excellent beta-carotene source and also contains Vitamin C, folate and potassium. However, its oxalic acid content may hinder the body's absorption of calcium and iron.

Both beetroot (beet) and spinach are thought to be rich in natural cancer-fighting agents. Fresh, raw beetroot juice is a concentrated vitamin and mineral source, but the vegetable also has a high sugar concentration.

SWISS CHARD

BEETROOT
(BEET)

SPINACH

LETTUCE FAMILY

Artichoke
Chicory
(Belgian endive)
Dandelion
Endive (chicory)
Lettuce
Salsify

Globe artichokes are good sources of potassium and folate. Lettuce contains useful amounts of folate, beta carotene, Vitamin C and calcium. Chicory (Belgian endive) and endive (chicory) both contain Vitamins A, K, the B vitamins and useful minerals.

Cynarin, found in the edible base of globe artichoke leaves, may improve liver function. Herbalists believe that lettuce has sedative properties. Dandelion is also a good detoxifier.

GLOBE
ARTICHOKE

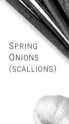

CHICORY
(BELGIAN
ENDIVE)

LETTUCE

Type	Nutritional value	Effects on health

ONION FAMILY

Asparagus
Chives
Garlic
Leek
Onion
Shallot
Spring onion (scallion)

Asparagus is rich in folate; it also contains beta-carotene, Vitamin C and Vitamin E. Leeks are a useful source of potassium and folate. Spring onions (scallions) and leeks contain Vitamin C.

Asparagus is a mild laxative and diuretic. Its high purine content means that it should be avoided by anyone with gout. Garlic has powerful antiviral and antibacterial properties. It may help to lower blood pressure and cholesterol levels, while the compounds it contains are good for the heart and high blood pressure. Onions are thought to help to prevent circulatory disorders and may even help to fight cancer.

ONIONS

SPRING
ONIONS
(SCALLIONS)

SHALLOTS

GARLIC

LEEKS

139

Type	Nutritional value	Effects on health

PARSLEY FAMILY

Carrot
Celeriac
(celery root)
Celery
Dill
Fennel
Parsley
Parsnip

Carrots are a first-rate source of beta-carotene, which the body turns into Vitamin A, and are a good fibre source. Celeriac (celery root) contains Vitamin C, soluble fibre and potassium, while celery is extremely low in calories as well as being a good potassium source. Fennel contains beta-carotene and folate. Parsnips are useful sources of starch and fibre, as well as containing Vitamins C and E. Parsley is an excellent source of iron and Vitamin C.

The beta-carotene level in carrots is so high that eating them improves night vision. Studies have shown that the anti-inflammatory agents in celery can reduce the symptoms of gout, while a sedative compound in it can help to lower blood pressure. In traditional medicine, fennel teas, made from the plant's seeds, are thought to aid digestion.

Type	Nutritional value	Effects on health

PEA AND BEAN FAMILY

Broad (fava)
bean
Green bean
Runner
(string) bean
Garden pea
Mangetout
(snow pea)
Sugar snap pea

Peas of all varieties are rich in thiamin and Vitamin C. They also contain protein, folate, fibre and phosphorus. Mangetout (snow peas) are excellent Vitamin C, beta-carotene and potassium sources. Because they are eaten whole – pod and all – they also supply the body with useful fibre. Broad (fava) beans are protein- and fibre-rich: they also contain iron, niacin, Vitamins C and E. Runner (string) beans contain Vitamin C, folate and iron.

Broad (fava) beans can produce side-effects when eaten by people taking MAOI antidepressant drugs. In such cases, medical advice is to avoid eating them. Runner (string) beans lose up to a third of their nutrients when they are cooked. The raw beans are a tasty salad addition, but their skins should be washed thoroughly to remove any pesticide traces.

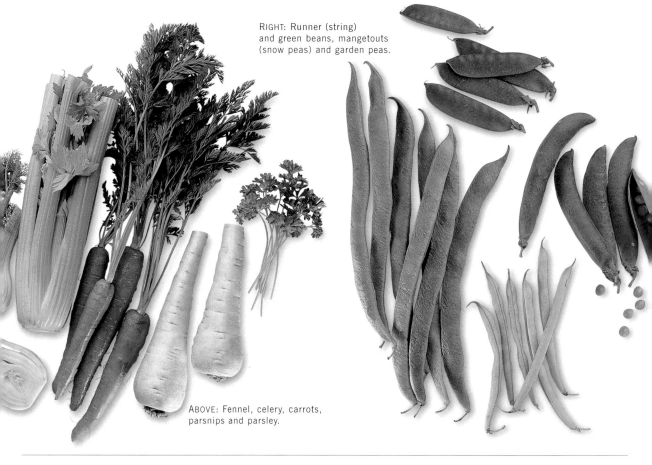

RIGHT: Runner (string) and green beans, mangetouts (snow peas) and garden peas.

ABOVE: Fennel, celery, carrots, parsnips and parsley.

Type	Nutritional value	Effects on health	Type	Nutritional value	Effects on health

POTATO FAMILY

**Aubergine
(egg plant)
Chilli pepper
Potato
Sweet (bell)
pepper
Tomato**

Sweet (bell) peppers are an excellent Vitamin C source: they contain useful amounts of beta-carotene and bioflavonoids. Chillies are rich in Vitamin C. Weight for weight, green (bell) peppers contain twice as much Vitamin C as oranges – and red (bell) peppers three times as much. Potatoes are high in carbohydrates, protein and fibre, while also containing significant amounts of Vitamin C and potassium. Tomatoes are good sources of carotenoids and potassium, and provide useful amounts of Vitamins C and E.

Aubergines (eggplant) can absorb large quantities of fat during cooking, so the best way to cook them is to bake them. The fierce heat of chillies comes from the capsaicin in their white ribs, flesh and seeds. Chillies can relieve congestion in blocked airways and are thought to have anticoagulant and cholesterol-lowering properties. The alkaloids in green and sprouted potatoes are toxic and some people are sensitive to tomatoes.

SQUASH AND PUMPKIN FAMILY

**Butternut
Courgette
(zucchini)
Cucumber
Marrow (large
zucchini)
Pumpkin
Squash**

Pumpkins and other squashes are all good sources of beta-carotene; they also provide the body with useful amounts of Vitamin E. Pumpkin seeds are rich in iron, magnesium, phosphorus, potassium and zinc. Marrow (large zucchini), cucumbers and courgettes (zucchini) are all low in calories.

Marrow (large zucchini) seeds have been used in folk medicine for centuries as a diuretic and as part of a treatment for tape worms. Most of the nutrient content of courgette (zucchini) is contained in the vegetable's skin. Cucumbers are good for the digestion and for gout.

BELOW: Courgette, (zucchini), cucumber, marrow (large zucchini) and squash.

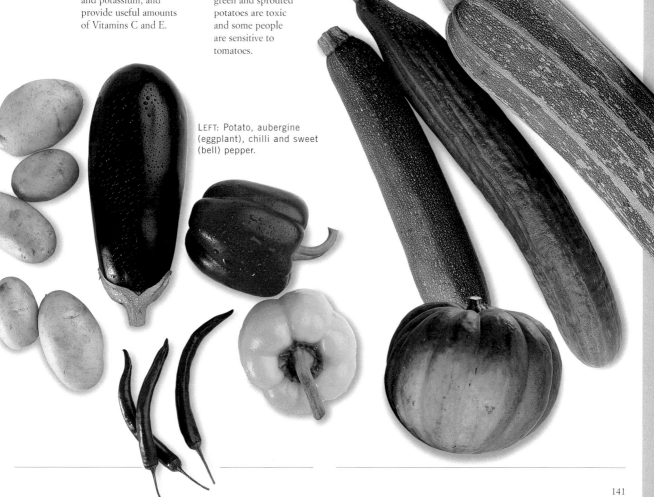

LEFT: Potato, aubergine (eggplant), chilli and sweet (bell) pepper.

PULSES, GRAINS, NUTS AND SEEDS

There is a host of pulses, grains, seeds and nuts to choose from, all of which make a healthy addition to the diet. Pulses, in particular, are high in starch and fibre, low in fat, and rich in valuable vitamins and minerals. Nuts and seeds are a good source of essential fatty acids, proteins, minerals and various vital vitamins, while wholegrains are an easy-to-assimilate source of carbohydrates. Beansprouts – sprouted pulses – are non-starchy alkaline foods that can be combined safely with anything.

LEFT: Grains are a good source of carbohydrate, minerals, vitamins and dietary fibre.

From the food combiner's view, pulses and beans present something of a problem. This is because nutritionally they are a mixture of starch and protein, which is one of the classic food combinations that experts advise avoiding. However, it should be borne in mind, that despite their protein content, the predominant nutrient in most pulses is starch; with the exception of protein in soy and flageolet (small navy) beans.

Essentially, this means that pulses and beans can be combined in moderation with other starches, as well as with salad and other non-starchy vegetables. They can also be combined with grains, again moderately, and preferably not daily. Pulses should not be mixed with foodstuffs that are protein rich, the obvious examples being poultry, meat, eggs and dairy products, such as cheese. Eating nourishing pulses and beans can bring manifold health benefits. They are high in fibre, low in fat and rich in complex carbohydrates, minerals, and important vitamins including B complex.

PREPARING PULSES CORRECTLY

Pulses are notorious for causing flatulence and bloating, which is particularly likely if you are not accustomed to eating them. These problems can be avoided. Often, they are the result of incorrect food combining. If not, it may be a matter of inadequate food preparation.

With the exceptions of lentils and split peas, you should soak all dried pulses in water for several hours – preferably overnight. Discard any pulses that float to the surface after the soaking and then rinse the remainder in fresh water. Thorough, careful cooking is essential to destroy the harmful toxins that pulses contain in their natural state. Boil the pulses for ten minutes or so, removing any white scum that rises to the surface, and then allowing them to simmer for 30–90 minutes. The alternative is to use a pressure-cooker, in which case the simmering time comes down to 5–20 minutes.

The exact timing depends on the type and quantity of pulses involved. When you eat them, always make sure that you chew them thoroughly, as this will help to break down the indigestible sugars that can otherwise cause indigestion and embarrassing wind (gas).

GRAIN GUIDELINES

All grains, with the exception of millet, are classed in food combining as acid-forming starches, combining well with any kind of vegetables, salad vegetables, seeds and herbs, but not with proteins. As well as being a good source of complex carbohydrates, they also provide some of the dietary fibre the body needs in order to keep the digestive tract healthy. Grains, which also provide minerals and vitamins, play an important part in keeping blood-sugar levels stable, as well as levels of blood cholesterol and blood pressure.

While some grains present possible health problems. Rice is easily digestible, and maize (corn), millet, buckwheat, quinoa and amaranth are all gluten-free. If you are allergic to gluten, switch to potatoes, pulses and nuts, use rice flour, soy flour or chestnut flour in cooking.

NUTS AND SEEDS

Rich in essential fatty acids, protein, minerals, and Vitamins E and B complex, nuts are excellent healthy foods. In food combining terms – with the exception of chestnuts – they are compatible with all other protein foods, but do not mix well with starch. Some people find the high nutrient content in nuts difficult to digest. The ideal way to eat nuts is on their own, like fruit, or in combination with other vegetables and salads. If eating them has led to digestive problems in the past, it is worth trying to recall what, if anything, you ate them with. It may have been the combination, rather than the nuts themselves, that was the cause.

Seeds, particularly sunflower and sesame seeds, are rich in essential fatty acids, minerals and the B vitamins. All are alkaline-forming. When using oils derived from seeds, the cold-pressed varieties are the most nutritious.

PULSES, GRAINS, NUTS AND SEEDS AT A GLANCE

Type	Nutritional value	Effects on health	Type	Nutritional value	Effects on health

PULSES AND BEANS

**Aduki
(adzuki) beans
Alfalfa
Black beans
Black-eyed
beans (peas)
Butter (lima)
beans
Chickpeas
(garbanzo)
Flageolet
(small navy)
beans
Haricot (navy)
beans
Kidney beans
Lentils
Mung beans
Pinto beans**

All beansprouts are good sources of Vitamin C, contain useful amounts of the B-complex vitamins, and provide the body with a source of easily digestible protein. Chickpeas (garbanzo beans) are a good manganese source. Flageolets (small navy beans) are a first-rate protein provider; they also contain folate, iron, phosphorus, potassium and zinc. Lentils are a good source of selenium, iron and manganese: in addition, they contain thiamin, Vitamin B_6, folate, phosphorus and zinc. Kidney beans are high in calcium and iron.

Sprouted beans are an ideal constituent of any food combining diet, since they are highly alkaline. They can be combined with practically any food. If kidney beans are eaten raw or undercooked, severe food poisoning may be a result of this.

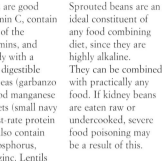

RIGHT: Lentils, black-eyed beans (peas), chickpeas (garbanzo beans), kidney, butter (lima) and soy beans.

GRAINS

**Amaranth
Barley
Buckwheat
Maize (corn)
Millet
Oats
Rice
Rye
Semolina
Quinoa
Wheat**

Rice is a good starch source; the starch is absorbed slowly, so helping to control blood sugar levels. Most of its nutrients are concentrated in the bran and germ. Brown rice is rich in B vitamins, calcium and phosphorus. Wheat is rich in B vitamins and in Vitamin E, while, as well as B vitamins and calcium, oats contain iron. The soluble fibre in both is thought to be helpful in lowering blood cholesterol levels. Millet has the highest iron concentration of all the grains while buckwheat is rich in calcium and contains Vitamin C.

Wheat grain is classified hard or soft, depending on the gluten content. The hardest and most gluten-rich is durum, used in pasta. Food combiners should stick to unrefined, whole grains, preferably ones that are completely additive-free. Rice is a treatment for a range of digestive disorders. Recent research shows that eating rice bran may reduce the risk of bowel cancer. Maize (corn), millet and buckwheat are gluten-free.

BROWN RICE

WHITE RICE

WHEAT

BUCKWHEAT

NUTS

**Almond
Brazil
Cashew
Chestnut
Coconut
Hazelnut
Peanut
(groundnut)
Pine nut
Pistachio**

With the exception of coconut, all types of nut are excellent Vitamin E sources with useful amounts of thiamin, niacin and other B vitamins into the bargain. Their mineral content includes phosphorus, iron, copper and potassium. Because of their omega 3 essential fatty acids, walnuts may help to reduce the risk of heart disease. With the exception of chestnuts and peanuts, nuts are good sources of protein.

Although nuts are high in fat, most of it is the healthy unsaturated type. Food combining classes peanuts as starch. Coconuts should be avoided on the whole. Although they are a useful source of fibre, they are very high in saturated fats and calories.

RIGHT: Brazil nuts, walnuts, almonds and hazelnuts.

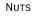

ALLERGY ALERT
Nuts in general and peanuts in particular are among the commonest of all food allergens. In exceptional cases, eating peanuts can result in anaphylactic shock – a rare and life-threatening allergic reaction. The condition lasts for life and cannot be cured. If you are allergic to peanuts, you must eliminate them, and any products containing even the slightest traces of them, including groundnut (peanut) oil, from your diet.

SEEDS

**Pumpkin
Safflower
Sesame
Sunflower**

Seeds are excellent protein sources, good sources of Vitamin E and contain all the B vitamins, with the exception of Vitamin B_{12}. They are also high in fibre and unsaturated fats. Pumpkin seeds contain iron, magnesium and zinc, while sesame seeds contain calcium. As well as Vitamin E, sunflower seeds are high in the linoleic acid which the body needs to make and maintain cell membranes.

All seeds should be eaten roasted or cooked as these processes destroy the protein toxins they contain. Salted seeds should be avoided because of their high sodium content. Some of the of the ingredients in sunflower oil mimic the effects of nicotine, which can make it useful for people who are trying to quit the habit of smoking.

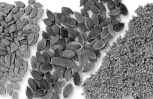

PUMPKIN SEEDS

SUNFLOWER SEEDS

SESAME SEEDS

143

FISH AND SHELLFISH

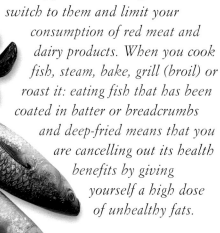

Their nutritional benefits make fish and shellfish good for you: they are packed with first-class proteins and many other health-giving nutrients. This is why food combining advice is to switch to them and limit your consumption of red meat and dairy products. When you cook fish, steam, bake, grill (broil) or roast it: eating fish that has been coated in batter or breadcrumbs and deep-fried means that you are cancelling out its health benefits by giving yourself a high dose of unhealthy fats.

LEFT: Fish and shellfish are packed with first class proteins.

Fresh oily fish, such as salmon and mackerel, is better for you because of the healthy omega-3 fatty acids they contain. These acids protect the body against heart problems and circulatory disorders. If you are pregnant, making sure that you eat food containing enough of the acids is particularly important, since the omega-3 fatty acids promote healthy foetal development, particularly of the eyes and the brain. It is recognized that oily fish, without question, is the best natural source of omega-3 fatty acids.

However, you can eat white fish as well, so giving your diet extra spice and variety. Whatever you select, the basic nutritional facts remain the same. One small portion of fish, say dieticians and other food experts, supplies up to a half of the protein intake adults require on a daily basis.

Most varieties of fish are rich in B vitamins, particularly Vitamin B_{12}. This is rarely found in food of plant origin and is a vital requirement for healthy nerve function as it helps to make myelin, the white protective sheath that surrounds the nerve fibres. Most fish also contains iodine, which the thyroid gland needs in order to function at peak efficiency. In addition to omega-3 fatty acids, oily fish, such as herring and mackerel, contain large quantities of Vitamin D, which some scientific authorities believe can help to relieve the symptoms of conditions such as psoriasis. Vitamin D is also vital for healthy bone structure and good teeth.

FISH SAFETY

For the Japanese, raw fish sushi and sashimi are favourite delicacies, but it is best to avoid raw fish unless you are confident that it is parasite-free and properly prepared. Many fish, particularly cod, are intermediate hosts for parasitic worms, which, along with their eggs, can be killed only through thorough cooking. Herring, mackerel and other oily fish should be cooked and eaten fresh as they spoil rapidly. If this happens, stomach upsets and skin rashes can result. Smoked and pickled fish present health problems as well, since there is scientific research to suggest that, if carried to extremes, the processes may lead to the production of potentially carcinogenic compounds.

Fish are also highly vulnerable to contamination by pollution. This particularly applies to freshwater fish, which can be contaminated by industrial and agricultural chemical spillage in their home streams and rivers.

SHELLFISH SENSE

Like white fish, most shellfish are extremely low in fat: crab being the exception to the rule. Crustaceans, such as crab, lobster, prawn (shrimp) and crayfish, have a high protein, calcium and Vitamin B_3 content, while molluscs, such as oysters, mussels, clams and scallops, contain these same nutrients, plus, in some cases, extra minerals as well. Oysters are the richest source of zinc of any food, while, out of the shellfish, lobsters contain the most selenium, although mussels, scallops and prawns (shrimp) are also good sources. Zinc is essential for growth, reproduction and for the immune system to work efficiently. Selenium, too, is also a particularly important trace mineral and an antioxidant. Like zinc, it works in conjunction with Vitamin E to stimulate body growth and promote fertility. Care must be taken when eating shellfish as they are highly perishable. They can cause allergies – the classic one being nettle rash – and must be checked carefully to make sure that they are healthy. Mussels and oysters are particularly vulnerable to contamination, since they are what is termed filter feeders. They can filter as much as 90 litres/20 gallons/24 US gallons of water daily. As a result they are easily contaminated. Such pollution can be extremely dangerous, especially where oysters are concerned, since it is customary to eat them raw.

Gout sufferers should avoid all shellfish. The purines they contain can raise uric acid levels and will increase the severity of the condition.

OYSTERS

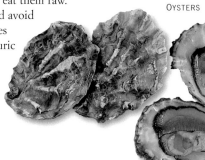

FISH AND SHELLFISH AT A GLANCE

Type	Nutritional value	Effects on health
WHITE FISH		
Bass **Cod** **Coley** **Flounder** **Haddock** **Hake** **Halibut** **Monkfish** **Mullet** **Plaice** **Skate** **Snapper** **Sole** **Turbot** **Whiting**	High in protein, but extremely low in fat. Contain valuable amounts of iodine, plus calcium and some of the B vitamins, notably Vitamin B_{12}.	Although eating smoked fish to excess may be potentially harmful, the smoking process in itself does not destroy the healthy nutrients in smoked haddock and cod.

GREY MULLET, HAKE AND PLAICE

Type	Nutritional value	Effects on health
MOLLUSCS		
Clams **Cockles** **Cuttlefish** **Octopus** **Oysters** **Scallops** **Squid** **Winkles**	High in protein, Vitamin B_{12} and minerals. Oysters contain zinc, mussels and scallops have useful supplies of selenium. Also have a very low fat content.	Some people are sensitive to them. Oysters and mussels are susceptible to contamination through water pollution and must be checked carefully for this.

OYSTERS

WINKLES

MUSSELS

OILY FISH

Anchovy **Herring** **Mackerel** **Salmon** **Sardine** **Swordfish** **Trout** **Tuna**	Excellent sources of omega-3 fatty acids, low in saturated fat and rich in protein, iron, some of the B vitamins and Vitamin D. Also a very valuable iodine source.	Whitebait, young sardines, anchovies and herrings are excellent calcium sources. Eat the easily digestible bones as well as the flesh. Smoking does not damage omega-3 or Vitamin D content, but avoid red-brown kippers (smoked herring) as the colour has been dyed.

MACKEREL AND HERRINGS

CRUSTACEANS

Crab **Crayfish** **Lobster** **Prawn** **Shrimp**	Rich in protein, Vitamin B_{12} and calcium. Contain useful amounts of iodine, iron and zinc. Lobsters contain more selenium than any other shellfish.	Can cause allergies. Although considered a delicacy by some gourmets, the green livers of lobster and the yellow ones of crab should not be eaten, as they could contain poisons (although this is very unlikely).

CRAB, CRAYFISH AND PRAWNS

MEAT AND POULTRY

Although in the past, some nutritionists argued that the benefits of eating beef and other red meats outweighed their disadvantages, food combiners, on the whole, would not agree. Meat is an excellent source of protein, B vitamins and minerals, such as iron, selenium and zinc, but it is also high in saturated fat, making up just under half of its fat total. In poultry much of the fat is in the skin, which can be removed before or after cooking.

LEFT: Red meat is extremely high in saturated fats.

If you do eat beef, make sure that the cut you choose is a lean one. Such cuts are now easier to find than they used to be, thanks largely to modern breeding techniques developed in response to commercial demand. Lean beef today, it is claimed, contains less than five per cent fat, although it should be noted that half of this is still saturated. It should be remembered that there is also scientific evidence to suggest that eating beef to excess can be linked to an increased risk of developing cancer of the colon.

In addition, unless the animals have been organically reared, there is the chance that the animals from which beef comes may have been fed growth-inducing hormones to get them to gain weight more quickly and to produce larger amounts of lean meat per animal. Although this practice has been officially banned in the EU since 1988, there is some evidence to suggest that the ban is being flouted to some extent, while feeding cattle growth hormones is still legal in parts of the US. Add to this the impact of BSE (see page 298) and it makes sense to follow the current food combining recommendation to buy organically reared beef – that is, if you buy beef at all.

Eating offal (variety meats), such as liver and kidneys, can also present health problems. In the past, eating liver was positively encouraged as part of the treatment for pernicious anaemia because of the large amounts of easily absorbed iron that liver contains. However, liver's high cholesterol levels are now considered to be a health hazard. Pregnant women and women trying to conceive are advised to avoid liver as there is the possibility that the extremely high levels of Vitamin A which liver contains can adversely affect the foetus in the uterus, possibly even causing birth defects.

Other health hazards from meat include bacteria, such as salmonella and Escherichia coli (E. coli), both of which can cause food-poisoning. For this reason, meat should be thoroughly cooked through – rather than merely cooked enough to serve it fashionably pink. This is especially important if it is to be eaten by young children, invalids, pregnant women or the elderly.

LAMB AND PORK

Fatty cuts of lamb are as high in saturated fat as beef. However, modern breeding methods are producing lamb that is much leaner than it used to be, the leanest cut being the leg. Top-quality early lamb can be distinguished by its pinky-brown, fine-grained flesh and its white fat. Summer lamb's meat is liable to be darker.

Pork is the leanest of meats, with a saturated fat content similar to that of poultry. Its bad health reputation stems from the fact that pork products – notably salami, sausages, spare ribs and streaky (fatty) bacon – are all rich in fat. It is the products, rather than the pork, that should be avoided. However, it is also vital to cook pork thoroughly to avoid the risk of parasitic infection.

You should avoid eating large amounts of cured pork, such as ham, bacon and gammon (cured ham), because of the additives that are used in the curing process. The standard ingredients include salt, sodium nitrate and sodium nitrite, with the possible additions of sodium polyphosphate, which helps the cured meat to retain moisture and gives it a juicier texture, and sodium ascorbate, which helps to accelerate the curing process itself. Sugar is sometimes added as well if the meat is sweet-cured. The process makes the sodium content of the cured meat extremely high, which can aggravate blood-pressure problems.

CHICKEN AND OTHER POULTRY

Like fish, poultry combines well with non-starchy vegetables, salads, seeds and herbs. It is an excellent source of protein, contains most of the B vitamins and supplies the body with some of the zinc it needs into the bargain. This makes poultry ideal for anyone who is not a vegetarian. It is also suitable for those following a low-fat diet.

Free-range birds are best. While the drugs used to treat factory raised poultry are said to be harmless, the fact remains that they are an unnatural addition to the food chain.

MEAT AND POULTRY AT A GLANCE

Type	Nutritional value	Effects on health

MEAT

Beef
Lamb
Pork
Veal

Rich in protein, Vitamin B complex, iron, selenium and zinc. High in fats, up to half of which are saturated fatty acids.

Rump (round) steak, stewing steak, silverside, (pot roast) shin (shank) and brisket are the least fatty cuts of beef. All meat should be cooked thoroughly to guard against the risks of food poisoning or parasitic infection.

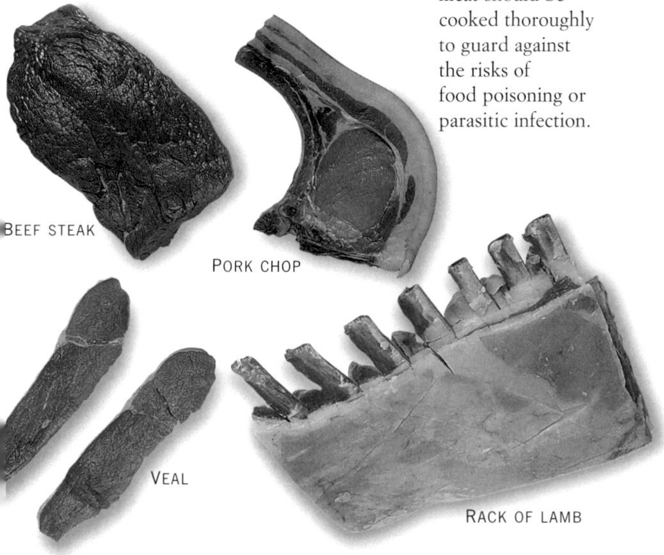

BEEF STEAK

PORK CHOP

VEAL

RACK OF LAMB

POULTRY

Type	Nutritional value	Effects on health

Chicken
Duck
Goose
Guinea fowl
Pigeon
(squab)
Quail
Turkey

Rich in protein, Vitamin B_2, Vitamin B_3, with some zinc. Low in saturated fat (this makes up no more than one-third of total fat content).

Fat content may be reduced further by removing skin. Cook thoroughly to avoid risk of unpleasant salmonella poisoning.

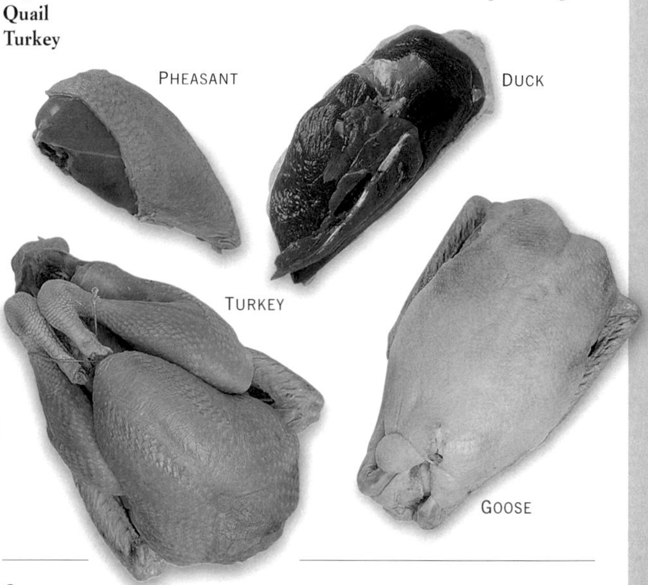

PHEASANT

DUCK

TURKEY

GOOSE

OFFAL (VARIETY MEATS)

Brains
Heart
Kidney
Liver
Sweetbread
Tongue
Trotter
(foot)

High in Vitamins A, B_2, B_3 and B_{12}, iron and zinc. Heart contains riboflavin. Liver is extremely rich in Vitamin A.

Highly perishable. High in cholesterol. Liver should be avoided during pregnancy because its high Vitamin A level may damage the foetus.

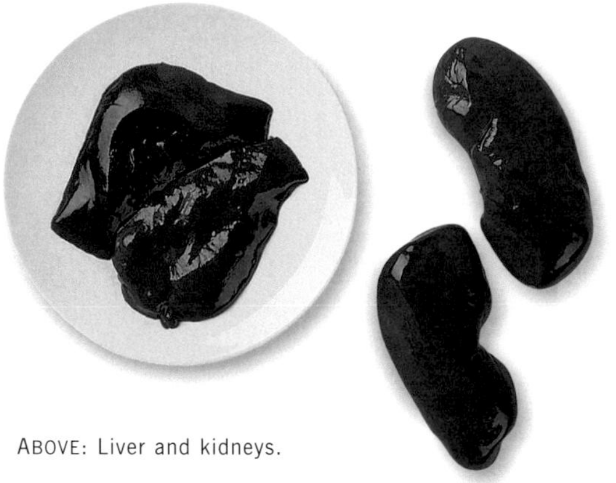

ABOVE: Liver and kidneys.

GAME

Grouse
Partridge
Pheasant
Rabbit
Venison
Wild boar
Wild duck
Woodpigeon

Good source of protein, the B vitamins, and minerals such as iron, selenium and zinc. High in fatty acids, but these are unsaturated.

Usually lower in fat than domestic equivalents.

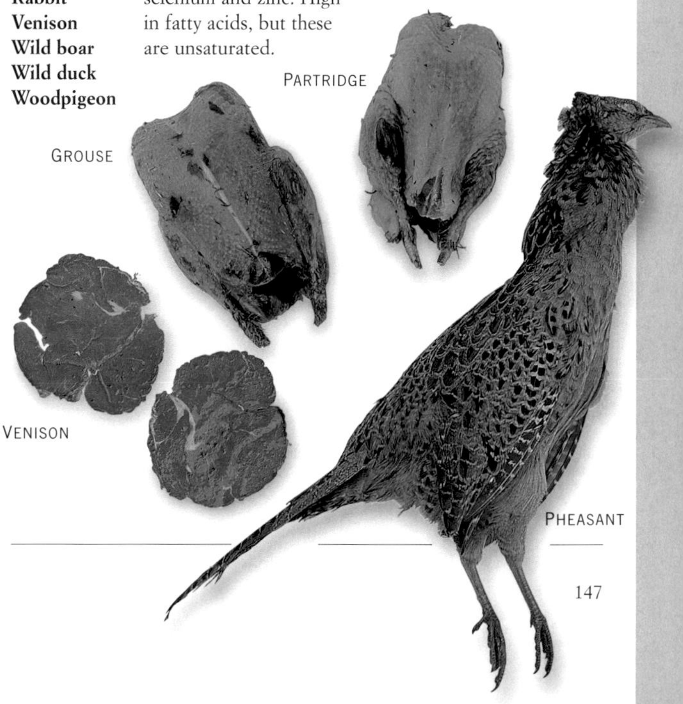

GROUSE

PARTRIDGE

VENISON

PHEASANT

147

DAIRY PRODUCTS AND EGGS

According to conventional nutritionists, there are few foods better for you than milk, but food combining experts do not necessarily agree. In fact, some believe that cow's milk is a potential allergen and recommend goat's milk, sheep's milk, buttermilk or natural (plain) live yogurt as healthier alternatives. While egg yolks are compatible with all types of food, which is why they are so useful in cooking, the protein in egg white can make eggs difficult to digest. Eat eggs only in moderation, in combination with other proteins.

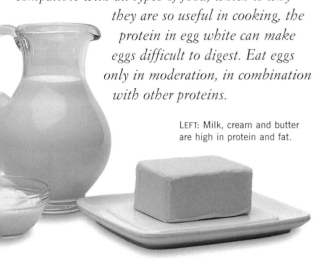

LEFT: Milk, cream and butter are high in protein and fat.

Milk, yogurt and cheese are all good sources of protein (cheese contains as much protein as meat), B vitamins, phosphorus and, above all, calcium. Milk, however, has its drawbacks. Whole milk, especially cream, is fat-rich, while all types of cow's milk contain lactose to which some people are intolerant. Goat's milk is a useful alternative, nutritionally similar to cow's milk and can be used in the same ways. If you suffer from a gastric problem, you may also find it lighter on the stomach and easier to digest. However, milk does not combine well: ideally, it should be drunk either on its own, or combined with fruits or non-starchy vegetables.

Skimmed (skim) milk – milk from which the fat has been largely removed – contains half the calories of whole milk, while retaining most of whole milk's nutrient value. Skimmed (skim) milk generally contains 0.1 per cent fat, as opposed to 3.9 per cent fat in full-cream (whole) milk: the semi-skimmed (low-fat) fat percentage is 1.6 per cent. For this reason, it is best to drink skimmed (skim) or semi-skimmed (low-fat) milk, rather than whole milk, although medical experts recommend that skimmed (skim) milk should not be given to children under the age of five.

IS BUTTER BEST?

Whether butter or margarine is better for you is a debate that has raged among food scientists for many years, but, as far as food combining is concerned, butter is the clear winner. Far too many margarines, food combining authorities state, are hydrogenated – that is packed with trans-fatty acids which result from the process that turns liquid oil, with its unsaturated fatty acids, into solidified margarine. Trans-fatty acids have as much potential to do you harm as saturated fats.

Attempts have been made to counter this, but even margarine high in polyunsaturates may not be the complete answer. Recent research indicates that high levels of polyunsaturates may predispose some people towards asthma. The food combining answer in either case is that, provided that it is not eaten to excess, butter is preferable as being the more natural product. If you are unhappy with the amount of saturated fat butter contains, you can try replacing conventional butter with a nut or seed alternative. For cooking purposes, all fat requirements can be satisfied with olive or sunflower oil.

FOODS AND SLEEP

Calcium is a potent sleep inducer. Experts say most of us get only a third of the daily amount of calcium that our bodies need, which can lead to increased tension and sleep disturbances. Drinking a glass of warm milk at bedtime can help to solve the problem, since milk is not only rich in calcium, but also contains L-tryptophan, a chemical compound that works in the brain to promote sleep. As an alternative, you could try a traditional Russian folk remedy, in which ground anise is mixed with warm milk and honey. If you suffer from regular bouts of sleeplessness, you should also adjust your diet, so that you are eating plenty of carrots, cheese, avocado, fish, lentils, peas, potatoes, spinach, sunflower seeds and wholemeal (whole-wheat) flour. All these foods contain Vitamin B_6, which the body needs in order to synthesise serotonin, another potent sleep-inducer. Researchers at the Massachusetts Institute for Technology have shown that eating a banana before bedtime may help to improve overall sleep quality.

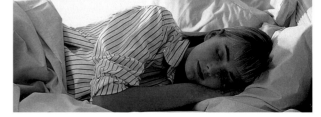

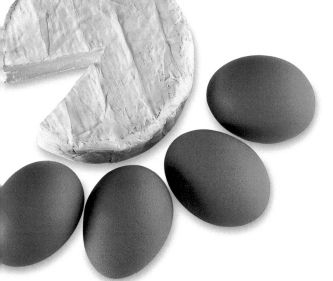

CHEESE AND EGGS

Cheese is a good source of protein, a rich source of calcium and, for vegetarians in particular, an important source of Vitamin B_{12}, which they otherwise find difficult to obtain. However, some cheeses are high in saturated fat and calories, and some contain large amounts of tyramine, a chemical that can trigger migraine attacks in the susceptible. As far as food combining is concerned, cheese is considered to be a protein food. This makes bread and cheese, for instance, a bad combination because it will disrupt the all-important acid-base balance within the body. You can rectify matters by adding salad or other non-starchy vegetables to the combination, which will help to restore the balance and make what you are eating easier to digest as a result. Cream cheese, however, is considered to be a fat, not a protein, and so is compatible with all other foods, always provided that the cream cheese you are eating is a genuine dairy product and not made of soy or any soy derivative. Processed, smoked and coloured cheeses should be avoided because of the additives they contain.

Eggs, too, are an excellent Vitamin B_{12} source, as well as being rich in other vitamins, minerals and protein. Their high cholesterol level, however, is a source of health concern: the official World Health Organization recommendation is not to eat more than ten eggs per week – a figure that includes eggs used in recipes for foods such as biscuits (cookies), cakes and mayonnaise. However, it should be remembered that dietary cholesterol from foods does not have a direct correlation with blood cholesterol in the body, which is thought to be raised more by eating saturated fat than by eating cholesterol-rich foods. Eggs on the whole are low in saturated fat: a large (extra large) egg contains, on average, less than 2 g. Generally speaking, egg cholesterol content is only a problem if the blood cholesterol level is already raised.

Like the celebrated curate's egg, immortalized in a 19th-century *Punch* magazine cartoon, food combiners find eggs a source of mixed benefits. Egg yolks are compatible with all foods, which makes them extremely useful in cooking. Egg whites, however, are protein rich – and the particular protein they contain can be difficult to digest.

DAIRY PRODUCE AND EGGS AT A GLANCE

Type	Nutritional value	Effects on health
DAIRY PRODUCE		
Butter **Cheese** **Cream** **Milk** **Yogurt**	All dairy products are rich in Vitamin A: milk yogurt and cheese supply the body with protein, Vitamins B_2, B_3 and B_{12} and calcium. Except for low-fat varieties, all are high in fat, two-thirds of which is saturated.	Cow's milk can be an allergen, especially if you suffer from lactose intolerance. Yogurt contains live bacteria, which helps to replace bacteria killed by antibiotics, and to boost the immune system. As well as aiding digestion, yogurt helps to prevent bad breath, diarrhoea, candidiasis and constipation problems.

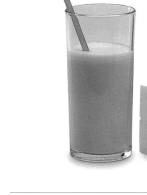

EGGS

Type	Nutritional value	Effects on health
Duck **Goose** **Hen** **Quail**	Contain protein, Vitamins A B_2, B_3, B_{12} and D, folic acid, iron and other minerals.	Although yolks are high in fat, food combiners class them as an all-purpose combining food. Children, pregnant women, invalids and the elderly should not eat any food containing raw egg, as salmonella poisoning could result.

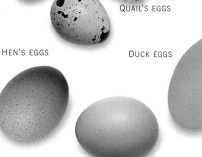

QUAIL'S EGGS

HEN'S EGGS   DUCK EGGS

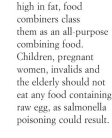

EVALUATING FOODS

Looking at the composition of a dish or menu, it should soon be possible to analyse whether it represents a good, bad or a problematic combination. Remember that it is the overall proportions of the nutrients in the foods that are the key to successful food combining. Although, in theory, protein together with starch is a bad combination, whether this is the case in practice depends very much on the amount of protein and the amount of starch involved.

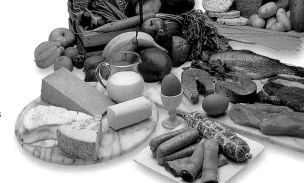

RIGHT: Take a look at the huge choice of foods that is available to us today. It is simple to combine them correctly for optimum health and digestion.

There are two methods of finding out about specific combinations of food. You can look at the comprehensive table (see pages 130–1) showing the names of particular foods grouped together according to the dominant nutrient. Alternatively, it is not difficult to judge for oneself whether a combination is favourable or not by finding out what the ingredients are, listing them and checking what group or groups of nutrients they should be classified with and in what proportion. Then reference to the food combining pentagon and the third chart here should provide enough information to decide whether the proposed combination is a good or bad one.

This third diagram presents a scheme that is slightly different from that of the pentagon. Protein can be combined with protein if it is of the same form, but different kinds of protein should not be combined and that is why there are two possibilities represented on the diagram. Similarly, fat combines easily with fat. It is also possible to mix different types of fat, although that is unusual. But if fat is added to foods that are already rich in fat, the overall proportion of fat may be too great, resulting in a problematical combination. However, starch with starch is a good combination, as is the combination of different kinds of sugar and also different kinds of acids.

INSTINCT AND INTUITION

As I have already stressed, with practice, if we look at the composition of a dish or menu, we should be able to analyse broadly if it is a good or bad combination. But to be correct in minute detail is a possibility that is really restricted to nutritional experts who have to apply such knowledge in order to prescribe diets for people who are ill. This is diet therapy and it can be an extremely complex business to apply.

In general, we should let intuition and instinct be our judge. It should be possible to come to a conclusion about the nature of a combination by observation. Statistics and measurements are useful at first in order to develop that intuition and instinct – to know what to look for. But after a while, we should have a very good idea of what can and cannot be combined.

	P	F	Su	St	A
A	–	✓	✓	–	✓
St	–	✓	–	✓	–
Su	–	–	✓	–	✓
F	–	✓×	–	✓	✓
P	✓	–	–	–	–

LEFT: This simple chart will help you see which combinations work well together and which do not.

THE IMPORTANCE OF PROPORTIONS

It cannot be emphasized enough that it is the overall proportions of a food's nutrients that are the key to food combining. Protein together with starch is a bad combination, but it is the amount of protein and the amount of starch that determine if the combination is good, bad or problematical. All foods, even farinaceous foods, contain protein. Combination is nonetheless possible, as long as permissible limits are not exceeded. The permissible limits can be determined in theory by analytical calculations, but in practice it is not that simple because other factors have a bearing, including a healthy acid-base balance, the actual quantity of food consumed, how well the food is chewed and the overall health and efficiency of the digestive system.

In evaluating a combination of foods, we start by assessing the capacity of the nutrients to combine in terms of their overall quantities. We need to know the quantities of nutrients because they determine the proportions of the nutrients in relation to each other and to the overall quantity of food. Remember, the proportions of the nutrients and the overall quantity of food are two separate elements that influence the digestive character of the combination.

A favourable nutrient ratio is essential. If the protein–starch ratio is 1:1, the combination is bad, if a dish contains 25 g/1 oz of protein and 25 g/ 1 oz of starch, digestion will be very difficult, but if the protein–starch ratio is 1:5, the combination is good and if a dish contains only 3 g/1⁄10 oz protein and 3 g/1⁄10 oz starch, digestion should be virtually smooth, even though the ratio is the same. It is vital always to keep a close eye on both the nutrient proportions and the quantities consumed.

EVALUATING DISHES AND MEALS

We evaluate the combination in each dish and, afterwards, the overall combination of the meal. In a dish, different foods are put together. They should be chosen to combine well together. And, indeed, the whole menu should be composed of dishes that combine well together – it is a waste of time, after all, to prepare dishes that each combine well, but react badly with one another. We should therefore not serve a high-protein appetizer if the main course is rich in starch, for instance. Even though the stomach fills itself in layers from the outside in and gastric digestion follows the same process, the whole of the stomach contents have to be taken into account: it is the composition of the entire stomach contents that is decisive for good food combining. A meal consists of one or more dishes, but should always be considered as a whole. There is no harm in eating several dishes consecutively so long as they do not disrupt the overall combination.

BELOW: A meal with separate courses should be evaluated as a whole.

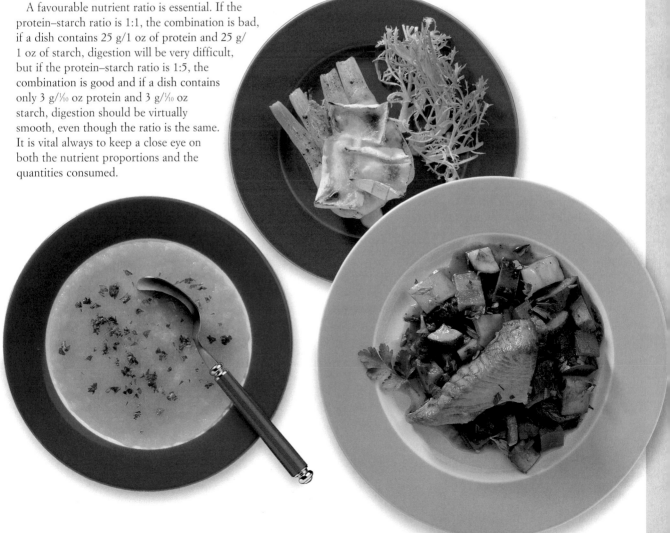

FOOD COMBINING GUIDELINES

To help you to find your way through the maze of statistics and measurements that food combining initially seems to involve, here are some practical tips. Of course, they represent ideas that have already appeared earlier in this book, but here *they serve as useful reminders. Start by choosing some conventional recipes and trying to adjust them so that they combine well. It is possible to be very creative with menu planning as long as the principles of food combining are borne in mind.*

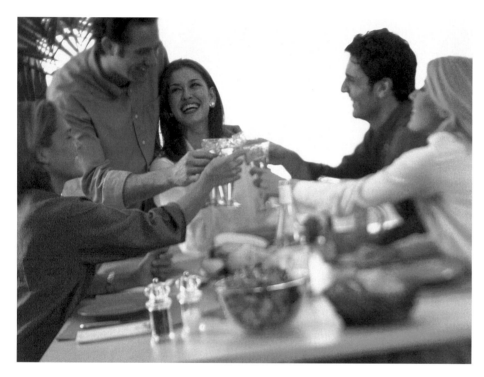

LEFT: Share your enthusiasm for food combining with your friends and allow them to discover and enjoy its benefits.

When you start food combining, it is recommended that any change of dietary regime should be gradual. Start by eliminating such combinations of food as protein with starch, and sugar with starch. That represents a great accomplishment in itself. As soon as you are feeling comfortable with that, you can begin to focus on the positive combinations.

Try also to avoid becoming fanatical about food combining. That would be perhaps the worst fate that could befall you. There should be a certain spontaneity about food and eating, and food combining should likewise have a spontaneous air, featuring dietary rules that are so reasonable you are glad to keep them, rather than being a rigid system that you feel you must obey, come what may. When you visit someone, do not refuse food that constitutes a bad combination – the

occasional mixed meal will not cause you a great problem and to do so might mean losing friends and other important social contacts. It is far better to talk to your friends about what you do at home and to share with them your enthusiasm for the benefits. Invite your friends to discover for themselves what food combining might do for them.

After some months of food combining, you will be more sensitive to bad combinations of food: you will experience digestive problems if you begin regularly to eat as you used to and you will quickly become aware that many distracting and irritating discomforts in former times were, in fact, the result of inappropriate combinations of foods.

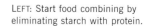

LEFT: Start food combining by eliminating starch with protein.

DIGESTION AND FOOD COMBINING

Good health begins with good digestion. Food combining is closely linked to digestion, helping the body to absorb and metabolize food. Consider the following points about food combining and digestion:

• Digestion is a complex process, which food combining helps to take place as smoothly and efficiently as possible.

• Those who do not practise food combining may have continuing digestive problems. They may feel that something is wrong, even while they are still eating. If food lies heavily on the stomach, the process of digestion is very unlikely to be smooth and efficient.

• Acid indigestion, wind (gas) in the stomach and intestines, flatulence, breathlessness, obesity and sometimes food sensitivities can all be caused by combining the wrong types of food.

• The breakdown of food inevitably produces wastes. Food combining makes sure that the build-up of these wastes is limited to a minimum. Toxins are removed more easily and accumulation should be impossible.

• Food combining means that you will need less food since you will digest it more efficiently. Digesting smaller quantities of food takes less energy.

• Digestion takes place in the mouth, the stomach, the duodenum, the small intestine and the large intestine.

• Starch is predigested in the mouth thanks to the salivary enzyme ptyalin, which can function only in a mildly acid environment. Acidic foods – foods with a low pH value – should not be combined with foods that are rich in starch as they will prevent ptyalin from doing its work properly.

• Protein undergoes its first digestive process in the stomach under the influence of the enzyme pepsin (in its eight or so forms), which works only in an acidic environment.

• All food is bathed in acid in the stomach and then comes into a more alkaline environment in the first part of the duodenum. The small intestine and the large intestine form a relatively alkaline chamber in which both fermentation and degradation of food are possible.

• If fat enters the duodenum, it causes the kneading movements of the stomach wall to slow down, with the result that any protein in the stomach is exposed to gastric acids for a longer period.

Combining fat with protein therefore helps the digestion of protein. However, if too much fat is added, the stomach's operation may become too slow.

• Acid also causes the gastric movement to slow down (acid inhibits acid) – so you should not consume too much acid with high-protein food that is also rich in fat as the stomach will slow down too much. However, a small quantity of acid with fat is always desirable, because acid has a favourable effect on the digestion of fat.

• With protein food that is low in fat, on the other hand, you should eat relatively more acid because the small quantity of fat has no effect on the overall proportions. The acid slows the gastric movement down, so that the high-protein food remains in the stomach longer and is better digested.

• Food entering the stomach stimulates the intestines into functioning. Some people experience a sudden urge to defecate immediately after a meal because of this, and may even be under the impression that the food they have just eaten is coming out again. The stimulus relayed by the stomach certainly can increase intestinal peristalsis (the wave-like movement of food through the gut), which is why we may experience flatulence or intestinal bloating during or after a meal. (The intestinal movement can encourage food to start to ferment as the natural process gets under way.)

• The gastric wall moves so that its acid can make good contact with the stomach contents. The movement also helps to press the stomach contents onwards down towards the duodenum.

• The stomach is not a blender that mixes everything together, and because digestion takes place layer by layer, the stomach does not have to be completely empty in order for you to eat again. The first part of the next meal simply joins the last part of the previous meal.

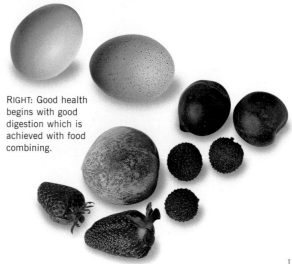

RIGHT: Good health begins with good digestion which is achieved with food combining.

153

THE BEST TIME TO EAT DIFFERENT FOODS

When is it best to eat a high-protein meal? That is a question which is frequently put to me. The digestion of protein demands considerable energy, which is why, particularly in English-speaking countries, a high-protein breakfast is often recommended. Because the stomach is completely empty and well rested in the morning, it is the time that is generally regarded as best for a high-protein meal. On the other hand, however, many people are not wide awake first thing in the morning and some have very little time for a decent breakfast. So a high-protein breakfast is not always sensible or practical.

For many years, I have been achieving good results with a light fruit breakfast. It has turned out to be a much better way to start a busy morning. To tell the truth, there is literally no good time to have a very large high-protein meal as the intake of high-protein food always should be restricted. But when you eat your high-protein meal does not really matter. It makes no difference whether it is as lunch or as supper. If you do insist on eating a lot of protein, though, it is best to eat it in the evening when you are relaxed.

If you go out to eat, remember that, all too often, the cuisine of other nations around the world violates the rules of food combining. Italian cooking, for example, is dominated by pasta and cheese, a protein-starch combination. It is best to add butter to the pasta: butter as a sauce is less acidic than tomato sauce. Spaghetti and other forms of pasta should be accompanied by vegetables, especially raw ones, so that the acid-base balance is maintained. To combine cheese or cheese sauce with spaghetti is horribly incorrect. A Greek salad, on the other hand, is a good example of how to eat cheese, particularly sheep's cheese. It is a good combination that works in favour of the acid-base balance.

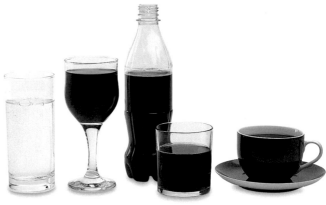

DRINKING

You may drink before, during, or after meals. The liquid does not dilute the gastric juice because it is filtered off quickly down the inner curved wall of the stomach. Drinking when the stomach is already full, however, can lead to an unpleasant sensation as the liquid cannot follow its usual rapid course through the stomach, remaining instead like a bubble at the bottom of the oesophagus or in the top of the stomach.

Acidic drinks like cola, coffee and carbonated mineral water render the saliva more acidic, which inhibits the predigestion in the mouth of foods rich in starch. Drinking coffee to excess can be particularly problematic, since the caffeine coffee contains stimulates the body's adrenalin production, making it difficult to relax. Sometimes, if the intake of coffee has built up over the day, it can be hard to sleep. If say, you are drinking 12 cups of coffee a day, your body is absorbing a gram of caffeine, the effects of which are more than enough to keep you awake. Cola drinks can have the same effect. It is also a mistake to drink alcohol to try to help get off to sleep, because, although it may appear to do the trick, the alcohol is actually destroying the B vitamins that are important for maintaining normal sleep rhythms.

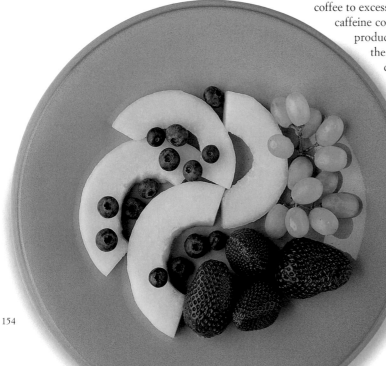

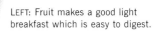
LEFT: Fruit makes a good light breakfast which is easy to digest.

FOOD COMBINING FACTS

Food combining can be successfully applied to any eating pattern. You do not have to be a vegetarian, for example, to benefit from favourable combinations of food. Here are some facts:

• Whether food is cooked or not makes no difference to food combining. However, in terms of how easy it is to digest, raw food cannot be compared with cooked food (but that is another subject altogether).

• All types of fruit (with the exception of melon) can be mixed together because they all contain acid and sugar. It is not possible to tell just by the taste whether a fruit contains a little or a lot of acid, as the sweet taste of fruit can mask a high acid content.

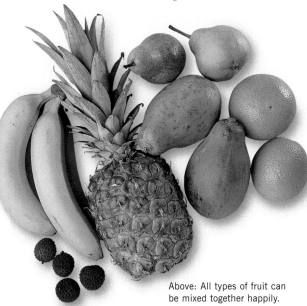

Above: All types of fruit can be mixed together happily.

• Fruit should be eaten before and not after a meal. Better still: eat fruit separately, as a meal in itself. People who know that they are subject to digestive problems should eat only one kind of fruit at any given time.

• When composing a menu, you should make sure that dishes that follow each other really do go together. The menu must have just a single dominant nutrient, and the acid-base balance must also be taken into consideration.

RIGHT: Both nuts and cheese are acid-forming foods.

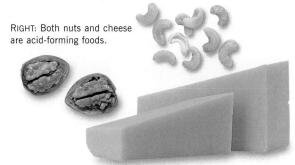

• Maintaining the body's acid-base balance is a critical element in food combining. If the balance is disturbed, digestion can be problematical even when eating a good combination of foods. Accordingly, you should always eat small quantities of high-quality foods in place of large quantities of low-quality foods. That is a simple, but extremely important rule.

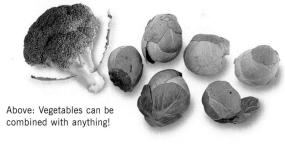

• The interval between meals is not critical, for the stomach is filled and emptied layer by layer. Whatever we eat first leaves the stomach first; whatever we eat last remains in the stomach the longest.

Above: The interval between meals isn't crucial – it's what we eat that is.

• Vegetables – apart from sauerkraut, those containing lactic acid, such as sweet and sour gherkins (dill pickles) or cocktail onions pickled in vinegar, and tomatoes (if they are vegetables at all) – may be combined with virtually any kind of food. Vegetables have a powerful alkaline effect and are good for the acid-base balance. It is for this reason that we should eat large quantities of vegetables with high-protein foods and foods rich in starch.

Above: Vegetables can be combined with anything!

• Some people believe food combining is a dieting method and think therefore that they should not food combine indefinitely. They are wrong. If you food combine, your body weight will return to what is normal for it – so fat people will become thinner and thin people will regain their normal weight If you are dieting, food combining can help you to return to your natural healthy weight.

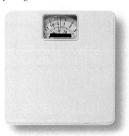

Right: Try not to treat food combining as a type of diet. You will regain your natural healthy weight.

CONTINUING DIGESTIVE PROBLEMS

There may be occasions when, despite having adopted food combining, you may still find yourself suffering from digestive and other related disorders that you had hoped were consigned to the past. You should not despair. Do not abandon food combining and revert to your old eating habits and patterns. The following pages will help you to identify other factors that may be causing you digestive discomfort and other problems.

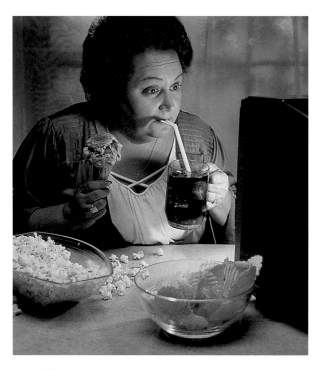

ABOVE: Over-eating is a common cause of indigestion. Eating little and often is a much healthier approach.

It is possible that, even after following to the letter the guidelines I have given, you may still be experiencing wind (gas) in the stomach and intestines, you may have neither lost weight nor gained it, you may still be suffering from stomach cramps, and you may still be suffering from food sensitivities. Do not condemn food combining roundly as an utter waste of time. Something else is likely to be causing your problems. Bad combinations of food can cause many gastrointestinal disorders, a good few of which may persist so obstinately that a thorough internal examination and a lengthy course of therapy may be required. Food combining always makes

sense and should always be applied, but its results depend on a number of factors. It is not a miracle cure and we should not expect it to work like one. At the same time, it is a fact that many people have been cured of their problems, miraculously or otherwise, by food combining. Here are nine factors that may contribute to digestive problems:

DISRUPTION OF THE ACID-BASE BALANCE

No matter how well you observe the principles of food combining, if you do not keep the necessity of preserving the body's acid-base balance firmly in mind, you will go on suffering from digestive problems as a result. Good food combining and the acid-base balance are inextricably linked. Here are two examples that prove the point. Although bread and cheese is a bad combination, if you add a large quantity of salad or other vegetables, it becomes easier to digest because the acid-base balance is restored. Meat and vegetables, by contrast, is a good combination, at least in theory. In practice, however, if you eat a large helping of meat with just a few vegetables, there will be little benefit from the good combination because the acid-base balance will have been destroyed.

EATING TOO MUCH AT A TIME

Over-eating can be one of your worst enemies. What is the point of going to the trouble of food combining, if you stuff your stomach to excess? It is very difficult for the stomach to function when it is full to bursting, even if you have confined yourself to eating food of only the one type. You simply must eat small quantities of food. Eating little and often is far better for you that eating one or two huge meals, especially if you are already experiencing digestive problems. The stomach is an organ that works systematically, processing layer after layer throughout the day and only emptying completely during the night.

EATING TOO QUICKLY

If we eat too fast, we do not chew the food sufficiently and so we swallow lumps of food that are simply too big. The purpose behind the stomach's peristalsis is not, as people often imagine, to grind food. Rather it is to keep the stomach contents in motion towards the pyloric sphincter and the duodenum. Large lumps of food cannot be digested completely: the protein and starch residues that are created as a result may thereafter ferment and degrade in the duodenum and intestines.

COPING WITH INDIGESTION

Indigestion occurs when excessive acid in the stomach causes discomfort, refluxing (flowing backwards) into the oesophagus, the tube that connects the stomach with the mouth. The result is heartburn and discomfort in the chest. Pregnant women often suffer from the condition as a result of the uterus pressing on the digestive tract as the baby grows. So, too, do people who are overweight.

Eating a healthy, fibre-rich diet, relaxing before and during meals, taking regular exercise and, of course, following food combining principles can all help to prevent indigestion. Food triggers may include acidic foods, such as pickles, meat extracts, fried food, hot, spicy foods, especially any containing chilli, and excessive eating of raw foods, such as onions, (bell) peppers and cucumber. If you are prone to indigestion, you should cut down on drinking alcohol, coffee and colas: alcohol increases stomach acidity, thereby helping to disrupt the all-important acid-base balance, coffee irritates the lining of the stomach wall, and carbonated drinks lead to wind (gas).

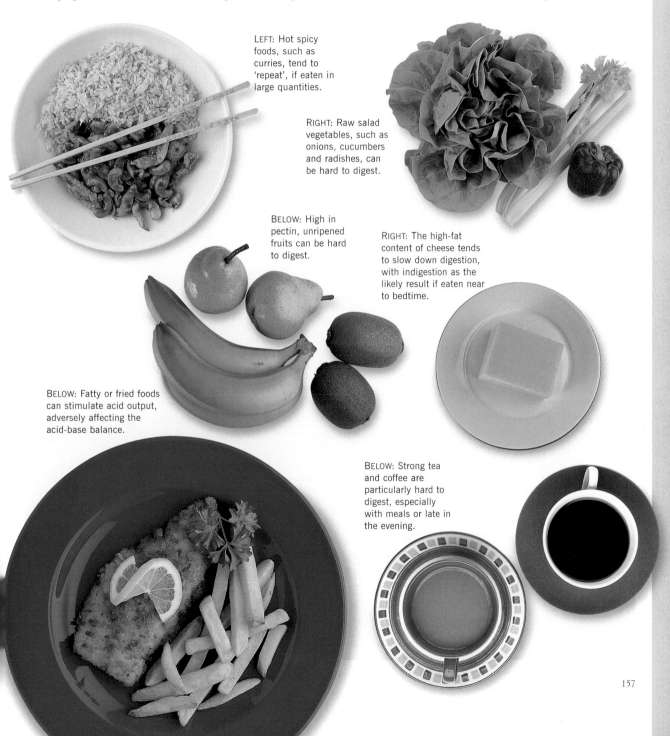

LEFT: Hot spicy foods, such as curries, tend to 'repeat', if eaten in large quantities.

RIGHT: Raw salad vegetables, such as onions, cucumbers and radishes, can be hard to digest.

BELOW: High in pectin, unripened fruits can be hard to digest.

RIGHT: The high-fat content of cheese tends to slow down digestion, with indigestion as the likely result if eaten near to bedtime.

BELOW: Fatty or fried foods can stimulate acid output, adversely affecting the acid-base balance.

BELOW: Strong tea and coffee are particularly hard to digest, especially with meals or late in the evening.

SWALLOWING AIR

It is impossible not to swallow some air while eating. But, if we eat too fast, we swallow a large amount of air, causing us to belch. Air bubbles trapped in the stomach attempt to rise back into the oesophagus. If gastric acid is present in quantity, some may also be brought up, causing the classic symptoms of acid indigestion.

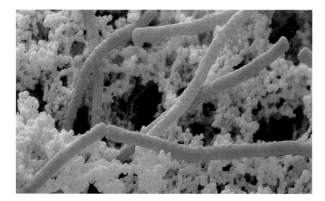

ABOVE: 'Friendly' bacteria – *lactobacillus bulgaris*. These inhibit the growth of more pathogenic bacteria in the human gut.

DISRUPTION OF THE INTESTINAL FLORA

At the very end of the small intestine and throughout the large intestine there is a multitude of bacteria which together continue the digestive breakdown of the pulpy chyme, between them digesting the protein and the sugars that remain in the liquid intestinal contents. When there is too much protein or protein residue, those bacteria responsible for breaking down the protein increase rapidly in number at the expense of those bacteria responsible for breaking down the sugars. This disrupts the balance of the intestinal flora.

Over time, food combining can beneficially influence the composition of the intestinal bacteria. But people suffering from acute intestinal problems need immediate solutions. For as long as their intestinal flora are out of action, they are bound to continue to suffer from intestinal problems. Yogurt with honey (an acid-sugar combination) can work well, helping to replace the flora temporarily, as the lactic acid bacteria take over the work of normal intestinal flora. Unfortunately, the effect is short-lived, because the lactic acid bacteria are unable to colonize the intestine: they cannot become the intestinal flora. They are a stop-gap solution only. The same is true of proprietary preparations based on intestinal bacteria. But yogurt together with such preparations can help the intestinal flora to function and flourish again.

The intestinal flora may also be attacked and destroyed by certain fungi that may invade the intestine. In such cases, a full gastrointestinal examination is essential.

CLOGGED INTESTINES

An intestine that has become befouled and partly clogged through years of eating the wrong food – and especially through eating the wrong things together – cannot be cleansed simply by food combining, although it may improve the digestion slightly in spite of the intestine's disgusting state. But such a slight improvement may disillusion some who have made a genuine effort to try food combining. These people really need to undergo a technique called colonic irrigation, which is a method by which the intestines can be cleansed thoroughly.

An apparatus introduces lukewarm water into the large intestine all the way from the rectum back to the ileo-caecal valve at the caecum. Then the water is drained out again while a form of intestinal massage is given. In this way, faecal matter that may have been stuck on the intestinal wall literally for years is washed off and evacuated through the anus. People who wish to try this technique should check that their practitioner is qualified to carry it out and that filtered water is used at all times during the process.

Colonic irrigation is essential for people who have been following an inappropriate diet for a number of years. Together, a clean intestine and food combining produce very good results.

BELOW: For some conditions it is advisable to consult an expert in how to cleanse the intestine.

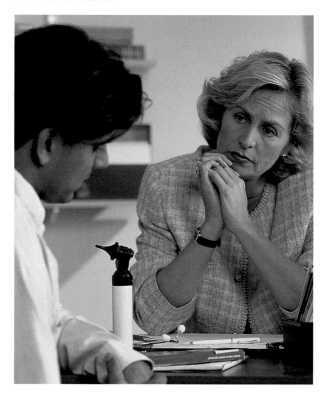

DIET AND STRESS

If you are stressed, your body needs greater amounts than usual of specific beneficial nutrients to fight fatigue and maintain a healthy immune system. It needs, for instance, more B vitamins, extra Vitamin C and more zinc, all of which you can supply easily by adjusting your food intake. To boost energy levels and beat the fatigue associated with the condition, vary your eating routine as well, trying to eat small meals every three hours or so. Eat slowly, relax and enjoy what you are eating. Here are particularly good foods for stress:

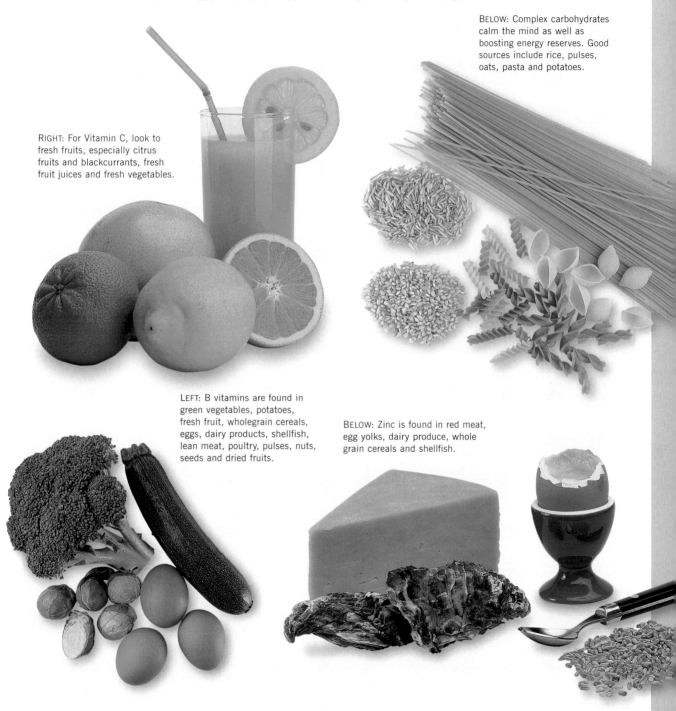

BELOW: Complex carbohydrates calm the mind as well as boosting energy reserves. Good sources include rice, pulses, oats, pasta and potatoes.

RIGHT: For Vitamin C, look to fresh fruits, especially citrus fruits and blackcurrants, fresh fruit juices and fresh vegetables.

LEFT: B vitamins are found in green vegetables, potatoes, fresh fruit, wholegrain cereals, eggs, dairy products, shellfish, lean meat, poultry, pulses, nuts, seeds and dried fruits.

BELOW: Zinc is found in red meat, egg yolks, dairy produce, whole grain cereals and shellfish.

REFLEXOLOGY AND STRESS

If stress is affecting your digestion, it may be worth trying reflexology. Practitioners believe that each part of the body is mirrored by a precise reflex point located on the hands and feet. By stimulating the appropriate reflex points, practitioners believe that they can clear away unwanted wastes that have accumulated in the respective organs, stimulate the flow of healing energy, open up blocked neural pathways

and improve the blood supply, so flushing away potential toxins. Reflexologists usually work with the feet because they are thought to be more sensitive, but, for self-help, the hands are usually more convenient. Before trying to administer the therapy yourself, you should always consult a qualified practitioner, who will advise you how best to proceed. The reflex points on the soles of the feet are shown here.

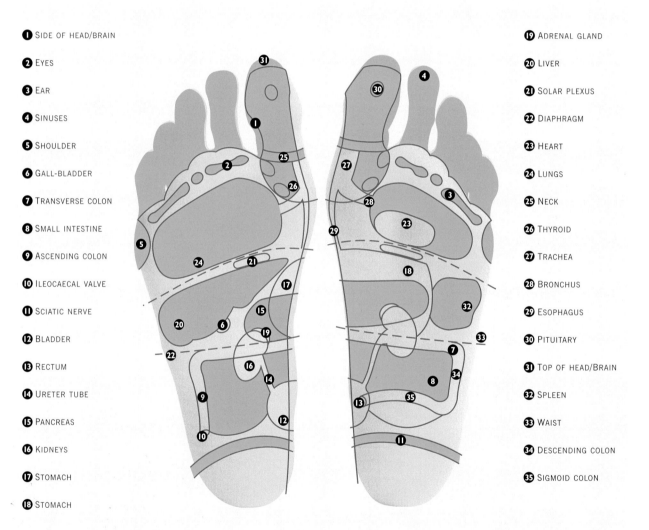

1 SIDE OF HEAD/BRAIN
2 EYES
3 EAR
4 SINUSES
5 SHOULDER
6 GALL-BLADDER
7 TRANSVERSE COLON
8 SMALL INTESTINE
9 ASCENDING COLON
10 ILEOCAECAL VALVE
11 SCIATIC NERVE
12 BLADDER
13 RECTUM
14 URETER TUBE
15 PANCREAS
16 KIDNEYS
17 STOMACH
18 STOMACH

19 ADRENAL GLAND
20 LIVER
21 SOLAR PLEXUS
22 DIAPHRAGM
23 HEART
24 LUNGS
25 NECK
26 THYROID
27 TRACHEA
28 BRONCHUS
29 ESOPHAGUS
30 PITUITARY
31 TOP OF HEAD/BRAIN
32 SPLEEN
33 WAIST
34 DESCENDING COLON
35 SIGMOID COLON

APPETITE DISRUPTION

The hypothalamus is the nerve centre in the brain responsible for appetite and for the sensation of fullness. Seeing, smelling, or even thinking about food stimulates the hypothalamus into action, helping to prepare the digestive system in readiness for eating. Such preparation is useful: if we eat when we are not hungry, the digestion hardly gets moving. We find ourselves automatically eating too much because we are not prepared for eating at all. All too frequently, digestive problems are caused by a digestion that is working too slowly because the appetite centre has not been stimulated. In addition, if the hypothalamus fails to register when we are full, we will inevitably eat too much. The digestive system then has problems coping with the excessive quantity of food. Food combining cannot redress problems with the hypothalamus immediately. Loss of appetite is usually the result of other factors such as stress, tension, emotional problems, or boredom. (See below.)

SERIOUS GASTROINTESTINAL DISEASES

Food combining can provide immediate relief from minor digestive disorders and will provide a long-term gastrointestinal balance, but we should not expect it to cure every problem. Serious intestinal diseases, such as Crohn's disease, peptic ulcers or a tumour in the colon, cannot be cured by food combining and these require expert medical diagnosis and attention.

NERVOUS TENSION AND STRESS

In many people, the effects of nervous tension are manifested in the stomach, the intestines or both. On occasion, the impact is restricted to those organs, but in most cases the entire digestive process is disturbed. People suffering from nervous tension may well endeavour to practise the principles of food combining, but for them results are pitifully meagre.

What such people are suffering from is not a nutritional problem, but a problem of stress. Eating good combinations of food will improve their digestive processes, but will do nothing to resolve the causes of stress. A possible solution in such cases is food combining in association with some carefully chosen relaxation therapy. I have found a form of therapy known as podosegmental reflexology to be an excellent method for dispelling tension in the stomach and intestines and for gently restoring the nervous system. As an indication of the factors of stress, the accompanying list prepared by psychologists at the University of Chicago rates life-changing events according to the degree of stress they are likely to cause. Several high- or highest-rated events at one time are likely to produce unmanageable stress and nervous tension with possible effects on the digestive process.

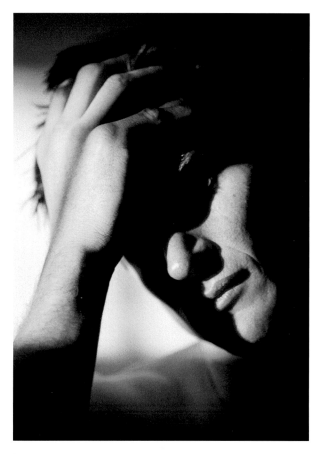

ABOVE: In some people stress and nervous tension manifest in the stomach or intestines, disturbing normal digestion.

HIGHEST
Death of partner
Divorce/separation
Prison sentence
Death of close relative
Personal injury/illness
Marriage
Redundancy/loss of job
Moving home

HIGH
Reconciliation with partner
Retirement
Serious ill health in family
Pregnancy
Sexual problems
New baby
Change of job
Financial problems
Death of close friend

MODERATE
Family disagreements
Financial commitments
New work responsibilities
Child starting/leaving school
Child leaving home
Difficulties with in-laws
Change in living conditions
Problems at work

LOW
Change in working conditions
Change of children's schools
Holidays
Change in contact with relatives
Minor legal offences
Joining/leaving social group
Christmas
Small loan

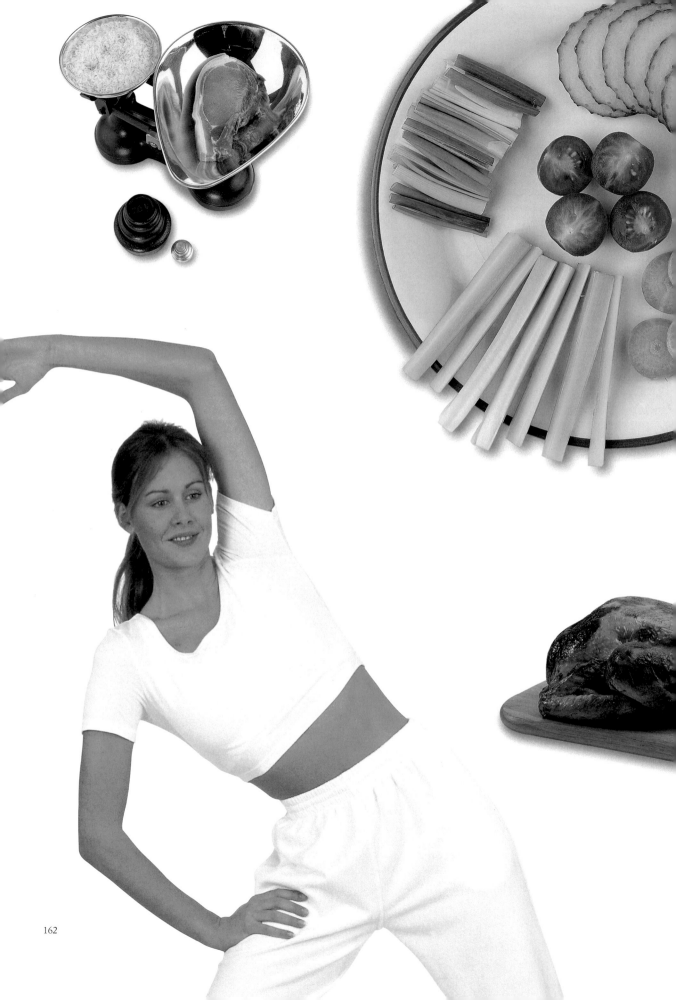

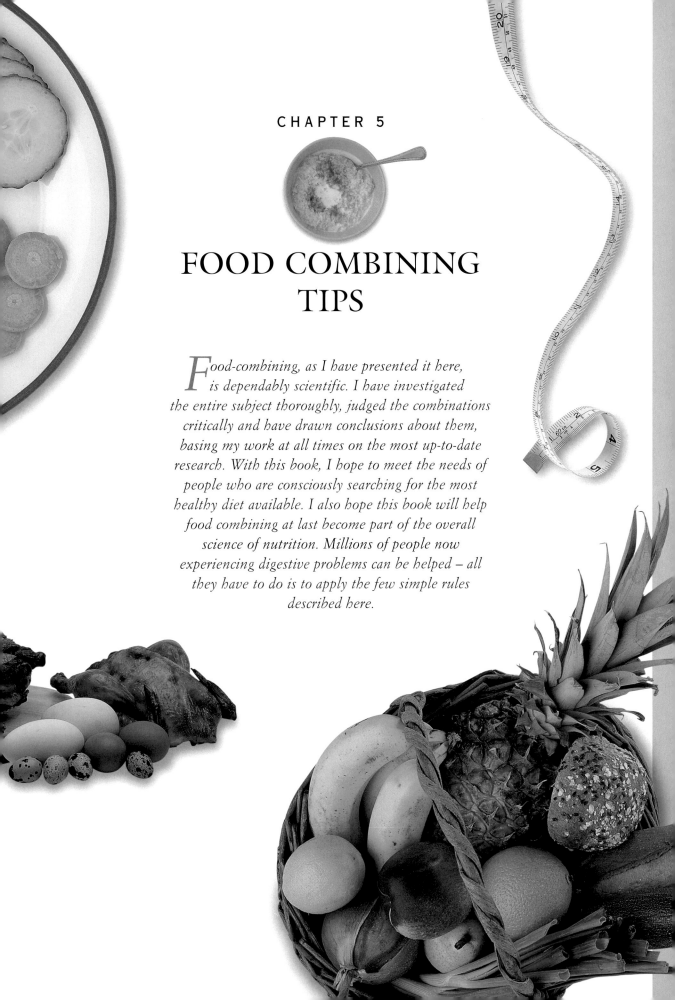

FOOD COMBINING TIPS

*F*ood-combining, as I have presented it here,
is dependably scientific. I have investigated
the entire subject thoroughly, judged the combinations
critically and have drawn conclusions about them,
basing my work at all times on the most up-to-date
research. With this book, I hope to meet the needs of
people who are consciously searching for the most
healthy diet available. I also hope this book will help
food combining at last become part of the overall
science of nutrition. Millions of people now
experiencing digestive problems can be helped – all
they have to do is to apply the few simple rules
described here.

HEALTHY FOOD

The human race has evolved with its own particular digestive system. Whatever eating pattern you adopt, you should always take into account what you know of food combining and of the acid-base balance. If you are healthy and do this, you will remain healthy. If you are in poor health, however, it is certainly in your interest to try to improve your diet. Even those in fair health can benefit from the extra protection against disease afforded by proper food combining.

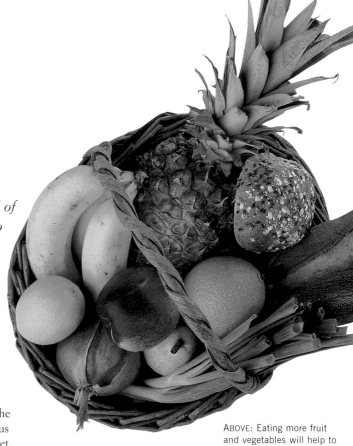

ABOVE: Eating more fruit and vegetables will help to guarantee a healthy diet.

There are almost as many ideas about what constitutes a healthy diet as there are experts on the subject. Some of the ideas are contradictory, but all are expressed with righteous fervour. Because food combining is supportive of every diet, I have chosen not to recommend any specific form of dietary regime. I am not trying to coerce you into eating in a new way. I am instead striving to reinforce the point that a healthy diet is more than just food combining. But food combining is a definite step in the right direction.

Food is individual to everyone. You must decide for yourself, and perhaps for your family, how far you are willing to go. The great value of food combining is that it can be incorporated into everyone's individual eating pattern.

'AGRICULTURAL' PRODUCTS

A large proportion of the problems to do with diet and health stem from today's exaggerated consumption of agricultural products (meat, cereals and dairy products). To a great extent, these products are foisted upon the consuming public because of their economic significance and are accordingly strongly defended in nutritional reference books. We now know, though, that these three foods are problematical in the extreme when combined. They have a seriously disruptive effect on the all-important acid-base balance.

If we really want a healthy diet, we must restrict our consumption of agricultural products to a minimum and we should eat more, much more, fruit and vegetables. By doing so, we will experience fewer problems with food combining and with maintaining the acid-base balance.

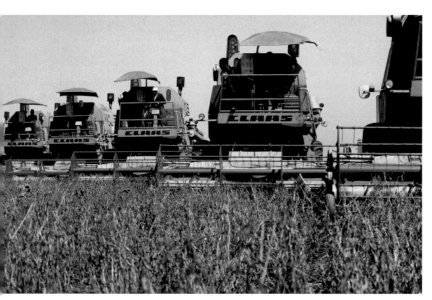

LEFT: Large-scale agricultural practices have greatly increased the consumption of cereals, meat and dairy products. Combining these foods can upset the acid-base balance.

LESS PROTEIN, MORE FRUIT

All nutritionists agree that people in advanced countries eat too much protein. Everyone needs a minimum of 15 g/½ oz of protein a day. This amount assumes that the protein is wholesome and contains all the essential amino acids. Because the quality of the protein cannot be guaranteed, 25 g/1 oz of protein per person each day should be regarded as the minimum. This is easily achieved and, if the food is combined well, this amount of protein can be digested efficiently.

However, it makes no sense to eat as much as 80–100 g/ 3–3½ oz or more of protein every day, since only a small part of it is going to be put to any real use. In any case, the greater part of it is damaged and wasted by preparation techniques, such as cooking. And, if put together in an inappropriate combination of foods, the protein may remain undigested in the body and degrade there, providing little or no nutritional value. Scientific studies have proved that vegetarianism is very healthy, ecologically sound, and much better from an ethical point of view. (Third World hunger could be wiped out if resources devoted to meat production were turned over to grain cultivation.)

In any case, humans are not really suited to eating meat or cereals: we are natural fruit-eaters. Fruit should be regarded as our most basic food. Large amounts of fruit combined correctly, or eaten separately, offer an inexhaustible source of energy. At the same time, we should bear in mind that tropical and subtropical fruits are comparatively rich and coarse in relation to fruits native to the temperate regions.

BELOW: Eating large amounts of fruit provides an excellent and easily digested source of energy for all the family

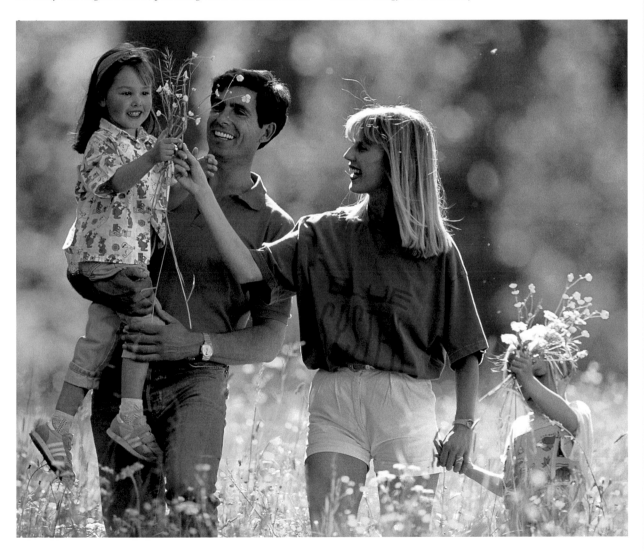

PLANNING YOUR MEALS

Proper eating is fundamental to good health, but most of us – at least in developed countries – ignore the rules in favour of a haphazard diet laden with meat, dairy produce, refined carbohydrates and processed foods. Planning meals the food combining way enables you to balance your food intake better. It does not mean cutting out all your favourite foods: rather, it shows you how, by thinking about what you eat, your diet will become more wholesome, packed with all the essential vitamins, minerals and nutrients your body needs.

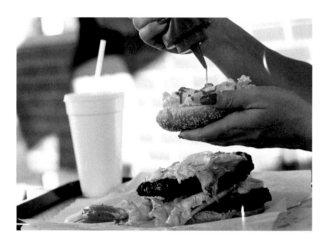

SMALL, FREQUENT MEALS

If practical, it is far better to eat several light meals a day, rather than a heavy lunch or dinner. It is hard to digest food eaten in this way and it can also make you sleepy, with the body's digestive processes slowing down accordingly. For this reason, you should try to eat an evening meal at least two hours before you go to bed. Similarly, you should give your body's metabolic system the chance to get into action in the morning before settling down to enjoy breakfast.

For many, if not for most people, breakfast consists of one dish. It is strange, then, that breakfast in hotels and motels is much more elaborate. In some tourist hotels, the breakfast buffet is an entire selection of different foods. From that ample provision, the right choice has to be made. Do not eat everything you see, but eat what goes well together. The complex carbohydrates in fruit, wholemeal (whole-wheat) toast and cereals, for instance, are much easier to digest than a high-protein cooked breakfast.

Most people eat one elaborate meal a day. Dinner, which is often postponed until late in the evening, frequently consists of several dishes: appetizer and/or soup, a main course and a dessert. At a dinner or formal lunch, there may also be side-dishes. Traditional cooking most commonly makes the main course a combination of protein and starch, such as meat with potatoes, chicken with rice, or fish and potato croquettes. According to the principles of food combining, protein and starch should be eaten separately. Meat with ordinary vegetables, or potatoes with the vegetables, would be fine. Vegetarians should also make the choice between a high-protein dish or a dish rich in starch.

CHOOSING THE COURSES

Although a meal is eaten in courses (which is a good thing, meaning that food is eaten slowly), from a food combining point of view, it can be seen as comprising a single gigantic dish. When it comes to a big meal, the choice of main course should determine the entire menu. A high-protein main course means that the dominance of protein must be taken into account. The same applies if the main course chosen is rich in starch. If we are planning a high-protein main course, it is easy to repeat the same combination in the other courses. A classic example is a meal made up thus: pea soup, followed by prosciutto, a meat main course and a dessert of cheese. As a combination of foods with similar nutrient ratios, this is an excellent menu, but it is rather too heavy. The acid-base balance would be badly disturbed: there is just too much protein. If a menu contains a high-protein dish, we should make sure that other dishes are as light as possible.

Let us improve on this example. The pea soup is replaced by a light vegetable soup. Instead of the ham, there might be a serving of raw vegetables, possibly supplemented with a little meat or fish, but only in small amounts. The main dish can stay, but it would be best to cut out the cheese altogether. There is no need for cheese following such high-protein dishes. If a dessert is really essential, all that is needed is a little creativity to produce new, healthier ones.

Soup, apart from varieties that are high in protein, has very little effect on the combination of dishes that follow it. The

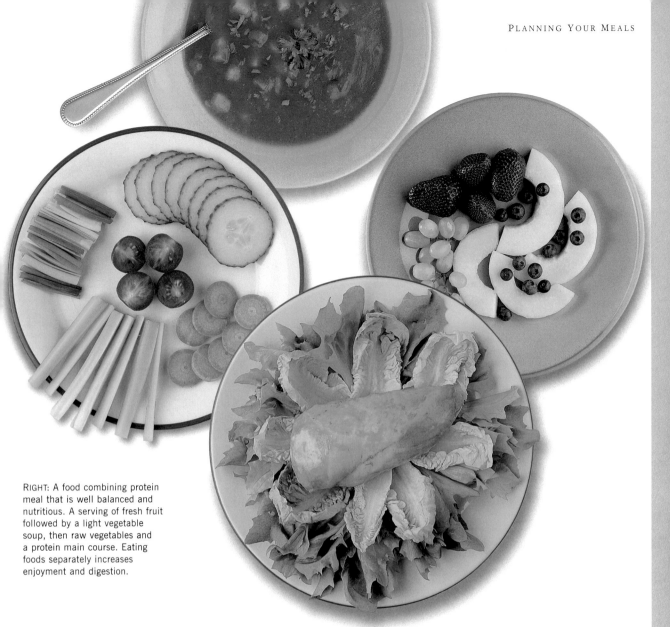

RIGHT: A food combining protein meal that is well balanced and nutritious. A serving of fresh fruit followed by a light vegetable soup, then raw vegetables and a protein main course. Eating foods separately increases enjoyment and digestion.

liquid part of the soup is filtered off quickly down the 'gastric passage' on the inner curved stomach wall and does not dilute the gastric juices. Only the solids in the soup are left deposited and waiting to be digested.

After the soup, we should not go straight on to a sweet appetizer. There is nothing wrong with having a sweet appetizer before the soup, however. A high-protein soup could be preceded, for instance, by half a honeydew melon, possibly filled with berries in a suitable sauce. The sugar will digest quickly, and, because the sweet appetizer is eaten first, it will leave the stomach first. Fruit can always be used as an appetizer. Dr Shelton rightly pointed out that fruit should be eaten before, and not after a meal.

The appetizer, however, has to be matched with the soup as much as possible. It should preferably be a small dish consisting of raw vegetables. If the main course is a high-protein dish, the appetizer should not be too acidic – sauerkraut, vegetables containing lactic acid or appetizers with sour cream in them are all examples – because acid inhibits acid. This would be a disaster when eating a meal in which plenty of gastric acid is needed to digest the high-protein main course.

Shelton claimed that fatty meat, full-fat cottage cheese and fatty fish form a better combination with acidic foods than meats, cheeses and fish that are low in fat. That is not correct, however. Fat and acid represents a good combination that lightens the digestion of high-fat and high-protein foods. Eating low-fat foods is to miss out on the function of the fat, which is to slow down the gastric peristalsis. High-protein foods that are low in fat are more difficult to digest than those that are rich in fat. By adding acid to low-fat foods, we effectively slow gastric movement.

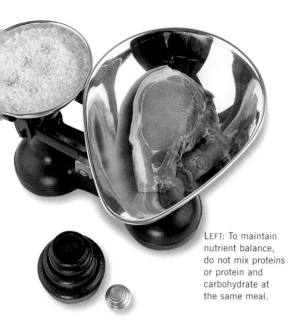

LEFT: To maintain nutrient balance, do not mix proteins or protein and carbohydrate at the same meal.

KEEPING NUTRIENTS IN BALANCE

We should be sure to eat only one form of protein at a meal. Acid should only be combined in moderation with protein (see pages 106–107). With foods that are high in protein but low in fat, we can use more acid than with foods that are rich in fat, since both the fat and the acid act to slow down gastric peristalsis.

If the proposed menu is rich in starch, the procedure is the same. But although sweet and acidic foods should not be combined with starch, both can precede a meal that is rich in starch. If we eat a sweet appetizer first, the sugar is stabilized by the gastric juice in the stomach and passes on fairly rapidly into the duodenum. The sugar has no effect on the starch that is to follow. In the final part of the stomach – the antrum – fermentation is not possible. If we eat an acidic starter, the acidity of the saliva is increased. But, as soon as we start on the dish that is rich in starch, a new type of saliva geared to treat the starchy food is produced.

A menu that contains dishes rich in starch must not also contain high-protein dishes. It is also important that the contents of the stomach are controlled by one dominant nutrient, whether it is protein, starch or sugar. Fat and acid are highly significant to digestion, but they cannot control the processing by the stomach. Fat is related to protein, acid to sugar.

What this all comes down to is the importance of combining dishes correctly, so that what you end up with is a truly balanced meal. As a natural consequence of this, you will find that you are automatically following official healthy eating guidelines by eating more fresh salads, vegetables and fruits, while simultaneously cutting down on potentially unhealthy sugars, fats and refined and processed foodstuffs. Salads, for instance, make excellent appetizers and side-dishes, always provided that they are not smothered in rich dressings and mayonnaise. A little oil and vinegar is a far healthier option. Other good appetizers include tomato or vegetable soups, or a mixture of raw vegetables. When it comes to main courses, grilled (broiled) or poached fish, poultry without its skin and lean cuts of meat – again, with any fat trimmed off them – are all safe recommendations. By finishing off a meal with a light dessert, rather than a rich one, you will leave the table without feeling bloated and with your digestion in good order.

GROWING UP THE HEALTHY WAY

It is never too early to introduce good food combining practices into young children's lives. You should be aware, however, that growth has its own specific nutritional requirements: children need extra supplies of certain nutrients to fuel their growing muscles and bones. In particular, children under the age of five need full-fat (whole) milk. The chart here sets out the basic daily requirements of key nutrients from 12 months to 18 years. Where there are two figures in a column, the first figure refers to male needs and the second to female ones. Good quality protein such as meat, fish, soy products and pulses, as well as wholemeal (whole-wheat) bread, pasta, potatoes, cereals and rice, and a wide range of vegetables, fruits, nuts and seeds will together provide a healthy balanced diet.

AGE	CALORIES	PROTEIN	CALCIUM	IRON
12 months	930/865	15 g	525 mg	7.8 mg
1–3 years	1230/1165	14.5 g	350 mg	6.9 mg
4–6 years	1715/1545	19.7 g	450 mg	6.1 mg
7–10 years	1970/1740	28.3 g	550 mg	8.7 mg
11–14 years	2220/1845	42.1 g	1000 mg	11.3 mg
				14.8 mg
15–18 years	2550/1940	55g/45 g	1000 mg	11.3 mg
				14.8 mg

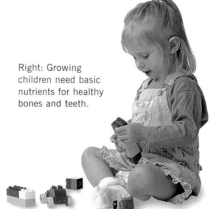

Right: Growing children need basic nutrients for healthy bones and teeth.

OLDER PEOPLE

Although the body's energy demands are normally reduced with age – scientists have calculated that, from the age of 40 onwards, energy requirements decrease on average, by up to five per cent per decade – older people's needs for vitamins and minerals actually increase with age. The table below shows you the nutrients each foodstuff provides. Remember that as you get older, you need plenty of fibre in the diet to help you avoid constipation and other digestive problems, which become more likely.

Turkey, chicken and duck, hen's and quail's eggs.

POULTRY AND EGGS
Chicken, in particular, is an excellent source of protein. You can cut down on its fat content – which is low in any event – by removing the skin before or after you cook it. Because eggs are high in cholesterol, consumption should be restricted to no more than three to four a week.

Plaice and trout.

FRUIT AND VEGETABLES
The official recommendation is to eat at least five servings of fruit and vegetables daily. Cabbage, spinach and other dark green leafy vegetables are important sources of Vitamin B_6, Vitamin E, Vitamin C and folate, with the added bonus of being rich in iron, magnesium and calcium. Potatoes, turnips and parsnips are particularly rich in carbohydrate and fibre. Citrus fruit, tomatoes and strawberries all contain valuable amounts of Vitamin C, while apples and pears provide useful soluble fibre. Bananas are a good source of carbohydrate and potassium.

Spinach and bananas

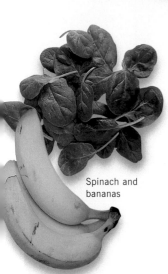

FISH
All types of fish are a good source of protein and B vitamins, with oily varieties providing essential fatty acids, Vitamin A and Vitamin D.

WHOLEGRAINS
Eat 2 servings a day of wholegrains, which supply the body with Vitamin B_6, folate and other essential nutrients, They are also an important source of insoluble fibre.

Wheat will supply the body with essential nutrients.

DAIRY PRODUCTS
Milk, cheese and yogurt are protein-rich. They also contain Vitamin A, Vitamin B_{12}, folate, riboflavin and niacin, and are a good source of calcium.

RIGHT: Freshly squeezed juice provides vitamins.

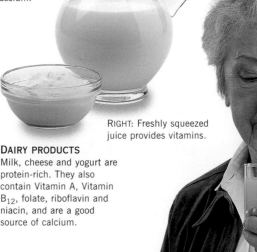

MENU PLANNING IN ACTION

Food combining revolves around a set of tried-and-tested nutritional principles that are easy to incorporate into regular and varied meal-planning, once you have grasped the fundamental basics. The suggestions here, based on some of the recipes given later in this book, are just some of the possibilities open to you and demonstrate that you will be sitting down to deliciously tempting meals and snacks that will not leave you feeling sated – or hungry and deprived.

LIGHT LUNCHES AND SUPPERS

Clear Vegetable Soup (page 207)
Herbed Mushroom Slices (page 198)

◆

Stuffed Artichokes (page 204)
Spicy Tomato Salad (page 242)

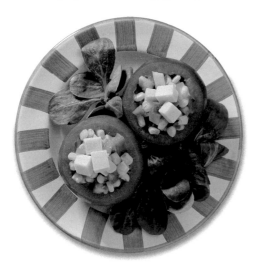

Mexican Stuffed Tomatoes

Minestrone (page 218)
Mexican Stuffed Tomatoes (page 202)

◆

Artichoke Bisque (page 218)
Steamed Vegetables (page 250)

◆

Minestrone (page 218)
Stuffed Bread Rolls (page 281)

◆

Avocado Soup (page 214)
Stuffed Bread Rolls with Leek Ragoût (page 282)

FRUIT FEASTS

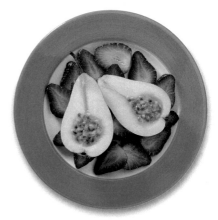

Stuffed Pear on a Bed of Strawberries

Fruity Cheese Sticks (page 307)
Stuffed Pineapple (page 314)

◆

Stuffed Pear on a Bed of Strawberries
(page 316)
Winter Pineapple (page 316)

◆

Cinnamon Apples (page 315)
Stuffed Pineapple (page 314)

◆

Citrus Salad (page 317)
Layered Fruit Salad (page 318)

◆

Stuffed Apricots (page 320)
Summer Fruits in Berry Sauce
(page 322)

◆

Poached Pears with Marjoram (page 326)
Pineapple Salad with Coconut (page 322)

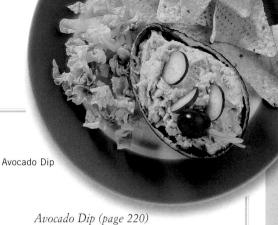
Avocado Dip

THREE-COURSE MEALS

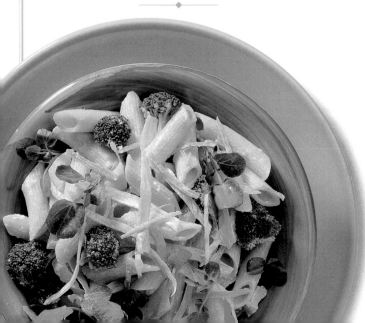
Refreshing Pasta Salad

SHOPPING FOR HEALTH

The first place to put food combining into practice and start reforming your diet, and that of your family, is in the food stores and supermarkets where you shop. Buying sensibly means that you will have a stock of fresh ingredients to inspire you and prevent you from relying on processed foods laden with chemicals and fats.

Before you go shopping, work out a list of priority food purchases and stick to it. It is all too easy to fall victim to the temptations of convenience and processed food products, especially the so-called 'healthy' varieties. These products may have a lowered saturated fat and calorie content, but their sodium levels can be higher than those of the standard versions. Salt (which is what sodium is) and sugar are both unnecessary additives and can be potentially harmful in excess. Since ingredients, by law, are listed on food labels by quantity, a handy rule of thumb is to avoid any product that has sugar or sodium high up the list. Sugar may be listed as glucose, fructose, dextrose, lactose, maltose, sorbitol and invert syrup.

In addition, convenience foods may save you time, but they rarely compare favourably in nutritional terms with the fresh, home-prepared alternative. In many instances, too, preparing them involves re-heating already cooked food, which further reduces the nutritional content – particularly of vitamins.

FRESH IS BEST

Buy the natural foods of a healthy diet: starchy foods, fresh vegetables, fruit, poultry and lean meat, fish, nuts and a judicious mix of dairy products. Wholegrain foods are preferable to those containing processed grains and, in general, eating whole foods increases both nutrient and healthy fibre intake. Seasonal fruit and vegetables, especially those locally grown, often taste better simply because they have not been stored for long or spent protracted periods of time in transport.

For this reason, frozen vegetables are often better buys if good fresh ones are unavailable. Frozen peas, for example, are frozen immediately after harvesting, preserving their

Vitamin C and thiamin content when only a little of their sugar has turned into starch. So-called 'fresh' vegetables that look tired and wilted should always be avoided. They are losing their vitamin content as they wilt. It is much better to buy fresh fruit and vegetables every few days to make sure of maximum nutritional benefits and to store them in a cool, dark place. Always use a sharp knife to prepare vegetables as blunt utensils will bruise the food, resulting in nutrient loss.

ORGANIC FOOD

The fresher the food and the less it has been processed or otherwise affected by chemicals, the more nutritious it is. The extra cost – because organic growing and farming produces smaller yields that do not keep so well as chemically treated produce – is well worth it.

Because of its freedom from pesticides, man-made fertilizers and artificial growth hormones, organic food is preferable to non-organic alternatives. This is particularly the case for organic meat and poultry. Many of the methods used in modern intensive farming are thought to be potentially unhealthy – in particular, there is scientific evidence to suggest that excessive use of antibiotics by farmers is having a knock-on effect, with an increase in human resistance to antibiotics being the end result. To qualify as organically reared, animals and poultry must be raised in natural conditions on organically farmed land. They must not be treated with antibiotics on a routine basis and the use of additives, such as artificial growth hormones, is banned.

SHOPPING SAFELY

By following a few basic rules of food safety, you can help to minimize the possibility of food poisoning.
*Avoid stores with poor hygiene practices, such as displaying raw and cooked meats together.
*Check that breakables, such as eggs, are not broken or damaged before you buy them.
*Reject any fruit with a bruised or punctured skin.
*Avoid items if their packaging is damaged or torn.

*Store cook-chill foodstuffs in the refrigerator as quickly as you can after purchase.
*Arrange your purchases so that raw meat or fish cannot drip blood and other juices on to other foods.
*Avoid dented or rusted cans.

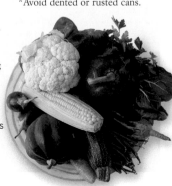

RIGHT: Fresh vegetables should be bought regularly, not stored.

READING FOOD LABELS

Knowing how to read a food label is essential shopping sense: for consumer protection, there are strict rules and regulations that govern what can and cannot be said and what information must be displayed. If a product has been processed, for instance, it must be clearly indicated, together with details of what processing method has been employed. Labels must also carry the name of the product, its weight or volume, a 'use by' or 'best before' date, and a list of ingredients, including any additives, plus nutritional information, detailing the calorie content and the amounts of protein, salt, sugar and so on. Additives are generally described by their function, followed by a name or code.

Safe storage information tells you how long you can use the food safely once it has been opened or thawed, and how best to store it over that time.

Nutritional information details calorie content and amounts of salt, fibre, fat and other substances an average serving of the food contains.

Weight and volume give an average amount of what is in each bottle or pack, so there may obviously be a slight variation.

Additives are listed with their function first, followed by their names and E numbers.

Manufacturing details must be given in full, together with a note of the product's country of origin.

Datemark tells you when you must use the product by, when it is 'best before' and, sometimes, the date up until when it should be displayed, after which it should be withdrawn from the shelves.

Illustrations must reflect what is actually in the product: a carton of yogurt flavoured solely with artificial additives cannot carry a picture of fresh fruit, for instance.

Statements such as 'reduced calorie' or 'low fat' cannot be made unless there is a significant, measurable difference between the version making the statement and the standard version.

Claims such as 'made with fresh eggs' must be supported by stating exactly how much has been used in the list of ingredients. Ingredients are listed in order of decreasing weight.

Below: Write a shopping list and stick to it.

ADDITIVE ALERT

The use of all food additives, other than artificial flavourings, is strictly regulated by law. Even so, there is some scientific evidence to suggest that the additives permitted in food can still be harmful to some young children, while asthmatics and other people with other types of allergies may react badly to them. There have also been claims that certain additives – notably the nitrates and nitrites – may be potentially carcinogenic. The table here shows you what the main types of additives are and how to identify them on food labels.

Artificial colouring
Tartrazine (E102), Quinoline yellow (E104), Sunset yellow (E110), Cochineal (E120), Indigo (E132), Carmine brilliant blue (E133), Beetroot red (E162), Caramel (E150).

Preservatives
Benzoaic acid and benzoates (E210-19), Sulphur dioxide and sulphites (E220-28), Nitrates and nitrites (E249-52).

Antioxidants
Butylated hydroxyanisole (E320 BHA), Butylated hydroxtoluene (E321 BHT), Ascorbic acid and ascorbates (E300-4).

Flavour enhancers
Monosodium glutamate (E621), Monopotassium glutamate (E622), Calcium glutamate (E623), Sodium inosinate (E631).

Emulsifiers, stabilisers and thickeners
Lecithin (E322), Guar gum (E412), Gum arabic (E414), Glycerol (E422), Pectins (E440), Cellulose (E460).

GOOD EATING HABITS

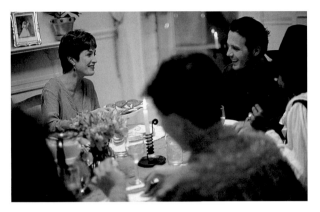

ABOVE: Regular 'family' meals encourage sensible eating habits.

Sitting down to a healthy nutritious meal with your family regularly on a daily basis can only help to encourage the growth of sensible eating habits. It also helps you to resist the unhealthy temptation to grab a quick bite to eat on the run or to eat excessively large amounts of food at inappropriate times of the day. Should you need to snack, there are lots of natural, healthy alternatives to junk food that do you far more good – and taste even better into the bargain.

Keeping yourself in good health, say food combiners, has more to do with increasing the quality of your nutrition – and, of course, combining its various elements correctly – than with obsessing about its quantity. Better health, they argue, is also hindered, rather than helped, by the modern tendency to eat sporadically, ignoring conventional mealtimes in favour of bingeing on high-fat snacks and relying more and more on unhealthy processed foodstuffs into the bargain. This is not Nature's way, nor is it the way of the practised food combiner. By following the clear, straightforward guidelines given in the previous chapters of this book, you can easily achieve that all-important nutritional balance. The aim is to make sure of the right intake of fruit, vegetables and dietary fibre, plus a sensible amount of healthy fats and oils. You should aim to eat one protein-based meal a day and another starch-based one, while, at the same time, being sure that you are getting enough alkaline food into your diet. This is vital if the correct acid-base balance within the body is to be preserved. Too much protein, for instance, and the balance will be skewed in favour of acid, with digestive problems as the likely result.

ABOVE: A nutritious and energy-boosting snack.

BENEFITS OF FOOD COMBINING

A healthy body works hard and constantly to detoxify itself. If, however, the digestion becomes overloaded and overstressed, then the natural consequence is for the body to become tired out as well. It can become a classic vicious circle. If you feel low in energy and unable to cope, you turn to food in an attempt to build up your vitality levels. But if you eat unsuitable food too frequently and at unsuitable times of the day, your body will be unable to function properly and you will continue to feel tired. The result is a nutritional impasse.

By putting the principles of good food combining to work and adopting healthy eating habits, you are enabling your body to work at peak effectiveness. Put simply, correct combining leads to competent digestion, which, in turn, means that all the nourishment in the food that you eat is being put to a properly effective use.

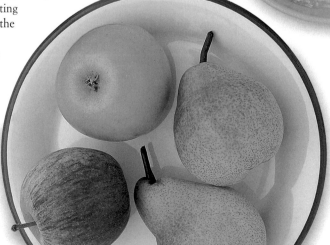

EATING THROUGH THE DAY

All nutritionists – not just simply food combiners – strongly advise spreading nutrient intake evenly throughout the day, with one wholesome main meal, one moderate one and one light one, plus, if you feel hunger pangs, nutritious energy-boosting snacks in the mid-morning and in the mid-afternoon. Preferably, the last meal of the day should be eaten at least two hours before you go to bed, as this gives the body the time to digest what has been eaten properly. If food is eaten too late in the evening, it has been shown scientifically that rather than being thoroughly digested, it is simply laid down as body fat during the night. People who regularly eat large meals late can be at more at risk of heart attacks into the bargain: statistics show that a significant number of heart attacks occur while their victims are in bed in the early hours of the morning.

Breakfast is definitely one meal that should not be skipped, since it enables the body to recharge its batteries, ready for the demands of the day ahead. Eating breakfast stimulates the metabolism, which falls while you are asleep: it also peps up the body's blood-sugar levels, with an increase in alertness as a result. Food combiners advise that breakfast is the ideal time to eat fruit: it is probably the one meal of the day when it makes the most sense to eat fruit on its own. You could try a fruit cocktail or a dried fruit compote, which is quick and easy to prepare in advance the night before and is delicious served with plain live yogurt. Or you could try some honeyed porridge – this sort of food is particularly recommended for diabetics, since it releases its energy slowly. For a protein-start to the day, try a delicious yogurt smoothie or some free-range scrambled egg but remember not to have toast. It is quite simple to remember what combines and what does not. Melon, for example, although delicious on its own, does not combine well with any other food – even any other fruit – because of the enzymes it contains.

LEFT: Breakfast is the best time to recharge the batteries, stimulating the metabolism and increasing alertness. To vary your breakfast meal try fresh or dried fruit, honeyed porridge or cooked eggs; served scrambled or poached and without toast.

HEALTHY SNACKING

Enjoying what you eat is obviously important, especially when it comes to the snacks that nutritionists and dieticians actively recommend you eat during the day. Research indicates that people who eat like this are more likely to take in a greater variety of essential nutrients. They are also, so it appears, less likely to eat unhealthy amounts of fatty foods.

This, of course, depends on not falling prey to an excessive intake of convenience or junk foods. Snacks become a healthy eating option only if the natural food balance is maintained. Starchy snacks, such as crispbreads and bananas, are perfect for slow, sustained energy release. Sweet biscuits (cookies), rich cakes and chocolate can be replaced by fresh or dried fruit, while, instead of crisps (chips), you can try a mixture of unroasted nuts, pumpkin and sunflower seeds, all of which taste just as good while being far better for you.

IMPORTANCE OF FLUIDS

In food combining, making sure that you are drinking enough and drinking the right liquids is almost as important as choosing the right food combinations and balancing your nutritional intake correctly. If you are just starting out on a food combining plan, you will need to drink plenty of fluids to help flush out of the system all of the toxins that may have accumulated in your body. You should drink at least 2 litres/3½ pints/8¾ cups of water a day, in addition to other liquids, such as fresh fruit and vegetable juices. The trick here is not to drink a lot with meals – fruit juices should always be drunk on their own in any event – and to drink plenty between meals. This aids the digestive process, whereas drinking solely at mealtimes can hinder it.

It is important to avoid becoming dehydrated. Cut back on alcoholic or strongly caffeinated drinks, which are diuretic and cause you to lose precious water through increased urination. Filtered water is preferable and bottled water is the obvious alternative, still, rather than sparkling, but check the label carefully. Some brands have an exceptionally high sodium content and should therefore be avoided.

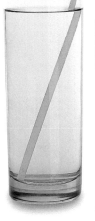
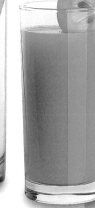

DIET WISE

Although many fashionable diets claim to be based on food combining principles, practitioners are at pains to point out that food combining is not a 'diet' in the accepted popular sense at all. Rather it is a healthy eating plan that should be followed for life – certainly not a quick fix weight-loss measure you can take up and drop when you feel you have achieved your goal. Food combining will help you to achieve your natural slim body weight, as well as building up your resistance to a host of potentially debilitating ailments.

In its initial stages, food combining will help you to lose weight slowly but surely, simply because you will be eating more fruit and vegetables at the expense of more calorific foods. Reducing the amount of fat in the diet is the most effective way of controlling the overall calorie intake: in the average diet, statistics show that fat provides more than twice as many calories as protein and carbohydrate. At the same time, you will be getting all the health-giving nutrients your body needs – indeed, you will be getting more because you will be substituting healthy foodstuffs for those that are relatively high in calories, but low in nutrients.

Contrast this with the effects of a typical crash diet, in which there is usually a dramatic weight loss at first because water and protein are being lost from the body. This is not the same thing at all as losing excess body fat. Once a normal eating pattern is resumed, the lost fluid is quickly replaced, with a quick weight gain as the inevitable result. In fact, you may even end up heavier than when you began. The dieting process becomes harder, rather than easier, as you have to start it all over again.

Dieticians call this phenomenon the 'yo-yo effect'. People who get trapped in a cycle of on-off dieting develop a tendency to compensate for the deprivations of dieting by bingeing when they start to eat normally again. The results are worse than useless, with consequent psychological damage to self-image and self-esteem to contend with, as well as possible physical side-effects.

LEFT: Improving the nutritional quality of your diet will assist weight loss.

SENSIBLE DIETING

If you want to diet the food combining way, the first step is to make an eating plan, starting by introducing foods of higher nutritional quality into your diet to replace ones of lower quality. The knowledge of food combining principles that you

---

WHAT SHOULD YOU WEIGH?

The traditional way of determining whether people were overweight relied on tables that related height to body weight. Doctors, dieticians and nutritionists now considered these to be old-fashioned and a far more reliable system has been devised. This features the body mass index (BMI), which medical professionals use to assess weight and health risks. To calculate your own, start with your current weight in kilograms (if your starting point is pounds, multiply by 0.45). Measure your height in metres (if you measure in feet and inches, divide the total number of inches by 0.39). To calculate your BMI, divide your weight in kilograms by your height in metres squared, rounding the numbers to a single decimal point. For example, someone who is 1.69 metres/5 feet 6 inches and weighs 64 kg/ 10 stone/140 lb has a BMI of 23 (64 divided by 1.69^2). If your BMI is 20 or below, you are considered to be underweight and you may be advised to bring your BMI up to between 20 and 25. A BMI of between 20 and 25 is the acceptable weight range, provided that your WHR (weight-to-hip ratio) is 0.80 or less. You calculate this by dividing your waist measurement by that of your hip. If your BMI is between 25 and 30, you probably need to lose some weight, particularly if you have excess weight concentrated around the waist. A BMI of between 30

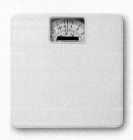

and 40 is considered to be obese (extremely overweight), while anything over 40 is very obese and potentially life-threatening if left unchecked.

have already gained from earlier on in this book will enable you to determine what goes with what, which combinations are problematic and which ought to be avoided at all costs. You should also bear in mind the order in which you eat different kinds of food during a meal: the foods that are the easiest to digest should be eaten first. Fruit, for instance, passes through the system more quickly than protein or starch and is digested far more efficiently if eaten on its own. You need to consider how much food you should eat as well, together with the best times for eating it. Some dieticians say that the rule here is to eat when you are hungry, not necessarily strictly by the clock.

What you have to do is develop a clear understanding of which foods are high in fats and sugars, so that you can avoid them. You also have to be sensible and not replace the loss by eating vast amounts of low-calorie foods as an alternative, since the body will still store any such excess as fat.

The key to the entire process is moderation. Eat when you are hungry and stop eating as soon as that hunger is satisfied.

CATABOLISM, STABILIZATION AND ANABOLISM

As a food combining regime starts to take effect, the body begins a process that the experts call 'retracing'. During the first phase, termed catabolism, the emphasis is on the breaking down and elimination of redundant substances. The body starts its own form of spring-cleaning, the aim being to remove the wastes and toxins deposited in all of its tissues. Because wastes are discarded more rapidly than tissue the physical sign of this process is loss of weight.

The second stage, called stabilization, follows once the spring-cleaning has been completed. The body weight now stays more or less the same, since the amount of waste material discarded by the body daily is roughly equivalent to what is being formed as a result of the new, more healthy nutrients the body is absorbing.

The third phase – a build-up period called anabolism – follows. In this period, your weight may increase, even though your diet is lower in calories than it was before. This is because the new tissue that has formed as a result of the improved diet is more durable and does not break down so easily. Also, new tissues are now being formed faster, thanks to better food assimilation made possible by the ceasing of incorrect food combining. As a result, the body's need for food – at least, the volume to which it was accustomed – decreases. Put simply, it is now possible to maintain a healthy body weight with less food, while, at the same time, being able to count on an increased energy supply.

You can help the body during this cleansing process by following a non-toxic diet. This means eating organic food whenever possible, drinking filtered water, practising food combining and rotating foods, especially common allergens

VITALITY BOOSTERS AND ROBBERS

Some substances are particularly important in helping to maintain the body's energy levels: others have a negative effect on your energy, or are of little or no nutritional value. The table here helps you to sort out the two.

VITALITY BOOSTERS

Beta-carotene Orange, red, yellow and dark green vegetables: sweet potatoes, pumpkins and squashes, tomatoes, broccoli, spinach, watercress, sweetcorn (corn), mangoes, apricots, peaches
Vitamin B_1 (thiamin) Sprouting seeds, brown rice, wholegrain cereals, peas, beans, Brazil and other nuts
Vitamin B_2 (riboflavin) Almonds and other nuts, wheatgerm, cheese, mushrooms, broccoli, beans, eggs, yogurt
Vitamin B_3 Beans, whole wheat, brown rice, barley, eggs, fish
Vitamin B_6 Soy, oats, wheatgerm, walnuts and other nuts, beans, bananas, avocado, wholegrains, fish, green vegetables, sweet potatoes
Vitamin B_{12} Egg yolks, cheese, milk, fortified soy milk
Vitamin C Most fresh fruit and vegetables: particularly oranges, red (bell) peppers, chillies, blackcurrants, parsley
Vitamin E Sunflower oil, nuts, seeds, avocados, asparagus, green vegetables, barley, soy beans, sweet potatoes, brown rice
Iron Wholegrains, nuts, eggs, leafy dark green vegetables, beans, seeds, wheatgerm, dried apricots
Magnesium All green vegetables, nuts, seeds, beans, fish, figs, bananas, brown rice
Zinc Wholegrains, fish, eggs, nuts, beans

VITALITY ROBBERS

Alcohol In excess (see page 107), this can interfere with the quality of sleep and can lead to dehydration.
Sugar With the exception of the calories it contains, white sugar is totally deficient in nutrients.
Caffeine Although popularly believed to be a stimulant, caffeine, long-term, is scientifically regarded as a vitality robber.
Tobacco The nicotine in tobacco, although an initial brain stimulant, actually acts as a depressant in the longer term. Smoking makes added demands on the liver, which uses up more of the B vitamins and Vitamin C as a result, and places an extra strain on the antioxidants that help to detoxify the body. It is also carcinogenic.

like milk products, eggs, wheat and foods containing yeast. Basically, your cuisine should be natural and seasonal, with plenty of fruit, vegetables, wholegrains, legumes, pulses and nuts and seeds. Omnivores can add some low-fat dairy products to this list, together with fresh fish (not shellfish) and organic poultry. Choose skimmed (skim) or semi-skimmed (low-fat) milk, low-fat yogurt and low-fat cheeses, such as cottage cheese and ricotta.

You should cut out or cut right back on red and cured meats, offal (variety meats), refined foods, canned foods, sugar, salt, saturated fats, coffee, alcohol and nicotine. Finally, should you need them you should substitute natural remedies, such as nutrients, herbs and homeopathic medicines, where possible, for over-the-counter pharmaceutical remedies. Other natural therapies can also be helpful.

THE IMPORTANCE OF EXERCISE

Food combining can undoubtedly help you to become more healthy, but it cannot guarantee that you expend more energy than you consume, which is the real answer to losing weight, should you need to do so. It is clear is that extremely low-calorie diets have the potential to cause more problems than they solve. For successful, long-lasting weight loss, you need to combine a healthy food combining regime with a regular exercise schedule, based around enjoyable, effective work-out routines.

If you eat more food than your body uses up in energy, the consequences are obvious. Your body stores the surplus calories you are eating as fat, which, every time you weigh yourself, will show up on the scales. While changing over to a food combining diet can help the body to detoxify itself, you need to help it by exercising regularly. This not only helps to shed the pounds: it will also help you to maintain

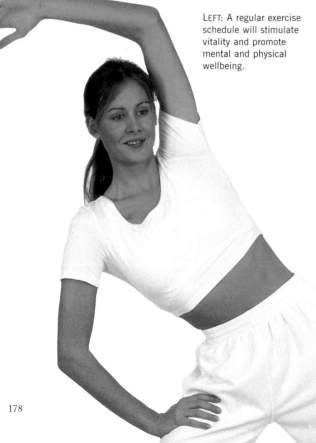

LEFT: A regular exercise schedule will stimulate vitality and promote mental and physical wellbeing.

your weight at its new, lower level. Exercise should also stimulate your overall vitality, since it triggers the release of chemicals called endorphins in the brain, which promotes a feeling of mental and physical wellbeing. You will feel more at ease with yourself, calmer and more clear-headed as a result of regular exercise.

This assumes, however, that the type of exercise you undertake is in tune with your current level of physical fitness and abilities. The golden rule is not to over-tax yourself right at the start, but rather to begin gently and build up slowly and surely, whatever form of exercise you decide suits you best. The cliché 'no pain, no gain' is simply not true. You should never work out until you are exhausted, since too much activity can be just as bad for you as too little. Take a leaf from the advice given to overweight middle-aged diabetics, for instance. They are told that a 20–30 minute walk three times a week will help to regulate their appetites, will help them to lose weight and will make them feel fitter overall into the bargain. If you start with this advice, you can always do more once you feel ready.

It is a good idea to choose more than one type of exercise. Variety will help to keep your exercise plan interesting. As far as what you eat and drink is concerned while on your exercise regime, you should cut down on sugary foods that contain few, if any, nutrients, and on alcohol and caffeinated drinks. You can eat healthy, energy-boosting snacks, such as bananas, dates, raisins and dried apricots and starchy foods, which will supply you with a slow, but steady, flow of energy, and, of course, fruit and vegetables.

TYPES OF EXERCISE

Basically, there are two types of exercise – aerobic and anaerobic. Both increase the rate at which the body burns up energy, so helping to reduce its store of surplus fat, but otherwise their benefits are different. All aerobic exercise boosts the heart rate, raising the level of oxygen in the blood. It helps to burn off calories by stimulating the body's entire metabolic system. Good forms include swimming, running, cycling and dancing. All four are beneficial for the heart and the circulation. They also stimulate the body to shed toxins and help to reduce the acidity in its tissues.

Anaerobic exercise builds muscle and strengthens bones; one good form is weight-training. For weight-watchers, the fact that anaerobic exercise helps to build muscle is particularly useful, as the more muscle there is in the body in relation to fat, the more the body's fat stocks are depleted to meet its increased energy requirements. (Muscle tissue burns up more calories, even at rest, than fat does.)

PLANNING AN EXERCISE SCHEDULE

Becoming your own personal fitness trainer is not so hard as it might seem, especially if you profit from the commonsense guidelines set out in the table here. There are all sorts of different, health-boosting activities that can be easily built into your routine.

BELOW AND RIGHT: Dancing and cycling are both excellent aerobic activities with the benefit of social interaction.

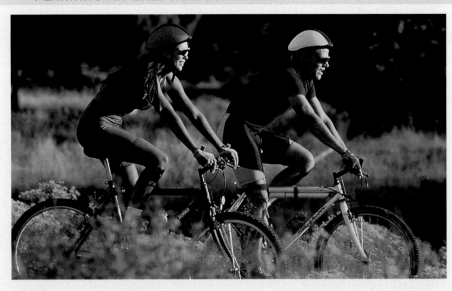

EXERCISE	ADVANTAGES	ACTION
Brisk walking	Stimulates heart, lungs, muscles and mind. Easy to fit into a typical lifestyle.	Start with 10–15 minutes three times a week, building up to 30 minutes.
Swimming	Exercises most of the major muscles and muscle groups, improving stamina, suppleness and strength with little risk of any physical damage.	Swim at least three times a week, but always wait for an hour after eating.
Dancing	Good for all levels of fitness with socialising as a bonus.	Barn dancing is a good form of aerobic exercise, while ballroom dancing aids general mobility. Some forms of dance, however, may be too physically demanding for people with joint problems.
Cycling	Regarded as one of the best forms of exercise, suitable for people of most ages and levels of physical fitness. Cycling tones the leg muscles and promotes muscular endurance.	Choose a bicycle that suits the type of cycling that you will be doing and one that is big enough for you. If you are cycling on roads, wear reflective clothing, a protective helmet, and a face mask to protect you against pollution.

An ideal exercise plan combines the two: you should start with up to three sessions of aerobic exercise a week, each session lasting around half an hour, and two shorter sessions of anaerobic exercise.

But do not think you have to invest in costly equipment – treadmills, rowing machines, exercise bikes, rebounders and the like – or join a gym or go to a class in order to exercise effectively; many simple forms of exercise, such as walking, are just as effective. You should slowly work towards increased activity levels. If you are unprepared, embarking on anything involving vigorous and excessive periods of exertion can lead to stress, strain and even physical injury.

179

TAI CHI, DEEP BREATHING AND EXERCISES

Aerobic exercise will help you to get into shape and reinforce the impact of your food combining nutritional plan. To complement your general exercise regime, you can try the ancient Chinese exercises of tai chi to relax the mind and tone the body simultaneously. Each day you should practise regular deep-breathing exercises to cleanse the body and as your exercise routine progresses, you can add specific exercises to shape up the hips, thighs, waist and stomach.

By combining movement with meditation, Tai chi chu'an – to give this ancient system of exercise its full name – helps to balance the body's yin and yang, thereby boosting its inner energy, or chi. Yin, according to Taoist philosophy on which the whole of tai chi is based, is dark, passive and feminine in character. It represents the body's interior and is concentrated in solid body organs, such as the liver. Yang, on the other hand, is light, active and masculine, representing the body's exterior and its hollow organs, such as the heart. The aim of the discipline is to achieve a balance between these two complementary forces. As a result, the body's chi, the healing life-energy that flows through internal channels called meridians, becomes more potent and focused, promoting good health and physical wellbeing.

EIGHT BASIC POSTURES

Tai chi tradition says that this set of movements was originally devised over a thousand years ago at the time of the Sung dynasty. Its purpose was to improve the health of soldiers in the Chinese imperial army. It can be used as a warm-up or as a complete tai chi form in its own right.

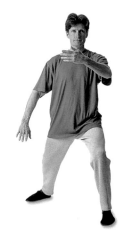

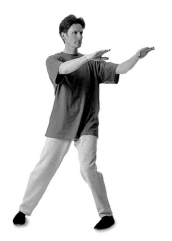

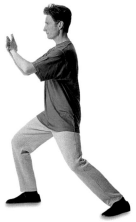

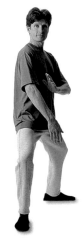

1 Ward off
Ward Off energy is sometimes likened to water supporting a boat. It is something that fills the entire body from the inside. It imparts a strong feeling of buoyant, natural strength and also creates space.

2 Pull
Pull tips the balance. Joining with the momentum of something, it adds just enough of its own energy to topple or upset the balance.

3 Press
Press is like a combination of Ward Off and Push: one arm wards off while the other pushes. It displays a bursting forward of energy up, down, or along, yet it retains a contained shape with which an incoming force may be met and repelled.

4 Shoulder
Shoulder stroke is a dynamic expression of solid earth strength, which uses the weight and momentum of the whole body through the shoulder and upper back. The last of the secondary postures, Shoulder makes you aware of your own physical strength.

LEARNING THE BASICS

Tai chi consists of a series of separate movements that link together to create what is termed a 'form'; each movement has its own symbolic meaning and name. Each form is circular, the aim is to develop muscular control, rather than muscular bulk. The exercises are not aerobic, so they should not boost your heart rate unduly, or leave you feeling puffed and out of breath. You may find yourself sweating, however, because of the heat generated by the *chi* as it makes its way around the body's meridians.

No special strength or exertion is required to practise tai chi, though, initially at least, the discipline is best learned from a qualified practitioner, who can ensure that you execute the exercises correctly with the body properly aligned. Such a teacher will also advise on the best warm-ups to follow before embarking on the exercise and how best to cool down once you have completed it. A tai chi session typically lasts for around 20 minutes and should be practised once a week.

In tai chi, the body's centre of gravity – the *tan tien* – is taken as being located just below the navel, slightly towards the spine. During movements, the latter should feel relaxed and vertical, almost as if you were suspended physically by a thread running from the top of the head. Remember, too, that the whole body is involved, not just the part that is actually moving. Your neck and shoulders should be relaxed, the elbows and knees flexible, the pelvis tucked in and the chin drawn back slightly. Start each movement with the feet placed a little wider apart than the hips. They should feel well-rooted on the ground.

Work through each movement of the form slowly, making sure that there is no pain or pulling in either muscles or joints. As you progress, you should feel your arms becoming longer and heavier, the chest broader, the back longer and the head higher, while your breathing should become relaxed and deep. You should focus on trying to sense the flow of healing *chi* spreading through the body. The traditional time to practise, according to tai chi teachers, is at sunrise or sunset.

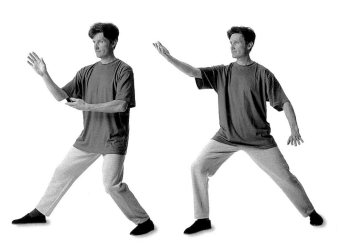 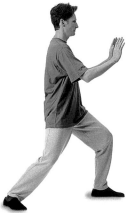 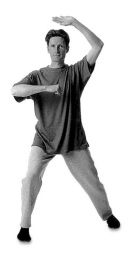

5 Rollback
Rollback is a protector that delivers a sense of choice. It actively invites incoming energy to the point where it exhausts itself. In neutralizing the incoming energy, Rollback creates a place of choice from where a counter movement or a letting go offer equal possibilities.

6 Split
The secondary posture Split is the explosive force that moves in opposite directions from the same central, spinning source.

7 Push
Push is a posture that sends energy outward. Always based on listening, it moves out through the hands and like fire, surrounding and consuming the space into which it moves.

8 Elbow
Short, sharp, and decisive, Elbow Stroke makes use of the energy generated as the arm folds at the elbow. The elbow is presented forward. As it unfolds, the fist is released to chop up or downward, and its movements can alternate with those of the elbow.

TONING EXERCISES

In addition to tai chi, you can integrate a few conventional exercises into your health plan. If you do, the starting point should be a few gentle stretches. As well as being useful warm-ups, which you should practise before embarking on any form of more strenuous exercise, they are also beneficial in their own right, since stretching is one of the most effective ways of helping to refresh your body. You should try to set aside ten minutes first thing in the morning to warm up your muscles, ready to meet the demands of the day ahead. Stretching at the end of the day is an ideal form of beneficial unwinding exercise. Here also are four routines to tone up the stomach, waist and hips.

MORNING STRETCHES

1. RIGHT: Standing straight with your feet parallel and about a shoulder-width apart, swing your right arm backwards in a circle, followed by the left arm. Repeat, this time swinging each arm forward in turn. Then try both arms together.

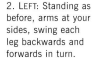

2. LEFT: Standing as before, arms at your sides, swing each leg backwards and forwards in turn.

3. BELOW: Lie down with your legs bent, making sure that your feet are flat on the floor. Raise your head and shoulders slowly until you can touch your knees with your hands. Lower yourself back to the floor again gently and repeat a couple of times.

EVENING STRETCHES

1. ABOVE: Lie down with your legs bent, feet flat on the ground. Roll gently from side to side. Bring your left hand over to the right side of the knee. Repeat several times on both sides.

2. BELOW: Remaining on the floor, lie with your legs bent and the sides of the feet flat to the ground. Spread out your arms and let your legs fall over to the right, feeling the stretch as they do so. Return to centre and then let them fall to the left. Repeat a few times.

3. BELOW: Lie on your back and stretch your arms above your head, feeling the stretch right through the body, from fingertips to toes. Lie back, relax and try to 'let go' of all your muscles, starting with the toes and working up the body, breathing deeply and evenly as you do this.

4. RIGHT: Get back on your feet and jog up and down on the spot for a minute or so. Then, while raising and clapping your hands above your head, jump out into a star shape. Repeat a few times.

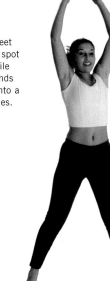

WAIST AND STOMACH

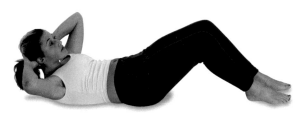

1. ABOVE: Lie on your back, with your knees bent and feet flat on the floor, your hands clasped loosely just behind your head, elbows wide. Consciously pull your stomach down towards the floor and then use the abdominal muscles to raise your head and upper part of the back off the floor. Come halfway down and raise yourself again, repeating the process up to 16 times – more, if you feel ready for it. Pause for breath, before you continue working.

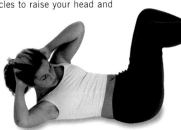

2. ABOVE: Lie on your back as before, this time raising your legs as high as you can, keeping your knees bent and crossing the ankles. Lift your right shoulder up and rotate it towards the left knee, bringing the left down slightly as you do so. This is good for the lower part of the abdomen. Lower your shoulder back to the floor and do the same thing with your other shoulder. Repeat eight times, working each shoulder alternately. (Avoid this exercise if you have back problems.)

HIPS AND THIGHS

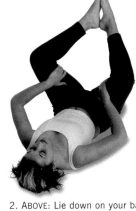

1. BELOW: You will need a chair or some other support for this exercise. Stand with your left hand resting on a chairback, your feet together and then, keeping your right leg straight with the knee relaxed, slowly raise your right leg outwards until you feel the raising in the right hip. Hold, then lower the leg back to its starting position. Repeat up to eight times, then do the same with the left leg.

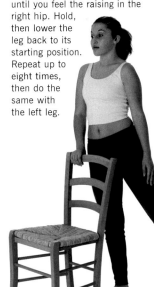

2. ABOVE: Lie down on your back and raise your legs in the air, feet together but letting your knees fall open so that you can place your hands on the inner part of the thighs. Bring the knees together as much as you can while pressing down with the hands. Release and repeat the exercise up to 16 times, keeping your stomach pulled in as much as you can throughout.

BREATHING FOR HEALTH

Deep breathing helps to relax, cleanse and alkalize the body. Because it improves the circulation and the efficient transport of oxygen and nutrients through the bloodstream, it is an essential adjunct to nutritional good health. You should practise this routine when you get up, before you go to bed, and when you have some free time during the day as well.

1. Lie on your back, making sure that you are comfortable, and let every part of your body grow floppy and relax.

2. Exhale completely, then breathe in slowly and deeply through your nose, counting slowly to ten. This will fill your lungs to their maximum capacity. Push your stomach out as you do this.

3. Hold the breath for a moment or two, then exhale through the mouth, counting to eight as you do so. Repeat the routine ten times.

4. You can follow this up by massaging the stomach area for a few minutes. Lubricate the skin with a good carrier oil – you can combine this with a suitable essential oil if you like – and then work across the abdomen, up and down and from right to left.

BELOW: Massaging the stomach can help the digestive system.

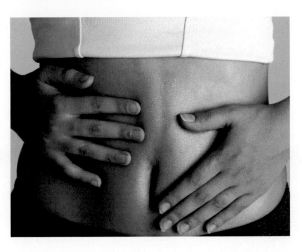

PREPARING, COOKING AND STORING FOOD

Every food combining authority will tell you that fresh food is best, but even food of the highest quality can lose some – and sometimes all – of its goodness if it is not prepared, cooked and stored correctly. The way food is handled before, during and after cooking can have a dramatic effect on its nutritional value. For this reason, you should never reheat food more than once. Not only does this encourage potentially harmful bacterial growth – it destroys still more health-giving vitamins into the bargain.

How your food is prepared can be just as important as what you eat: choosing the wrong cooking techniques can all-too-easily turn what started out as healthy food into an unwholesome meal. As the recipes that follow demonstrate, there are simple ways of creating tasty, appetizing dishes that will satisfy even the heartiest of appetites or the most fussy feeders without destroying nutrients or adding harmful quantities of fats, sugar and salt into the bargain.

It is now a generally held nutritional opinion – not one simply confined to food combiners – that people as a whole need to eat a radically different, more wholesome type of diet, which is rich in plant produce and grains and much lower in proteins, fats and sugars than they are used to. This means concentrating on starchy foods, such as potatoes, rice and pasta, and on fresh fruits and vegetables. Although we can still eat fish, poultry and some lean meat, we should be eating less of them and less dairy produce as well. Indeed, some food combiners argue that cow's milk, in particular, is best avoided, as it can cause digestive difficulties, especially when mixed with other foods. They suggest substituting goat's or sheep's milk, buttermilk or plain live yogurt for cow's milk.

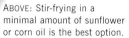

ABOVE: Stir-frying in a minimal amount of sunflower or corn oil is the best option.

BEFORE YOU COOK

When it comes to the preparation of food, the priority in every kitchen should be hygiene. It is vital to stop food from becoming contaminated with harmful bacteria, as stomach upsets and, in extreme cases, food poisoning may result. To avoid the risk of transmitting the bacteria that raw meat and fish carry to other foodstuffs, you should wash your hands and thoroughly clean knives, chopping boards and any other kitchen utensils you have been using, between preparing each type of food.

Storing food correctly before cooking, is just as important. You should always transfer perishable food to your refrigerator as soon as possible after its purchase. Make sure, too, that you do not over fill the refrigerator so that the cold air on which the preserving process relies is unable to circulate freely. If this happens, the food will not be chilled properly. The optimum working temperature at which you need to maintain a refrigerator to guard against the risk of bacterial contamination is 0–5°C/32–41°F, and no higher.

Statistics show that fresh soft fruit and green vegetables can lose as much as 15 per cent of their Vitamin C content in a single day if they are kept at room temperature. To minimize this loss, you should ideally leave their washing, peeling, cutting or grating to just before cooking or eating. Some vegetables, like potatoes, are more nutritious if left unpeeled, since more vitamin loss occurs if the surface is exposed to the air.

FRYING FOODS

Although you may have bought the freshest-possible produce, if your cooking methods are not healthy, the finished dish will not be as nutritious as it might have been. Especially when time is at a premium, the temptation is to turn to the quickest, most convenient cooking option which is often the least healthy method.

Potatoes are a classic example. Eaten baked, they are an excellent source of dietary fibre and Vitamin C. If, however, you decide to chop and deep-fry them in oil, the fat they will absorb (ranging from around seven per cent for freshly cut potatoes up to a staggering 20 per cent for frozen ones) turns

BELOW AND LEFT: Lightly steaming fresh vegetables maximizes nutrient retention and flavour.

them from a healthy to an unhealthy eating option.

If deep-fat frying is something a recipe specifically calls for – and there is no healthier alternative – the trick is to make sure that the cooking oil is hot enough to seal the outside of the food quickly, leaving the inside to steam, rather than fry. Otherwise the food can be permeated deeply by fats from the oil. The optimum temperature, where practical, for the hot oil is around 180°C/350°F but you should always wait until the oil is really hot before adding the food. Cooking oil of any variety should not be reused, because reheating may spark off a chemical reaction, creating harmful free radicals, which will be absorbed by the food you are cooking.

Stir-frying, one of the staple methods in Asian cooking, is always a better option. This requires only small amounts of oil, with, traditionally, a little water added. Stir-fried ingredients tend to absorb only small amounts of fat as a result.

If you are frying food, use small amounts of oils like sunflower oil or corn oil, as these predominantly consist of polyunsaturated fats. An alternative is to use an oil of monounsaturated fats, such as rapeseed (canola), groundnut (peanut) and virgin olive oil. These types of cooking oil are far healthier than saturated fats, such as butter or margarine.

BOILING, STEAMING AND MICROWAVING

All cooking methods inevitably result in the loss of some nutrients, the boiling of vegetables being a notable example. However, thorough cooking destroys harmful bacteria, particularly those found in fish and meat. It also destroys the toxic substances that are a natural constituent of some vegetables, such as kidney beans. From the food combiner's point of view, one of its most important attributes is that cooking makes the starch in rice and potatoes digestible. When vegetables are boiled, many water-soluble vitamins – particularly C and the B vitamins – simply leach away into the cooking water, particularly if the vegetables are over-cooked. For this reason, it is good practice to reserve the cooking water, rather than throwing it away. It can be turned into a nutritious vegetable stock to make soups, sauces and gravy.

Cabbage is a vegetable that needs handling with particular care if its nutrients are to be preserved. It is an excellent source of vitamins when raw, but more than half its Vitamin C content is usually lost if the vegetable is boiled until very soft, rather than a crisp, crunchy delight to the taste buds. Boiling broccoli, too, almost halves the amount of Vitamin C it contains. The way to minimize such nutrient loss is to bring the water to the boil before adding the vegetables, or, as in the case of potatoes, by boiling them in their skins, peeling them, if desired, once they are cooked. Many other vegetables can be cooked and eaten in this way, but remember that the skins should be cleaned scrupulously before boiling. Even then, there is the possibility that they may still contain residues of pesticides, moulds and some naturally-occurring toxins.

For vegetables, light steaming, stir-frying and microwaving are healthier cooking methods, since they all maximize nutrient retention. When broccoli is steamed, only 20 per cent of its Vitamin C content is lost, while stir-fried vegetables retain most of their nutrient content as well as their crispness. If you are cooking fruit, simmering gently and reserving the juice, or baking it, destroys the least number of nutrients that it contains.

Microwaving is considered to be the most nutrient-retentive cooking method, as well as retaining much of the moisture and colour of vegetables. However, as the method involves radiation, healthy living authorities believe that microwaves should be used with caution.

GRILLING (BROILING) AND ROASTING

Both grilling (broiling) and roasting are staples of any food combining regime.

When it comes to cooking fish and healthy cuts of meat, grilling (broiling) is a first-rate cooking option, particularly as far as the latter is concerned. This is because much of the fat from the meat simply drips down into the tray of the grill (broiler) pan. As an alternative, most meat and fish, along with healthy vegetable accompaniments, can be casseroled slowly, while many types of fish can be baked, wrapped in a parcel, roasted, poached or stir-fried.

RIGHT: Grilling (broiling) is the healthiest method of cooking chops, steaks and thin cuts of meat.

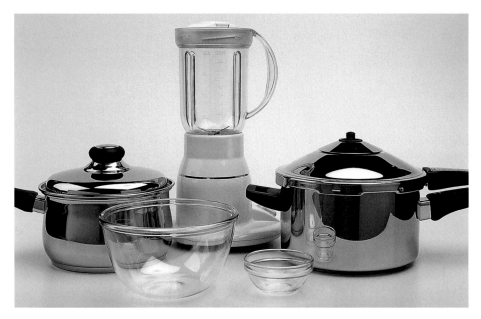

LEFT: Basic kitchen equipment for food combining might include a blender for making soups and juices, a pressure cooker to speed up the cooking times for pulses, and pans with well-fitting lids and suitable for an expandable steamer. A wok for stir-frying and a food processor for slicing vegetables quickly are particularly useful additions.

For larger cuts of meat and poultry, oven-roasting is still probably the most convenient and effective method. The healthy way to do this is to place what you are cooking on a rack in a roasting tin (pan), so that the fat can drain off. Roasting poultry in its skin will help to retain its natural moisture – although, like roast meat, it should be basted from time to time as it cooks – but it is healthier to remove the skin before serving. Doing this can reduce the saturated fat content in an average portion of chicken by as much as 60 per cent.

Many vegetables, too, can be roasted – classic examples include root vegetables, such as parsnips and turnips, as well as potatoes. It is best, however, to roast them on their own, rather than packing them into the roasting tin (pan) and cooking them in the fat that is dripping down from the poultry or meat.

KITCHEN EQUIPMENT

Cooking the food combining way does not mean throwing out all your existing kitchen utensils, cooking trays, or your cherished collection of pots and pans. However, there are a few items of kitchen equipment that you might consider buying if you have not already got them, as they can help make your cooking healthier – and life in the kitchen easier.

As far as cooking utensils are concerned, nothing can beat stainless steel or glass cookware. For steaming, you should look for an expandable metal steamer designed to fit into any size of pan, while, for stir-frying, a wok is an essential working tool. So, too, is a food-processor. Food combining means that you will be eating lots of vegetables and salads and the device is ideal for chopping the ingredients quickly. A blender or a purpose-designed juicer is a good idea if you intend to create your own fruit and vegetable juice drinks.

FREEZING AND THAWING: THE GOLDEN RULES

This chart shows you at a glance how to freeze and thaw some food staples safely. With the sole exception of green vegetables, it is vital to make sure that all frozen food is completely thawed before you cook it. Once it has thawed, you should never refreeze it.

FOOD	USE WITHIN	THAWING TIME
Butter	3–8 months	12 hours (refrigerator) 1–2 hours (room)
Whole white and oily fish	3–6 months	6–10 hours (refrigerator) 3–5 hours (room)
Fish steaks	3–6 months	6–10 hours (refrigerator) 3–5 hours (room)
Apples	9 months	7–8 hours (refrigerator) 4 hours (room)
Green vegetables	12 months	
Meat and poultry	4–6 months	5 hours (refrigerator) 2 hours (room)

Note: Unsalted (sweet) butter can be stored for longer than salted butter. You should scale and fillet fish before you freeze it and note that oily fish can be frozen for a maximum of three months. Apples should be washed, peeled, cored, sliced and blanched before freezing. Green vegetables should be washed, trimmed, blanched and drained.

Pressure cookers are first-rate for preparing quick soups or dishes based on pulses – the latter are excellent substitutes for animal protein. You need to to destroy the toxins pulses contain in their natural state, which means boiling them in fresh water for ten minutes. The water is thrown away and they are then cooked in the pressure cooker for 5–20 minutes more, depending on the type of pulse. Slow cookers are also useful; they are perfect for succulent, slow-cooking casseroles and stews, based on healthy low-fat ingredients and nutritious stocks. Finally, a microwave can be a good investment: cooking fish in a microwave means that you can avoid the use of fat; it also takes far less time to bake potatoes in a microwave than it does to bake them in a conventional oven.

STORING FOOD IN THE FREEZER

You need to take just as much care in the storing and preserving food as you did in its initial preparation. Many foods are quick to spoil for a variety of reasons, chief of which are the growth of micro-organisms within the food, internal enzyme action, oxidation, and temperature fluctuations. Bacterial growth, for instance, is at its most prolific at temperatures of 7–60°C/45–90°F: if you are reheating left-overs, you should make sure that the temperature reaches at least 150°C/300°F. Not only should you make sure that frozen food is totally thawed before you cook it – you should

never refreeze it once it has thawed. Take care about what you wrap food in as well, as there is research to indicate that the plasticizers and other chemicals used in some types of clingfilm (plastic wrap) may have the potential to be harmful.

Freezing food is now part of the average family's way of life. It not only slows down the enzyme activity that can lead to food spoilage, but checks bacterial growth as well. The freezing process makes it impossible for the bacteria to gain access to the moisture they need in order to multiply. Most foods freeze well, but not all. For example, some soft fruits, which have a high water content, may turn into a mush when thawed. Other foods that do not freeze well include milk, cream, mushrooms and cucumber.

When stocking or restocking a freezer, you should wrap what you intend to freeze carefully in freezer bags and label the latter clearly. The labels should indicate what is in each bag and the date on which the bags were frozen. Pack the food as closely together as possible, as this is a more efficient use of space as well as being more economical.

Some freezers come with a self-defrosting facility: others need to be manually defrosted. To do this, empty the freezer of its contents and wash it out with a mixture of warm water and bicarbonate of soda (baking soda), which will clean the freezer effectively without leaving a lingering smell. You should get the freezer's temperature down to at least -18°C/ -15°F) before you refill it.

Stocking a refrigerator the healthy way
The following tips will help to preserve your food in optimum condition:

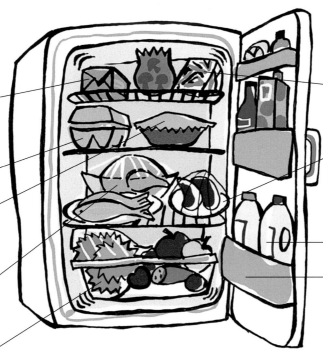

Dairy products, such as butter and cream, should be kept covered. Otherwise they tend to absorb the flavours and smells of other foods.

Do not store eggs in egg trays in the door. Rather, they should be stored in the main part of the refrigerator, where they will keep for up to three weeks.

Store cooked meats on a separate shelf from raw meats.

Raw meat and fish should be stored as low as possible in the refrigerator to stop them dripping on to other foods. Store poultry giblets separately.

To retain their freshness, store salad vegetables in plastic bags in the salad drawer. Store mushrooms in a paper bag so that they do not sweat.

Store cheese in foil, not clingfilm (plastic wrap). The latter is not suitable as wrapping material for food with a high fat content.

Discard the polystyrene (Styrofoam) trays that meat may be supplied on, as they will slow down cooling. Drain off any fluid and cover the meat loosely.

The warmest part of any refrigerator is its door. Only non-perishable items should be stored here, or ones that will be used quickly, such as milk, bottled water and fruit juice.

The optimum refrigerator temperature is 5°C/41°F or less.

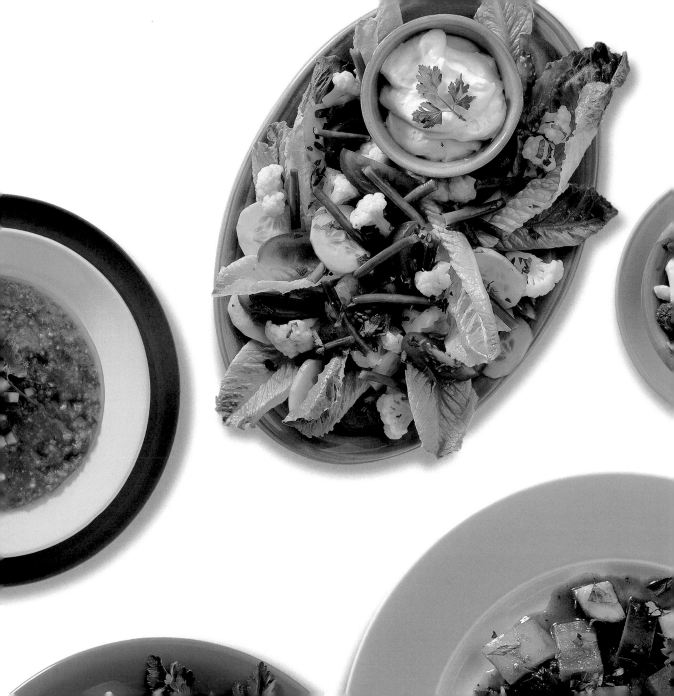

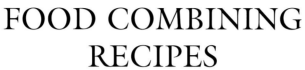

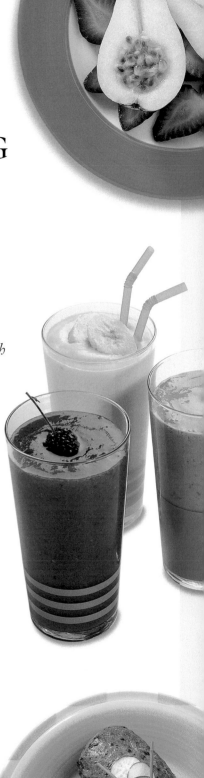

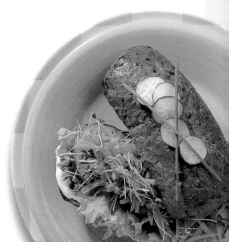

CHAPTER 6

FOOD COMBINING RECIPES

*M*y *daughter Inge's delicious recipes
from around the world are an
inspiration, showing you how to put food-
combining theory into practice. Through them,
you will become familiar with the types and
combinations of food that are good for you, which
will bring relief to your digestive system and
thereby improve your overall health. (Inge did
not write any of the recipes that contain meat,
fish, poultry or game.)*

BEFORE YOU START

The recipes in this book give quantities in metric and imperial
and standard cup measures. Remember to follow only one set of
measures in a recipe: *they are not interchangeable.*
The recipes refer to imperial pints, as used in the UK.
An imperial pint contains 20 fl oz, whereas the US pint is 16 fl oz.
Throughout, too, tablespoons refer to the UK standard.
The UK and US tablespoon holds 15 ml. Teaspoons contain 5 ml.

SAUCES AND DRESSINGS

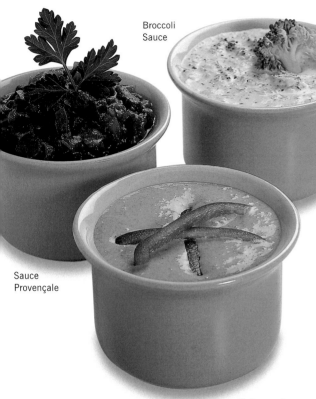

Broccoli
Sauce

Sauce
Provençale

Creamy Red (Bell) Pepper Sauce

Sauces and dressings can make all the difference to the taste of a dish, especially if they are fresh and homemade. Their chief drawback is that they usually contain more than their fair share of fats. This has been taken into account in the creation of the healthy recipes in this section. Try combining these sauces and dressings with other dishes in this book, or with dishes of your own devising.

SAUCE PROVENÇALE

Ingredients
½ green (bell) pepper
1 tbsp olive oil
½ onion, peeled and finely chopped
3 beefsteak (beef) tomatoes
2 dried bay leaves
1 pinch each dried oregano, basil and mixed herbs
1 tsp stock granules or bouillon powder
pinch of paprika
freshly ground black pepper

Preparation time: 10–12 minutes
Cooking time: 3–4 minutes

1. Deseed the green (bell) pepper and chop finely.
2. Heat the olive oil in a pan over a low heat and gently cook the onion and the (bell) pepper until soft.
3. Skin, quarter and deseed the tomatoes. Add to the pan with the bay leaves, herbs and stock granules or bouillon powder.
4. Simmer the mixture over a low heat. Season with the paprika and pepper before serving.

SPICY RED SAUCE

This sauce goes well with grilled (broiled) vegetables. Choose a tomato ketchup that is free from artificial additives.

Ingredients
125 ml/4 fl oz/½ cup tomato ketchup
1 tbsp creamed horseradish
1 tsp French mustard
½ tbsp white wine vinegar
½ tbsp lemon juice
3 drops Tabasco sauce
1 spring onion (scallion), finely chopped
freshly ground cayenne pepper, to season
pinch of paprika, to season

Preparation time: 5 minutes

1. Combine the tomato ketchup, horseradish, mustard, wine vinegar, lemon juice and Tabasco.
2. Add the spring onion (scallion) to the mixture. Blend the sauce well and season with cayenne pepper and paprika.

BROCCOLI SAUCE

Ingredients
200 g/7 oz broccoli
125 ml/4 fl oz/½ cup cream
freshly ground black pepper
1 tsp stock granules or bouillon powder

Preparation time: 10 minutes
Cooking time: 6 minutes

1. Wash the broccoli, cut into pieces and steam until tender (about 6 minutes).
2. Purée the steamed broccoli.
3. Add the cream and season with the pepper and the stock or bouillon powder.

Cocktail
Sauce

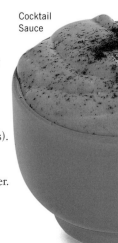

MUSTARD SAUCE

This sauce makes a good accompaniment to boiled or steamed asparagus.

Ingredients
3 tbsp wholegrain mustard
2 tbsp Mayonnaise (see page 192)
1 tbsp lemon juice
2 tbsp sour cream
2 lemon balm leaves, finely chopped

Preparation time: 4–5 minutes

1. Thoroughly combine the mustard, mayonnaise, lemon juice and sour cream.
2. Stir in the chopped lemon balm leaves.

COCKTAIL SAUCE

Serve with salads, as a dip or with cold stuffed tomatoes.

Ingredients
4 tbsp Mayonnaise (see page 192)
2 tbsp tomato ketchup (additive-free is best)
1 tsp paprika
freshly ground black pepper

Preparation time: 3–4 minutes

Mix the mayonnaise with the tomato ketchup and the paprika. Season with pepper.

ISTANBUL GARLIC SAUCE

Ingredients
4 tbsp Mayonnaise (see page 192)
2 tbsp Greek (plain strained) yogurt
2 garlic cloves, peeled
¼ cucumber, peeled, deseeded and shredded
salt and freshly ground black pepper
1 tbsp chopped fresh chives, to garnish

Preparation time: 5–8 minutes

1. Mix the mayonnaise with the yogurt.
2. In a separate dish, crush the garlic on to the cucumber shreds, then add to the sauce.
3. Season the mixture with salt and pepper and garnish with the chopped chives.

CREAMY RED (BELL) PEPPER SAUCE

Ingredients
2 red (bell) peppers
1 shallot
1 tbsp butter
125 ml/4 fl oz/½ cup cream
salt and freshly ground black pepper

Preparation time: 8–10 minutes
Cooking time: 3–4 minutes

1. Clean and deseed the (bell) peppers. Finely chop the (bell) peppers and the shallot.
2. Melt the butter in a pan on a low heat.
3. Sauté the (bell) peppers and shallot in the butter until soft.
4. Transfer the vegetables to a blender. Add the cream and season with salt and pepper.
5. Blend until smooth. Serve the sauce hot.

TOMATO SAUCE

Ingredients
4 beefsteak (beef) tomatoes
½ onion, peeled and finely chopped
1 tbsp oil
freshly ground black pepper
1 tsp stock granules or bouillon powder
1 tbsp chopped fresh basil

Preparation time: 10 minutes
Cooking time: 3–4 minutes

1. Skin, quarter and deseed the tomatoes.
2. Heat the oil in a pan on a low heat and cook the tomato and onion until soft.
3. Purée the mixture in a blender, then strain. Season with the pepper, stock granules or bouillon powder and the basil.

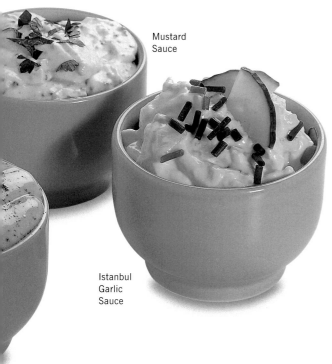

Mustard
Sauce

Istanbul
Garlic
Sauce

AIOLI

A classic accompaniment to crunchy raw vegetables, aioli also goes well with other foods, especially cold potatoes.

Ingredients
1 egg or 1 egg yolk
1 tsp mustard
250 ml/8 fl oz/1 cup olive oil
juice of ½ lemon
2 garlic cloves, peeled

Preparation time: 5–8 minutes

1. Combine the egg and the mustard in a blender, unless you are beating by hand, in which case, use the egg yolk.
2. With the motor running or beating constantly, add the oil little by little, followed by the lemon juice.
3. Squeeze in the juice from the garlic and mix well.

MAYONNAISE

This recipe may used on its own or as a base for many other sauces and dressings.

Ingredients
1 egg or 1 egg yolk (see Aioli method)
1 tsp mustard
250 ml/8 fl oz/1 cup vegetable oil
juice of 1–2 lemons
salt and freshly ground black pepper

Preparation time: 5–8 minutes

1. Combine the egg or the egg yolk and the mustard in a blender.
2. With the motor running or beating constantly, add the oil little by little, followed by the lemon juice.
3. Season with salt and pepper and blend again until smooth.

VINAIGRETTE

To vary this vinaigrette, make it as described here, but omit the chopped onion. Instead add two tablespoons of tomato purée (paste), mix well and season with oregano and paprika.

Ingredients
1 tsp mustard or ground mustard seeds
125 ml/4 fl oz/½ cup oil
4 tbsp wine vinegar, cider (apple) vinegar or lemon juice
pinch of spices and chopped fresh herbs to taste, such as paprika and oregano
½ onion, peeled and finely chopped

Preparation time: 4–5 minutes

1. Mix the mustard with the oil.
2 Add the wine vinegar, cider (apple) vinegar or lemon juice and mix until well combined.
3. Season with spices, herbs and the chopped onion.

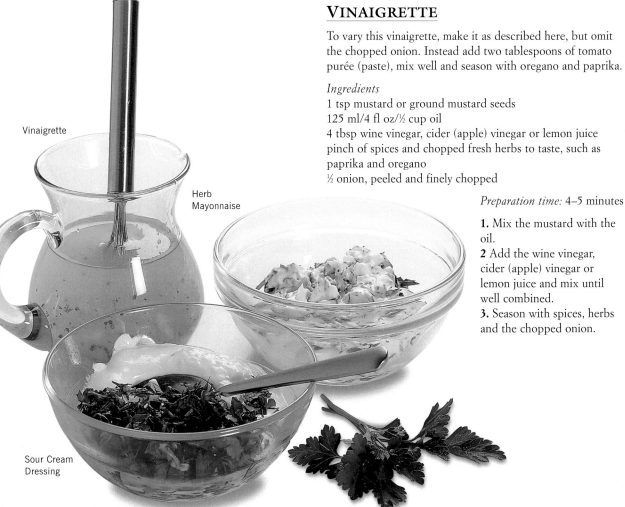

Vinaigrette

Herb
Mayonnaise

Sour Cream
Dressing

CREAM SAUCE

Ingredients
25 g/1 oz/2 tbsp butter
1 tbsp flour
125 ml/4 fl oz/½ cup vegetable stock (see page 206)
125 ml/4 fl oz/½ cup cream
pinch each nutmeg, salt, freshly ground black pepper and paprika to taste

Preparation time: 5 minutes
Cooking time: 8–10 minutes

1. Melt the butter in a pan. Gradually add the flour, stirring constantly.
2. Add the vegetable stock. Continue to stir until the sauce has thickened.
3. Add the cream and season with the nutmeg, salt, pepper and paprika.

YOGURT DRESSING

Ingredients
2 parts Mayonnaise (see opposite)
1 part live yogurt or buttermilk
chopped fresh or dried herbs, to taste
1 garlic clove, peeled and crushed
a little finely chopped onion

Preparation time: 4–5 minutes

1. Blend the mayonnaise with the yogurt or buttermilk.
2. Season the dressing with the chopped herbs, crushed garlic and chopped onion.

HERB MAYONNAISE

Ingredients
2 tbsp Mayonnaise (see opposite)
1 tbsp finely chopped fresh herbs

Preparation time: 2–3 minutes

Blend the mayonnaise with the fresh herbs.

SOUR CREAM DRESSING

Ingredients
200 ml/7fl oz/scant 1 cup sour cream
1 tbsp finely chopped fresh garden herbs, such as dill, chives, parsley, basil or peppermint, to taste

Preparation time: 2–3 minutes

Mix the sour cream with the herbs.

LOUISIANA SALAD DRESSING

Chill this dressing for a few hours before serving. It goes well with a mixed salad.

Ingredients
3 tbsp Aioli (see opposite)
2 tbsp sour cream
2 tbsp tomato ketchup
1 tsp lemon juice
1 tsp spicy mustard
2 spring onions (scallions), finely chopped

To season:
freshly ground cayenne pepper
2 drops Tabasco sauce
pinch of grated horseradish
salt

Preparation time: 4–5 minutes

1. Combine the aioli, sour cream, tomato ketchup, lemon juice and mustard.
2. Add the chopped spring onions (scallions) to the aioli and cream dressing and mix well.
3. Season with cayenne pepper, Tabasco, horseradish and salt.

DIET DRESSING

Ingredients
4 beefsteak (beef) tomatoes
½ tbsp lemon juice
½ tbsp chopped fresh basil
½ tbsp chopped fresh oregano
freshly ground black pepper

Preparation time: 10 minutes

1. Plunge the tomatoes briefly into boiling water and remove the skins. Deseed, quarter and purée them.
2. Mix the puréed tomatoes with the lemon juice.
3. Season with basil, oregano and pepper.

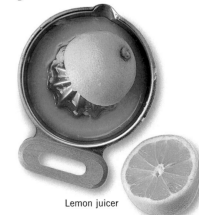

Lemon juicer

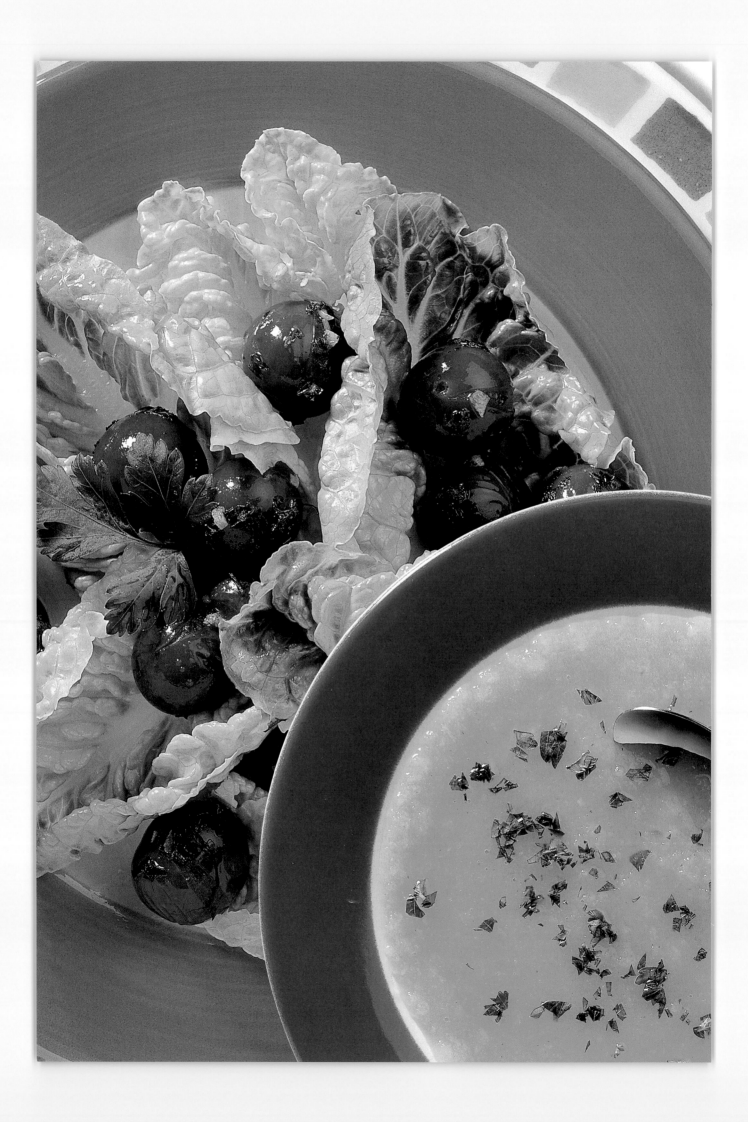

APPETIZERS AND SOUPS

One of the most enduring myths about food combining is that achieving the necessary balances in the diet is time-consuming and difficult. Another is that successful food combining means adopting a somewhat restricted diet, cutting out lots of your favourite treats and comfort foods. As the recipes in this chapter show, nothing could be further from the truth. Here, you will find plenty of nourishing appetizers that taste as good as they look and take only a few minutes to prepare. They can be eaten as part of a main meal or on their own as healthy snacks. The soups that feature in this chapter are equally nutritious. Soup can be a filling and nourishing meal in itself, while the way in which it is cooked means that its ingredients retain most of their healthy nutrients. If you can, it is always better to use fresh stock, rather than stock (bouillon) cubes. The latter are not only high in sodium – one cube can contain up to a teaspoon of salt – but can also contain monosodium glutamate and other additives.

STUFFED MUSHROOMS

(SERVES 4)

Ingredients
20 large, closed cup mushrooms
20 g/¾ oz/4 tsp butter, plus extra butter for grilling (broiling)
1 shallot, peeled and finely chopped
1 garlic clove, peeled and finely chopped
3 fresh basil leaves
1 fresh parsley sprig
8 fresh chives
freshly ground black pepper
60 g/2¼ oz/generous 1 cup fresh white breadcrumbs
mixed salad leaves (greens), to serve

Preparation time: 10–15 minutes
Cooking time: 6–8 minutes

1. Wipe the mushrooms clean. (Mushrooms should never be washed, because they absorb water and become spongy.) Remove the stalks (stems) and chop them finely.
2. Melt 20 g/¾ oz/4 teaspoons of butter in a pan on a low heat. Sauté the chopped mushroom stalks (stems), shallot and garlic until soft.
3. Wash the basil, parsley and chives, pat them dry and chop finely. Add to the mushroom mixture and season with pepper.
4. Stir in the breadcrumbs, then fill the mushroom cups with the mixture.
5. Place a knob of butter on each mushroom and cook under a medium grill (broiler) until golden brown.
6. Serve on a bed of mixed salad.

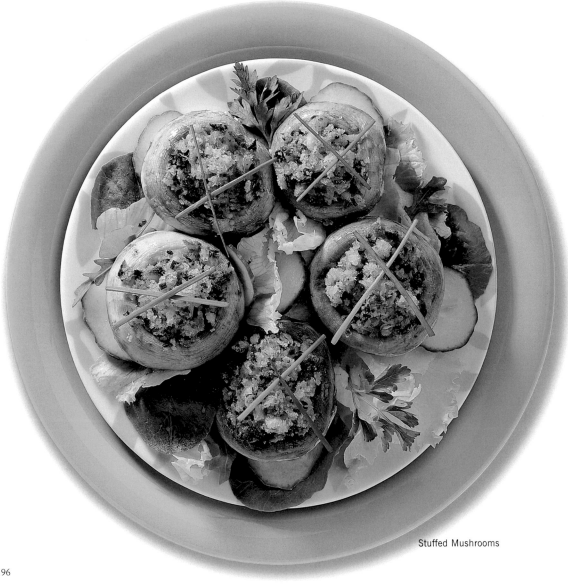

Stuffed Mushrooms

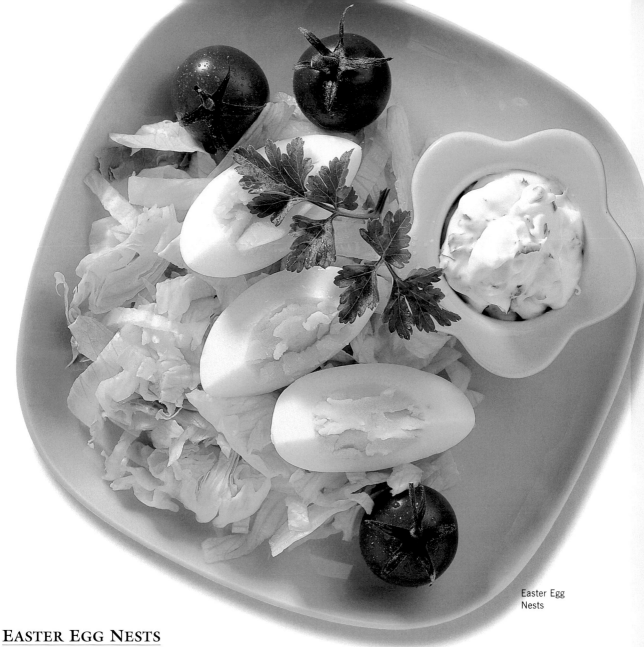

Easter Egg
Nests

EASTER EGG NESTS

(SERVES 4)

Ingredients
½ medium head of lettuce
3 eggs
12 cherry tomatoes
4 tbsp Herb Mayonnaise (see page 192), to serve

Preparation time: 5–10 minutes plus 30 minutes cooling
Cooking time: 10–12 minutes

1. Wash the lettuce, dry the leaves and cut into strips. Form four individual lettuce 'nests' on four plates.
2. Hard-boil (hard-cook) the eggs. Let them cool, remove the shells, and slice lengthways into four. Fill each lettuce nest with three slices of egg.
3. Wash and dry the cherry tomatoes, then divide them among the nests.
4. Serve with Herb Mayonnaise.

SOUTHERN TOMATOES

(SERVES 4)

Ingredients
4 small tomatoes
1–2 mozzarella cheeses
4 large, crinkly lettuce leaves
12 fresh basil leaves, to garnish

Preparation time: 5–10 minutes

1. Wash the tomatoes and cut into slices.
2. Slice the mozzarella cheese, with an egg slicer if possible.
3. Place a lettuce leaf on each of four dessert plates. Arrange alternate slices of cheese and tomato on each leaf.
4. Garnish each portion with the basil leaves.

AVOCADO STUFFED WITH RAW VEGETABLES

(SERVES 4)

Ingredients
2 ripe avocados
1 tbsp lemon juice
4 leaves red lettuce
4 mushrooms
10 cm/4 inches cucumber, peeled
4 radishes, chopped

For the dressing:
1 tbsp vegetable oil
½ tbsp lemon juice
pinch finely chopped fresh mixed herbs

Preparation time: 10 minutes

1. Cut the avocados in half, remove the stones (pits) and sprinkle the flesh of the fruit with lemon juice to prevent discoloration. Put each half on a separate plate.
2. Wash the lettuce, pat dry, cut into strips and fill each avocado with them.
3. Wipe the mushrooms clean and slice thinly. Slice the cucumber thinly.
4. Arrange the mushroom and cucumber slices on top of the avocado halves.
5. Garnish with the radishes.
6. For the dressing, combine the oil, lemon juice and herbs. Whisk together, then pour over the avocados.

HERBED MUSHROOM SLICES

(SERVES 4)

Ingredients
4 slices of wholemeal (whole-wheat) bread
4–6 tbsp Herb Mayonnaise (see page 192)
4 lettuce leaves
125 g/4½ oz/1¼ cups mushrooms
juice of ½ lemon
mixed fresh herbs, finely chopped, to garnish

Preparation time: 5–8 minutes
Cooking time: 2–3 minutes

1. Toast the bread.
2. Spread the toast with the Herb Mayonnaise.
3. Wash the lettuce, pat dry, then cut it into strips and place on the toast.
4. Wipe the mushrooms clean, slice thinly and arrange on top of the lettuce.
5. Squeeze the lemon over the mushroom toasts and garnish with the chopped herbs.

ALL ABOUT AVOCADOS

A ripe avocado not only tastes delicious: it has positive health benefits. Its flesh is a rich source of Vitamin E and potassium and it also contains useful amounts of Vitamin B_6, Vitamin C, riboflavin, manganese and monounsaturated fats. The only drawback is that avocados, particularly certain Californian varieties, are high in calories. Just one pear may contain up to 400 calories.

* Avocados have the highest protein content of any fruit.
* They can be round, pear-shaped, no bigger than a hen's egg, or weigh up to 1 kg/2¼ lb.
* Depending on the variety, skin colour can vary from dark green and crimson, to yellow and near-black.
* Unlike most other fruits, avocados start to ripen only after they have been harvested. If you buy an unripe avocado, keep it for a few days at room temperature – this will allow it to mature, and the flesh will soften.
* Although avocados were discovered in the Americas by Spanish explorers as long ago as 1519, it took until the 1900s for the fruit to win widespread popularity. In the years in between, most people dismissed it as having no flavour.

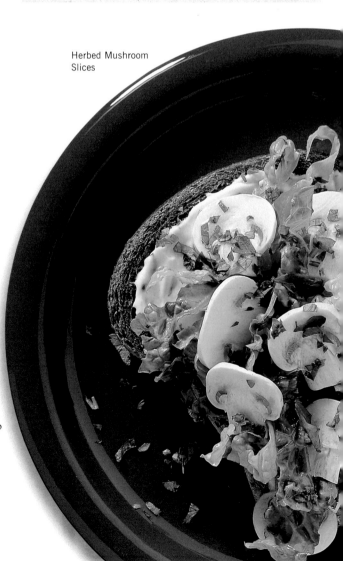

Herbed Mushroom Slices

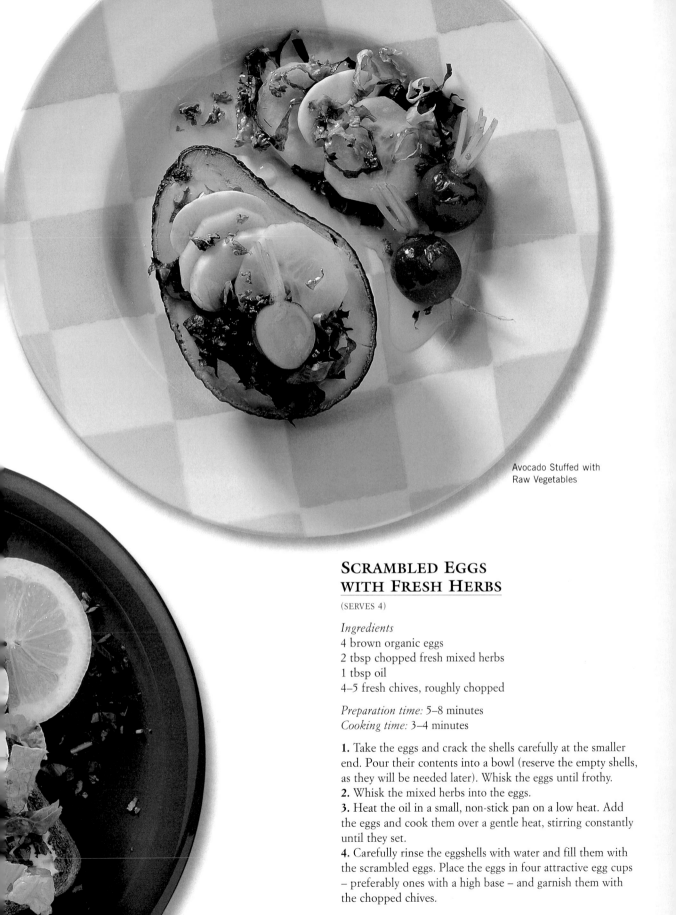

Avocado Stuffed with
Raw Vegetables

SCRAMBLED EGGS WITH FRESH HERBS

(SERVES 4)

Ingredients
4 brown organic eggs
2 tbsp chopped fresh mixed herbs
1 tbsp oil
4–5 fresh chives, roughly chopped

Preparation time: 5–8 minutes
Cooking time: 3–4 minutes

1. Take the eggs and crack the shells carefully at the smaller end. Pour their contents into a bowl (reserve the empty shells, as they will be needed later). Whisk the eggs until frothy.
2. Whisk the mixed herbs into the eggs.
3. Heat the oil in a small, non-stick pan on a low heat. Add the eggs and cook them over a gentle heat, stirring constantly until they set.
4. Carefully rinse the eggshells with water and fill them with the scrambled eggs. Place the eggs in four attractive egg cups – preferably ones with a high base – and garnish them with the chopped chives.

199

SPICY AVOCADO

(SERVES 2)

Ingredients
1 ripe avocado
1 green celery stick (stalk), chopped
1 tbsp lemon juice
1 tsp curry powder
4 red lettuce leaves
2 lemon slices and 2 black olives, to garnish

Preparation time: 8–10 minutes

1. Cut the avocado in half and remove the stone (pit).
Carefully scoop out the flesh with a spoon and purée with the
celery in a blender. Reserve the avocado skin halves.
2. Add the lemon juice, which prevents discoloration, and the
curry powder. Mix well.
3. Wash the lettuce, pat dry and divide between two plates.
Fill the avocado halves with the avocado purée.
4. Place the avocado halves on the
lettuce and garnish with the
lemon slices and olives.

OYSTER MUSHROOMS COATED WITH BREADCRUMBS

(SERVES 4)

Ingredients
400 g/14 oz/5⅔ cups small oyster mushrooms
1 egg white
3–4 tbsp fresh white breadcrumbs and/or sesame seeds
1 tbsp vegetable oil or butter

Preparation time: 10 minutes
Cooking time: 4–6 minutes

1. Wipe the mushrooms clean.
2. Beat the egg white and pour into a soup plate.
3. Spread the breadcrumbs and/or sesame seeds over one or
two plates as required.
4. Coat the mushrooms first in the egg white, then dip them
in the breadcrumbs and/or sesame seeds.
5. Heat the oil or butter in a frying pan (skillet). Cook the
mushrooms on a medium heat, turning them so they cook
evenly, until they are golden brown.

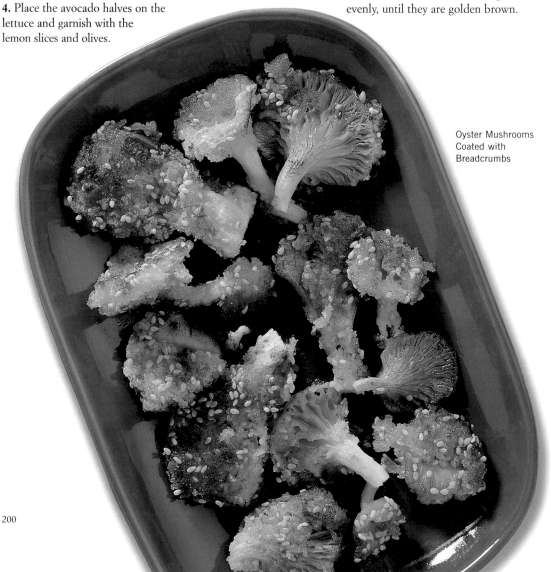

Oyster Mushrooms
Coated with
Breadcrumbs

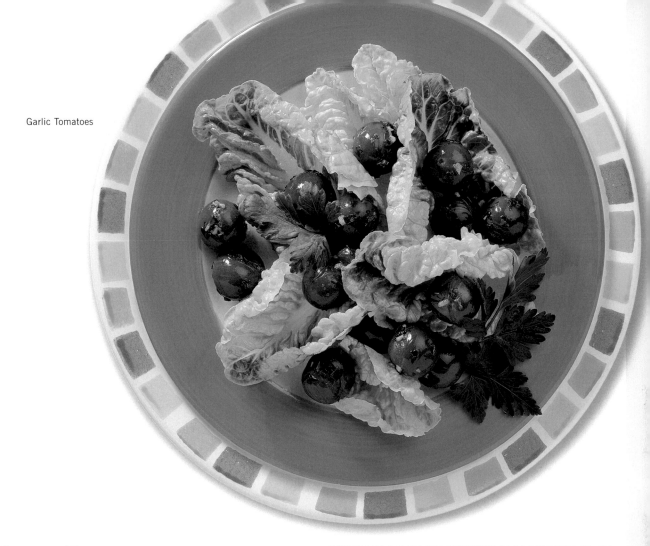

Garlic Tomatoes

GARLIC TOMATOES

(SERVES 4)

Ingredients
300 g/11 oz cherry tomatoes
1 tbsp oil
1 garlic clove, peeled and finely chopped
3 fresh parsley sprigs, finely chopped
3 fresh basil leaves, finely chopped
shredded lettuce, to serve

Preparation time: 5 minutes
Cooking time: 3–4 minutes

1. Wash and dry the tomatoes.
2. Heat the oil in a non-stick frying pan (skillet). Sauté the tomatoes for 5 minutes, sprinkling the garlic and herbs on to them as you do so, shaking the pan frequently to brown them evenly.
3. Serve on a bed of shredded lettuce.

GARLIC: THE MIRACLE BULB

Modern science has now confirmed what herbalists and naturopaths have been proclaiming for many years – garlic is a life-enhancing plant. The bulb's antiviral and antibacterial properties are now recognized and supported by evidence from clinical studies. Scientists have demonstrated that the sulphur compounds in garlic are good for the heart – eaten daily, the compounds will help to lower blood pressure, check excessive cholesterol production and raise the amount of beneficial lipoproteins the blood contains.
* Raw garlic is a good remedy for a cold, helping to reduce nasal congestion and fight infection.
* In herbal medicine, garlic is prescribed as a remedy for many complaints, ranging from asthma to arthritis.
* Studies in China suggest that eating garlic regularly may help the body to protect itself against the development of stomach cancer.
* Garlic is best eaten raw, since many of its health-giving properties are lost through cooking.
* The herb's main drawbacks are that it makes the breath smell, and in susceptible people it can trigger allergies and migraines. Touching peeled cloves has also been known to cause dermatitis.

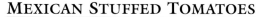

FENNEL AU GRATIN

(SERVES 4)

Ingredients
2 medium bulbs fennel
pat of butter, for greasing
freshly ground black pepper
paprika
4 medium slices Camembert
frisée lettuce, to garnish

Preparation time: 5 minutes
Cooking time: 6–8 minutes

1. Cut the fennel bulbs in half, trim, then steam for
2–3 minutes until just tender.
2. Put the halved bulbs in a greased, flameproof shallow dish.
Season with pepper and paprika.
3. Place the Camembert slices over the fennel and cook under
a medium grill (broiler) for 3–5 minutes until browned.
4. Serve on individual plates, garnished with frisée.

FENNEL SEEDS: SPICE AND MEDICINE

Aromatic fennel seeds are not only one of the world's oldest-known spices, they double up as one of folk medicine's most ancient healing remedies. In India, fennel seeds have long been chewed after eating to prevent bad breath, while in classical Greece and Rome the seeds were believed to prevent obesity. There are two varieties of the vegetable itself – Florence fennel and garden fennel. The former has a hard, bulbous, fleshy base with a crunchy texture, while the latter has dark green spindly stems and feathery leaves. Florence fennel, with its delicate, but distinctive, liquorice taste is frequently eaten raw in salads or served as a side vegetable, either boiled or braised.
* Both types of fennel contain beta-carotene, which the body turns into Vitamin A, and folate, which is needed for red blood-cell formation.
* Drinking tea made from fennel seeds can help to ease a wide range of digestive problems, from hiccups and colic to flatulence and bloating.
* Hippocrates, the ancient Greek physician, and Nicholas Culpeper, the 17th-century British herbalist, both recommended that breastfeeding mothers should drink fennel teas to stimulate milk production. However, because the seeds are thought to encourage the muscles of the uterus to contract, it is best to avoid drinking fennel tea during pregnancy.

MEXICAN STUFFED TOMATOES

(SERVES 2)

Ingredients
4 large tomatoes
¼ green (bell) pepper
60 g/2¼ oz/⅓ cup cooked sweetcorn (corn)
60 g/2¼ oz) medium-fat cheese, such as Cheddar
lamb's lettuce (mâche), to serve

Preparation time: 15 minutes

1. Wash the tomatoes, cut off the tops and scoop out the flesh. (Reserve the flesh for use in another recipe.)
2. Wash the green (bell) pepper, remove the seeds and finely chop the flesh.
3. Mix together the sweetcorn (corn) and finely chopped (bell) pepper.
4. Dice the cheese and add to the vegetable mixture. Make sure they are well combined.
5. Fill the tomato shells with the cheese and vegetable mixture and arrange them on a bed of lamb's lettuce (mâche).

STUFFED EGGS

(SERVES 4)

Ingredients
4 eggs
1–2 tbsp Mayonnaise (see page 192)
1 tsp curry powder
4 lettuce leaves
cress, to garnish

Preparation time: 8–10 minutes plus 30 minutes cooling
Cooking time: 10 minutes

1. Hard-boil (hard-cook) the eggs. Let them cool, then remove the shells and cut the eggs in half. Carefully scoop out the yolks.
2. Mash and blend the egg yolks with the mayonnaise and curry powder.
3. Put the lettuce leaves on a plate and arrange the egg halves on them.
4. Using a piping (pastry) bag, fill the egg halves with the yolk mixture. Garnish with cress.

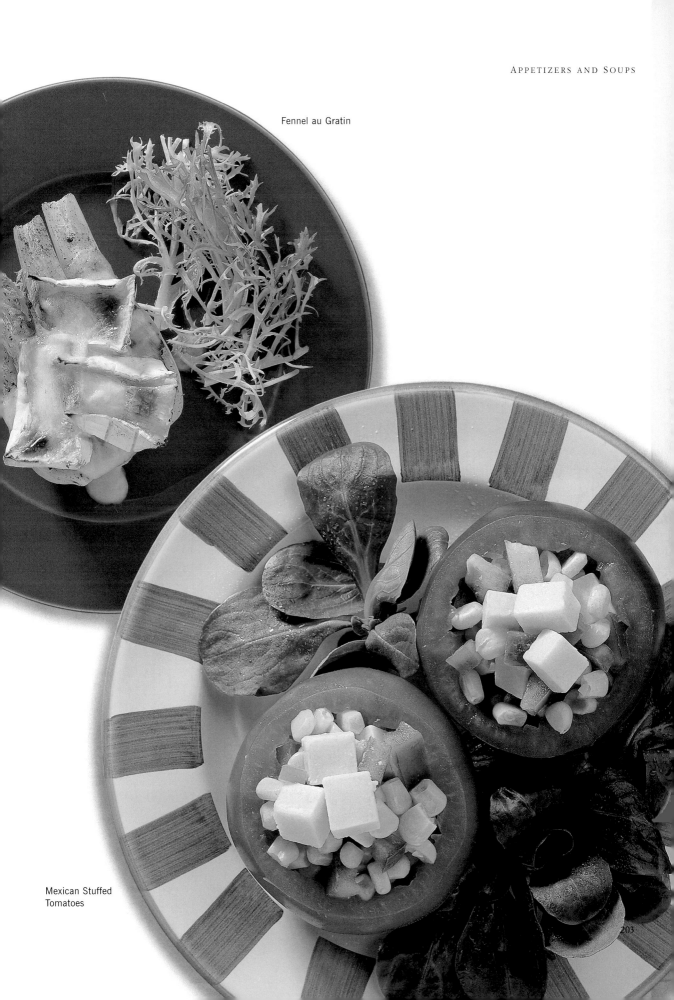

Fennel au Gratin

Mexican Stuffed
Tomatoes

ARTICHOKES: HELPFUL HEALERS

Whether served hot or cold, with their leaves or stripped down to their hearts, globe artichokes are excellent sources of folate and potassium. There is also scientific evidence to support the theory that the cynarin in the vegetable's edible base has useful healing powers. This view is promulgated by many herbalists, who often prescribe artichoke-based preparations for gallstones and other conditions. Research studies in Germany have shown that the cynarin artichokes contain can help to reduce blood cholesterol levels and improve liver function and that it also has a beneficial effect on the gallbladder, particularly if gallstones develop. Artichokes are also valuable because they are among the foods that seldom, if ever, trigger allergic reactions. (Other non-allergenic foods include pears, peaches, lettuce, apples, carrots and brown, white and wild rice.)

* Artichokes are rich in folate, a group of compounds derived from folic acid, which the body needs for cell division, the formation of DNA and RNA and for protein synthesis. Folate is also vital for the healthy growth of a baby during pregnancy and for the formation of the blood protein haemoglobin, which carries oxygen from the lungs to the other tissues of the body.

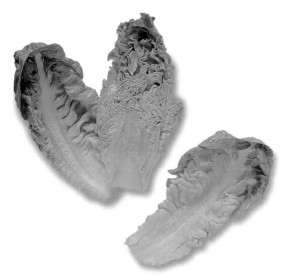

* Artichokes are thought to limit the rise in blood sugar levels after eating, and is often recommended to help diabetics.
* Globe artichokes are not related to the Jerusalem artichoke.

STUFFED ARTICHOKES
(SERVES 4)

Ingredients
4 medium-size globe artichokes
3 tbsp Mayonnaise (see page 192)
1 tbsp natural (plain) yogurt
2 tbsp chopped fresh mixed herbs
2 pickled gherkins (cornichons), finely chopped
1 shallot, peeled and thinly sliced
salt and freshly ground black pepper
paprika

Preparation time: 15–20 minutes plus 30 minutes cooling
Cooking time: 40–45 minutes

1. Wash the artichokes thoroughly and cut off their stalks. Cook them in a pan of boiling water for 40–45 minutes. (An artichoke is fully cooked when its base can be pierced easily with a fork.) Remove from the water and set aside to cool.
2. Remove the middle part – the small leaves – from the artichokes, so that the hearts are visible. Then remove the stalks and cut a slice off the bottom of each to level them, so that they will stand upright.
3. Blend together the mayonnaise, yogurt and herbs.
4. Add the gherkins (cornichons) and shallot to the sauce and blend well.
5. Season with salt, pepper and paprika.
6. Fill the hollow of each artichoke with the sauce and serve. Peel off the leaves one by one and dip them in the sauce. The lower part of each leaf is edible and so is the delicious base.

SOUR STUFFED TOMATOES
(SERVES 2)

Ingredients
4 tomatoes
4 tbsp finely chopped pickled vegetables
1 pickled gherkin (cornichon), finely chopped
1 pickled onion, finely chopped
4 lettuce leaves, to serve

Preparation time: 10–15 minutes

1. Wash the tomatoes, cut off the tops, scoop out the flesh (reserve this for later use, such as soup) and place the shells upside down to drain.
2. Mix all the pickled vegetables together, then fill the tomatoes with the mixture.
3. Place the lettuce leaves on a plate and arrange the stuffed tomatoes on top.

TASTY CROISSANTS

(MAKES 6)

Ingredients
375 g/13 oz frozen puff pastry
1 tbsp vegetable oil
6 mushrooms
1 garlic clove, peeled and finely chopped
freshly ground black pepper
2 shallots, peeled and finely chopped
3 fresh parsley sprigs, chopped
8 fresh chives, chopped
3 tbsp chopped vegetables, such as onion, carrots
and broccoli

Preparation time: 20–25 minutes
Cooking time: 20–25 minutes

1. Preheat the oven to 190°C/375°F/Gas Mark 5.
2. Thaw the pastry 15 minutes before it is needed.
3. Cut the pastry into 3 equal rectangles, then halve each one diagonally to make six triangles.
4. Heat half of the oil in a non-stick frying pan (skillet). Wipe the mushrooms clean, slice them, then add them to the pan with the garlic and season with pepper. Sauté them until soft.
5. In a separate pan, sautée the shallots until golden, adding a pinch or two of the fresh parsley and chives.
6. In a wok, stir-fry the vegetables in the remaining oil until they are soft.
7. Fill the pastry triangles first with the mushroom mixture, then with the shallots, followed by the stir-fried vegetables. When you have finished, roll the stuffed pastry into croissants.
8. Place the croissants on a baking (cookie) sheet and bake for 10–15 minutes, until golden.

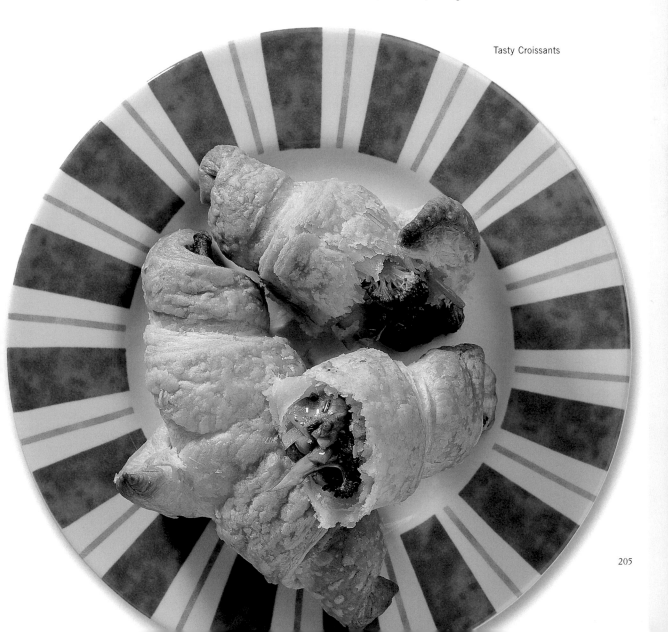

Tasty Croissants

ALL ABOUT STOCKS

A good homemade stock is the ideal basis for any nourishing soup. However, if you are pressed for time, the fresh stock you can find on sale in most supermarkets and food stores is a good, convenient alternative. The secret behind almost any stock recipe, including the one given here, is the time taken to cook it: the long, slow simmering it undergoes, which concentrates its flavour. Stock (bouillon) cubes should be avoided, if possible, because they are usually high in sodium (salt) and contain artificial flavour-enhancers and thickeners.

Although instant vegetable stock granules or bouillon powder are useful for quick stocks – they can also substitute for salt when it comes to seasoning a dish – their use, on the whole, is second best. As well as containing highly concentrated extracts of beef, chicken, mushroom and other vegetables, commercial stock cubes harbour many additives, such as monosodium glutamate, sugar, salt, yeast extract and thickeners. Monosodium glutamate can trigger headaches and the thickeners are often derived from wheat, which can adversely affect those with gluten intolerance.

Stock and soup hints and tips
* Although a toothsome fish stock can be made from almost any clean fish trimmings, such as bones and skin, it will start to smell strongly if overcooked, and will taste bitter into the bargain. Simmer it for only around 20 minutes, which is usually sufficient cooking time.
* Chilling meat and chicken stocks before using them is a good practice. You can easily lift off and discard the solid layer of fat that rises to the surface, exposing the layer of nutritious, soft, fat-free jelly underneath.
* Carton soups are next best to homemade soups, because they use fresh ingredients that have retained most of their nutrient content. Unlike canned soups, carton soups are pasteurized rather than heated to very high temperatures.
* Generally speaking, packet soups contain fewer nutrients and more additives than their homemade or canned equivalents.
* Gout sufferers should avoid meat stocks. The purines such stocks may contain can raise uric acid levels in the body. (If this happens, the acid can crystallize, resulting in painful joints.)

Freezing stock
Homemade stock usually freezes well: it will last for up to six months. After this time it should be thrown away for health reasons. Therefore, you should make sure that any stock you freeze is labelled and dated. Chilled stock should be discarded after a week.

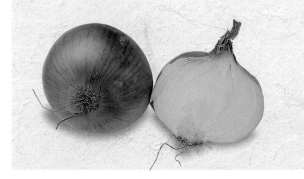

VEGETABLE STOCK

Ingredients
1 celeriac (celery root)
2 onions
1 carrot
2 leeks
3 litres/5¼ pints/13 cups water
2 garlic cloves, peeled and finely chopped
2 bay leaves
freshly ground black pepper
1 tbsp salt

Preparation time: 10–15 minutes
Cooking time: 2 hours

1. Clean all the vegetables thoroughly, then chop them into small pieces.
2. Heat the water to boiling point in a large pan. Add all the vegetable pieces, the garlic and bay leaves. Season well with pepper and salt.
3. Lower the heat, cover and simmer for 2 hours.
4. Remove from the heat, then strain the stock and use as required. The stock can be frozen for up to 6 months or kept in the refrigerator for up to 1 week.

RAW VEGETABLE SOUP

(SERVES 4)

Ingredients
1 carrot, peeled
½ shallot, peeled
½ small celeriac (celery root), peeled
10 cm/4 inches cucumber, peeled
1 litre/1¾ pints/4 cups Vegetable Stock (see above)
1 tbsp finely chopped fresh parsley

Preparation time: 10–15 minutes
Cooking time: 3–5 minutes

1. Wash and slice the vegetables.
2. Heat the stock to simmering point and then pour it into a blender with the vegetables. Blend until smooth.
3. Serve the soup, either hot or cold, garnished with finely chopped parsley.

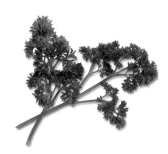

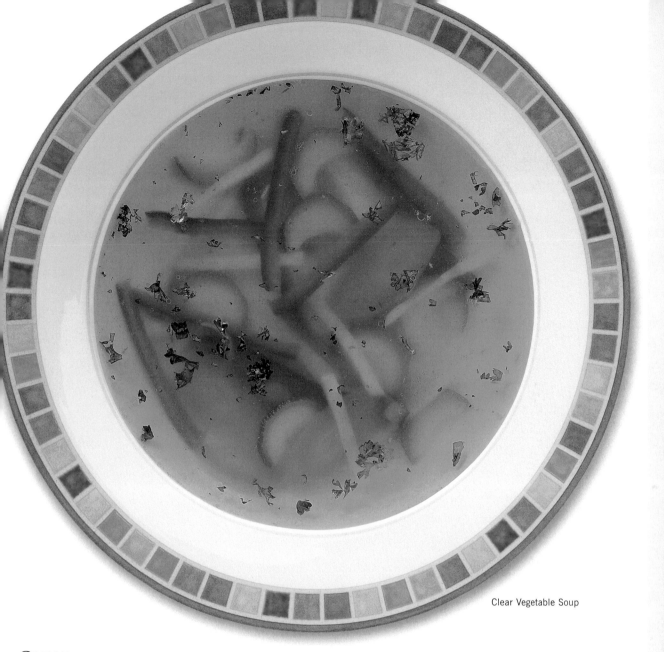

Clear Vegetable Soup

CLEAR VEGETABLE SOUP

(SERVES 4)

Ingredients
1 large carrot
½ small celeriac (celery root)
1 red (bell) pepper
1 small courgette (zucchini)
1 shallot, peeled
1 tbsp vegetable oil
1 litre/1¾ pints/4 cups Vegetable Stock (see opposite)
1 tbsp finely chopped fresh parsley, to garnish

Preparation time: 10–15 minutes
Cooking time: 6–8 minutes

1. Peel the carrot and cut into slices.
2. Peel the celeriac (celery root) and cut into strips.
3. Wash the red (bell) pepper, remove the seeds and cut the flesh into strips.
4. Wash the courgette (zucchini), halve and remove the seeds with a small melon scoop or teaspoon, then slice.
5. Thinly slice the shallot.
6. Heat the oil in a non-stick pan on a low heat and sauté the shallot slices until soft. Add the rest of the vegetables and cook gently. Add the stock and bring to the boil, but make sure the soup does not boil for more than 2 minutes.
7. Lower the heat, simmer for 2 minutes, then strain.
8. Serve in bowls, garnished with finely chopped parsley.

CREAMY CUCUMBER SOUP WITH DILL

(SERVES 4)

Ingredients
1 large cucumber
1 tbsp butter
2 tbsp flour
1 litre/1¼ pints/4 cups Vegetable Stock (see page 206)
3 fresh dill sprigs, finely chopped
swirl of single (light) cream, to garnish (optional)

Preparation time: 10 minutes
Cooking time: 5 minutes

1. Peel the cucumber, cut it into pieces and purée in a blender, adding a little water if necessary.
2. Heat the butter in a deep, non-stick pan and stir in the flour to make a roux.
3. When the butter has absorbed the flour completely, pour in the stock, a little at a time, stirring constantly.
4. Add the cucumber purée and heat the soup through until it becomes creamy, stirring occasionally.
5. Just before serving, add the dill to the soup.
6. For a special occasion, add a swirl of cream to the soup just before serving.

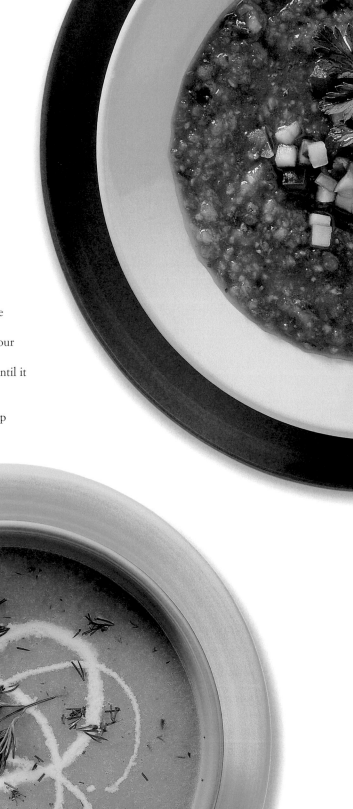

Creamy Cucumber
Soup with Dill

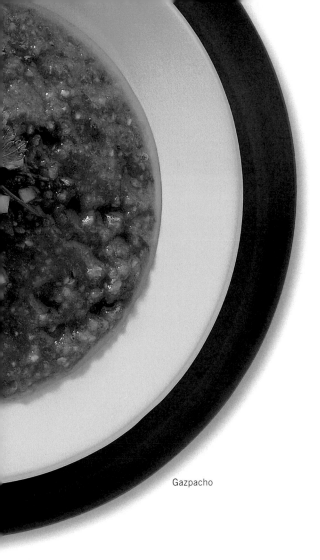

Gazpacho

LEEK SOUP

(SERVES 4)

Ingredients
3 leeks
25 g/1 oz/2 tbsp butter
1 tbsp flour
1 litre/1¼ pints/4 cups Vegetable Stock (see page 206)
freshly ground black pepper
1 tbsp chopped fresh lemon balm leaves, to garnish

Preparation time: 15 minutes
Cooking time: 15 minutes

1. Remove the dark green part from the leeks, cut off the base, including the roots, and discard. Wash the rest thoroughly and slice into rings.
2. Melt half the butter in a pan. Add the leeks and cook gently until soft.
3. Heat the remainder of the butter in another pan and stir in the flour to make a roux.
4. When the butter has absorbed the flour completely, pour in the stock, little by little, stirring constantly. Add the leeks and heat the soup through for a few minutes.
5. Season with plenty of pepper. Just before serving, garnish with the chopped lemon balm leaves.

GAZPACHO

(SERVES 4)

Ingredients
1 cucumber
1 red (bell) pepper
3 large beefsteak (beef) tomatoes
1 shallot, peeled and finely chopped
2 garlic cloves, peeled and finely chopped
½ tbsp olive oil
finely chopped (bell) pepper, cucumber and parsley, to garnish (optional)

Preparation time: 10–15 minutes plus 1–2 hours chilling

1. Peel and roughly chop the cucumber.
2. Deseed the red (bell) pepper, quarter, and roughly chop.
3. Skin the tomatoes (plunge them into boiling water for 2 minutes first), then quarter, deseed and chop.
4. Put all the vegetables (including the shallot and garlic) in a blender, together with the oil. Blend until the desired consistency is reached.
5. Serve the soup cold, garnished with finely chopped (bell) pepper, cucumber and parsley, if you like.

LEEK LORE

In traditional medicine, leeks were used to treat a wide variety of ailments: the ancient Egyptians, Greeks and Romans all set great store by what they believed to be leeks' therapeutic properties. Roman doctors advised eating leeks as a cure for a sore throat, and leeks were also thought to be useful in treating conditions such as gout and kidney stones. Modern nutritionists now know that leeks are useful sources of folate, needed to help the body make haemoglobin, and of potassium, which encourages the kidneys to function more efficiently. Leeks are also effective diuretics. Their main drawback is that they may cause wind (gas).
* One leek provides an eighth of the daily potassium requirement for an adult, while a portion of the cooked vegetable contains around a third of daily folate needs.
* Roman historians record that the Emperor Nero ate large quantities of leeks in an attempt to improve his voice.
* Leeks must be cleaned thoroughly before cooking, because their layered structure can retain a good deal of gritty soil.

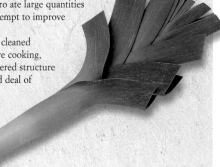

209

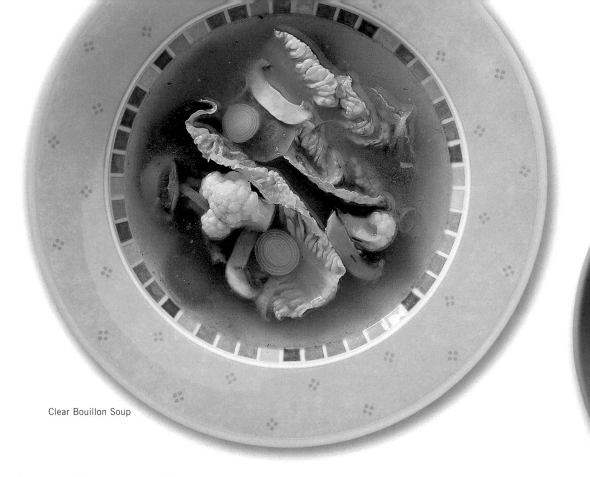
Clear Bouillon Soup

CLEAR BOUILLON SOUP

(SERVES 4)

Ingredients
1 carrot
125g/4½ oz/1¼ cups mushrooms
6 small cauliflower florets
1 leek
1 tbsp vegetable oil
1 litre/1¼ pints/4 cups Vegetable Stock (see page 206)
freshly ground black pepper
1 tbsp soy sauce
8 lettuce leaves

Preparation time: 8–10 minutes
Cooking time: 10–12 minutes

1. Peel the carrot and cut into slices as thinly as possible.
2. Wipe the mushrooms clean, remove the lower part of the stalks (stems) and slice. Wash the cauliflower florets.
3. Wash the leek carefully to remove grit, remove and discard the dark green parts and roots and slice into rings.
4. Heat the oil in a large pan and sauté the vegetables until just cooked, but do not overcook.
5. Add the stock and simmer the soup for 2 minutes (no longer in order to maintain the crispness of the vegetables). Season with pepper and soy sauce.
6. Just before serving, place two lettuce leaves in the base of each soup bowl. Pour the broth over the lettuce and serve hot.

MUSHROOM SOUP

(SERVES 4)

Ingredients
250 g/9 oz/3⅔ cups mushrooms
1 tbsp butter
1 tbsp flour
1 litre/1¼ pints/4 cups Vegetable Stock (see page 206)
freshly ground black pepper
chopped fresh parsley

Preparation time: 10 minutes
Cooking time: 10 minutes

1. Wipe the mushrooms clean, then slice them.
2. Melt the butter in a pan on a low heat. Add the mushrooms and sauté until soft.
3. Add the flour and cook, stirring constantly. When the butter has absorbed the flour completely, gradually stir in the stock, adding a little at a time.
4. Simmer the soup for a few minutes until hot and then season with black pepper.
5. Remove from the heat, pour into four soup bowls and garnish with chopped parsley before serving.

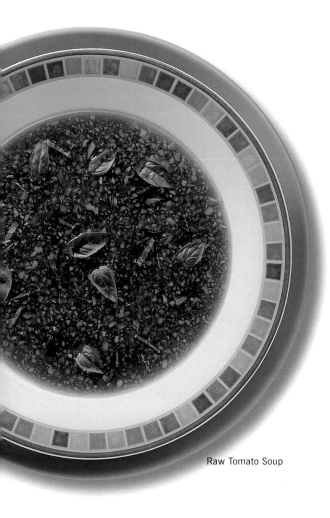

Raw Tomato Soup

WHAT'S IN SOUP?

Depending on how it is made, the nutritional content of soup can vary quite significantly, as this table comparing different types of tomato soup shows. While the protein content is more or less the same in each soup, the homemade version contains the most fat and calories and the canned variety contains the most sodium. The packet soup is the winner in terms of being low in calories, but it also contains the smallest amount of nutrients.

HOMEMADE TOMATO SOUP

PROTEIN: 2.5 G
FAT: 14.9 G
SUGAR: 4.9 G
SODIUM: 213.5 MG

CALORIES: 179.1

TOMATO SOUP (CARTON)

PROTEIN: 1.8 G
FAT: 4.2 G
SUGAR: 7.5 G
SODIUM: 900 MG

CALORIES: 88

TOMATO SOUP (TINNED)

PROTEIN: 1.8 G
FAT: 1.3 G
SUGAR: 5.7 G
SODIUM: 1.01 G

CALORIES: 121

TOMATO SOUP (PACKET)

PROTEIN: 1.3 G
FAT: 1.1 G
SUGAR: 7.7 G
SODIUM: 858 MG

CALORIES: 68

RAW TOMATO SOUP

(SERVES 4)

Ingredients
3 medium-size tomatoes
20 cm/8 inches cucumber, peeled and chopped
½ shallot, peeled and finely chopped
1 celery stick (stalk), finely chopped
1 litre/1¾ pints/4 cups Vegetable Stock (see page 206)
pinch chopped fresh basil, to season

Preparation time: 15 minutes

1. Skin the tomatoes, quarter, deseed and chop.
2. Put the tomatoes, cucumber and shallot in a blender. Process briefly. Add a little water if needed.
3. Add the celery and blend with the other vegetables.
4. In a large pan, bring the stock to the boil. Stir the vegetables into the stock.
5. Season the soup with chopped basil and serve immediately.

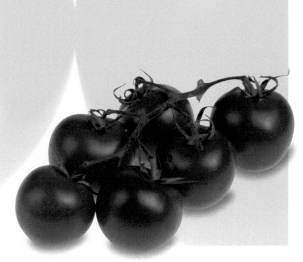

CAULIFLOWER AND BROCCOLI SOUP

(SERVES 4)

Ingredients
½ small cauliflower
1 small head of broccoli
1 carrot
1 shallot
1 tbsp vegetable oil
1 litre/1¼ pints/4 cups Vegetable Stock (see page 206)
freshly ground black pepper
pinch chopped fresh mixed herbs to garnish

Preparation time: 10 minutes
Cooking time: 4–5 minutes

1. Wash the cauliflower and broccoli and separate into florets.
2. Peel the carrot and cut into fine strips. Peel the shallots and chop finely.
3. Heat the oil in a large pan. Gently sauté all the vegetables together for 2 minutes.
4. Add the stock. Bring to the boil, then reduce the heat and summer the soup for 2–3 minutes. (Do not overcook, or the cauliflower and broccoli will not remain crisp.)
5. Season with pepper and serve garnished with the chopped mixed herbs.

BROCCOLI BASICS

In common with cauliflower, cabbage and sprouts, broccoli contains a significant number of beneficial phytochemicals, notably indoles. These are nitrogen compounds that some experts think may protect against cancer because they stop harmful carcinogens from attacking the body's DNA. One portion of the cooked vegetable also provides slightly more than half of the daily requirement of Vitamin C, beta-carotene, folate, iron and potassium. The way in which the vegetable is prepared is important: boiling broccoli almost halves its Vitamin C content, so it should be lightly steamed or stir-fried.
* Broccoli's tender florets are richer in beta-carotene than the vegetable's stalks, and the deeper the colour of the florets, which can range from green to deep blue-green and purple, the more Vitamin C and beta-carotene they contain.
* The beneficial phytochemicals in broccoli retain their powers when it is frozen or cooked.
* The vegetable is believed to have originated in the Mediterranean in Roman times; its name comes from the Latin word *bracchium*, meaning 'branch'.
* One of the most popular varieties of broccoli is calabrese, which comes from Calabria in Italy, where the vegetable has been cultivated since the 1500s.

FINE HERB CREAM SOUP

(SERVES 4)

Ingredients
½ leek
1 bulb fennel
1 celery stick (stalk)
½ medium onion
1 tbsp butter
1.5 litres/2½ pints/6¼ cups Vegetable Stock (see page 206)
2 tbsp chopped fresh mixed herbs, such as tarragon, fennel, chervil, chives and basil
cream, to serve (optional)
fresh basil leaves to garnish

Preparation time: 8–10 minutes
Cooking time: 10 minutes

1. Clean the leek thoroughly, removing any roots and green parts. Trim the fennel, removing the feathery leaves. Chop the leek, fennel and celery. Peel and finely chop the onion.
2. Melt the butter in a large non-stick pan. Add the leek, fennel, celery and chopped onion and sauté until soft.
3. Pour in the stock and bring to the boil. Add the herbs.
4. If a smooth texture is preferred, blend the soup. Just before serving, stir in some cream and garnish with a few leaves of basil.

CELERIAC (CELERY ROOT) SOUP

(SERVES 4)

Ingredients
1 celeriac (celery root)
1 large potato
2 medium-size carrots
1 onion
1 tbsp oil
1.5 litres/2½ pints/6¼ cups Vegetable Stock (see page 206)
1 bay leaf
fresh parsley sprigs, to garnish

Preparation time: 15 minutes
Cooking time: 35 minutes

1. Peel the celeriac (celery root), potato, carrots and onion, then dice them into small cubes.
2. Heat the oil in a large, non-stick pan on a low heat. Sauté the vegetables for 3–4 minutes.
3. Add the stock and the bay leaf and bring to the boil. Cook the soup for 30 minutes until the vegetables are tender.
4. Purée the soup in a blender until smooth. Serve garnished with sprigs of parsley.

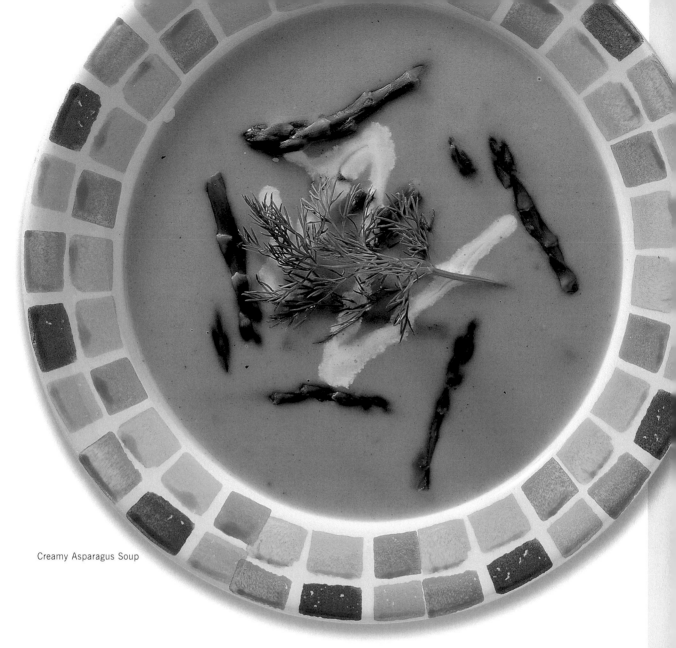

Creamy Asparagus Soup

CREAMY ASPARAGUS SOUP

(SERVES 4)

Ingredients
1 bundle of asparagus
1 litre/1¾ pints/4 cups Vegetable Stock (see page 206)
1 tbsp butter
1 tbsp flour
2 tbsp cream
small handful fresh dill, roughly chopped

Preparation time: 5–10 minutes
Cooking time: 10 minutes

1. Wash the asparagus, removing the fibrous lower part, and cut the stems into equal pieces. If you are making stock specially for this recipe, add the asparagus parts you have discarded to it. Cut off the asparagus tips and set them aside.

2. Heat the butter gently in a large pan, then stir in the flour to make a roux.
3. When the butter has absorbed the flour completely, stir in the strained stock, a little at a time, and the asparagus pieces. Let the soup cook until these are well done.
4. About 3 minutes before serving, add the asparagus tips.
5. When the soup is ready, swirl in the cream and garnish with the dill.

NOTE: GOUT VICTIMS BEWARE!

Although asparagus is a rich source of beta-carotene, Vitamin C, Vitamin E and folate – a single serving will supply three-quarters of the body's daily folate needs – those with gout should avoid it. This is because asparagus is one of the few vegetables that contain large amounts of compounds known as purines. Doctors link a high intake of these with a subsequent build-up of uric acid crystals in the joints of the body (gout).

AVOCADO SOUP

(SERVES 4)

Ingredients
2 ripe, medium-size avocados
1 litre/1¾ pints/4 cups Vegetable Stock (see page 206)
freshly ground black pepper
small handful chopped fresh mixed herbs, to garnish

Preparation time: 10–15 minutes

1. Halve the avocados, remove the stones (pits) and peel, then cut the flesh into pieces.
2. Bring the stock to the boil, add the avocado to it and transfer to a blender.
3. Blend the soup to the desired consistency. Season with pepper and serve garnished with fresh mixed herbs.

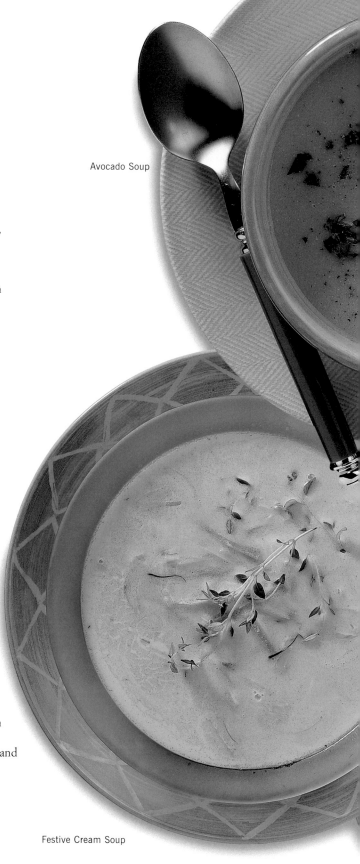

Avocado Soup

FESTIVE CREAM SOUP

(SERVES 4)

Ingredients
1 medium-size leek
1 fennel bulb
1 celery stick (stalk)
1 carrot
1 shallot
1 tbsp butter
1 litre/1¾ pints/4 cups Vegetable Stock (see page 206)
pinch saffron
3 fresh thyme sprigs
125ml/4fl oz/½ cup cream

Preparation time: 8–10 minutes
Cooking time: 15–20 minutes

1. Clean the leek thoroughly, removing any roots and the green parts. Trim the fennel bulb, removing the feathery leaves. Shred the leek and fennel.
2. Peel and shred the celery and carrot. Then peel and finely chop the shallot.
3. Melt the butter in a large, non-stick pan. Add all the vegetables and cook them gently for 2–3 minutes.
4. Add the stock, saffron and thyme.
5. Increase the heat to bring the mixture to the boil, then simmer for 5–10 minutes.
6. Just before serving the soup, remove the thyme sprigs and swirl in the cream.

Festive Cream Soup

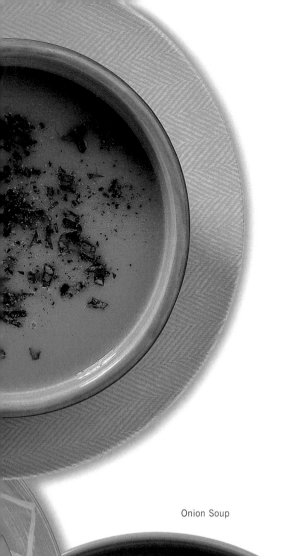

Onion Soup

ONION SOUP

(SERVES 4)

Ingredients
2 potatoes
1 tbsp butter
4 large onions, peeled and finely chopped
1 litre/1¼ pints/4 cups vegetable stock (see page 206)
2 bay leaves
1 tbsp each chopped fresh chives and croûtons, to garnish (optional)

Preparation time: 10 minutes
Cooking time: 20 minutes

1. Peel the potatoes and dice into cubes.
2. Heat the butter in a large pan and sauté the onions and the potatoes on a low heat until golden.
3. Add the stock and the bay leaves.
4. Simmer the soup for 10 minutes, then blend in a food processor if a smoother consistency is preferred.
5. Garnish each serving with chives and crûtons if you like.

ONIONS: NATURE'S CURE-ALL

For centuries, onions have been a powerful weapon in the herbalist's armoury. Now, modern science is seriously investigating whether this wonder vegetable actually possesses healing properties. Evidence from studies indicates that eating raw onion may indeed help to reduce abnormally high cholesterol levels and combat the harmful effects that eating fatty foods can have on the blood. It is also thought by some experts that the sulphur compounds that onions contain may possibly help to prevent the growth of cancer cells. (It is these compounds that give onions their flavour and strong smell.)

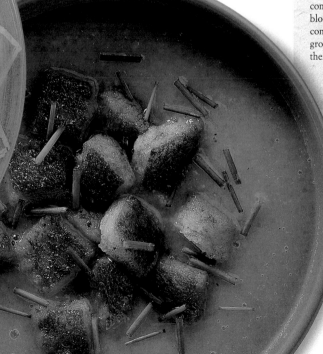

COLD CUCUMBER SOUP

(SERVES 4)

Ingredients
1 cucumber
500 ml/18 fl oz/2¼ cups natural (plain) yogurt
juice of ½ lemon
3 fresh mint leaves, chopped
½ tbsp chopped fresh chives
1 garlic clove, peeled and crushed
1 fresh parsley sprig, finely chopped
chopped fresh chives and fresh parsley sprigs, to garnish

Preparation time: 5–10 minutes plus 2–3 hours chilling

1. Peel the cucumber and shred or purée the flesh.
2. Add the yogurt and the lemon juice and blend thoroughly.
3. Season with the mint, chives, garlic and parsley, cover and chill in the refrigerator.
4.Garnish with some chopped chives and parsley sprigs and serve cold.

CHINESE VEGETABLE SOUP

(SERVES 4)

Ingredients
2 spring onions (scallions)
½ red (bell) pepper
150 g/5½ oz/2¼ cups beansprouts
1 carrot
1 tbsp vegetable oil
1 tbsp soy sauce (see note below)
1 litre/1¾ pints/4 cups Vegetable Stock (see page 206)
2 Chinese (cabbage) leaves, shredded
freshly ground black pepper

Preparation time: 10 minutes
Cooking time: 5–6 minutes

1. Clean the spring onions (scallions), removing and discarding the roots and any withered green parts. Slice the white parts, then finely chop the fresh green parts separately. Set them to one side – they will be needed later as a garnish for the soup.

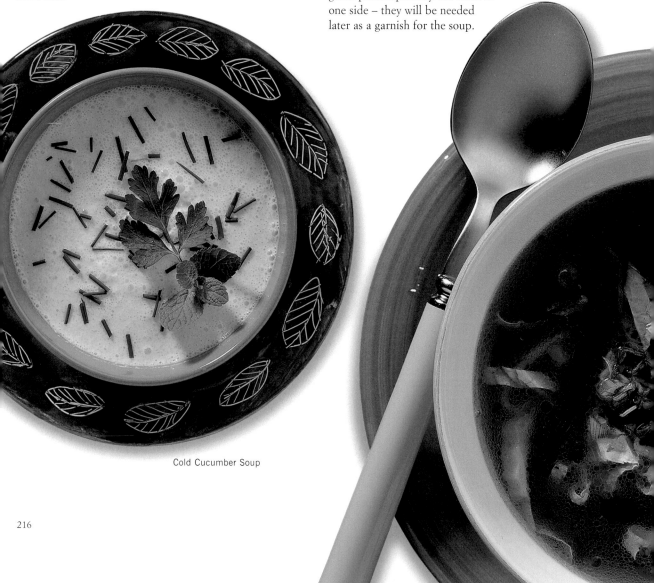

Cold Cucumber Soup

2. Wash and deseed the red (bell) pepper and cut the flesh into thin strips.

3. Wash the beansprouts and remove the dark roots.

4. Peel and thinly slice the carrot.

5. Heat the oil in a large, non-stick pan. When hot, stir-fry the vegetables for 3–4 minutes.

6. Add the soy sauce and the stock and bring to the boil. Simmer for 5 minutes.

7. Just before serving, add the shredded Chinese (cabbage) leaves to the soup and season with pepper. Serve garnished with the finely chopped spring onion (scallion) greens.

NOTE: SOY SAUCE CAUTION

Made from fermented soy beans, soy sauce should be used only in moderation because it is an extremely concentrated source of sodium (salt). It also contains wheat, so it should be avoided by anyone with a gluten or wheat intolerance. Black and yellow bean sauces, also used widely in Asian cooking, are made from soy beans, which have either been salted or allowed to ferment. Their sodium content, too, may be unhealthily high as a result.

Chinese Vegetable Soup

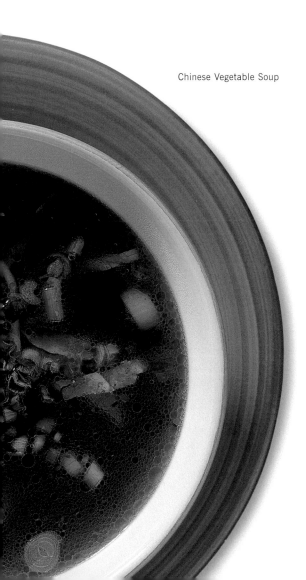

NUTRIENT-PACKED BEANSPROUTS

Beansprouts are outstandingly nutritious. As soon as the beans germinate, the oils, starches and other nutrients they contain start turning into vitamins, enzymes and other useful forms of proteins, minerals and sugars. Commonly available varieties include mung sprouts, with their translucent white shoots, tapering roots and pale-green pods; alfalfa, which produces fine, pale green spindly shoots; lentils; aduki (adzuki) beans; chickpeas (garbanzo beans); and soy beans. The last two must be cooked before eating in order to soften the chickpeas (garbanzo beans) and remove the toxins in the soy beans.

* The sprouting process increases the Vitamin C content of the bean 600 times. It also uses up indigestible sugars, so that eating beansprouts means producing less wind (gas) than after eating beans that have not sprouted.

* A serving of freshly sprouted mung beans contains around three-quarters of the average daily Vitamin C requirement.

* Sprouting also increases the Vitamin B content of beans, particularly that of thiamine, folate, biotin and Vitamin B_6.

* Beansprouts are low in calories and are an excellent source of easy-to-digest protein.

* Caution: beansprouts can sometimes trigger allergic reactions, particularly among people suffering from lupus, a rare disorder of the immune system.

Growing your own beansprouts
Beansprouts are cheap and quick to grow at home. You can buy a commercial sprouter if you like, but glass jars are just as easy to use and are equally effective propagators.

1. Check through the beans; discard any that are discoloured or damaged. Leave the beans to soak in lukewarm water for around 12 hours or overnight.

2. Drain and rinse the beans and place them in glass jars, leaving enough room in each jar for the sprouts to grow. Cover the jars with muslin (cheesecloth) or cotton tops, securing these with elastic bands, and store them somewhere dark and warm. Avoid anywhere that is too hot or too cold, because this will discourage sprouting. Avoid bright sunlight as well.

3. Rinse the growing beansprouts gently in lukewarm water 2–3 times each day. Depending on the type of bean, they are ready to eat after 2–6 days.

PUMPKIN SOUP

(SERVES 4)

Ingredients
1 small pumpkin
1 tbsp vegetable oil
1 onion, peeled and sliced
1.5 litres/2½ pints/6¼ cups Vegetable Stock (see page 206)
1 tbsp chopped fresh parsley

Preparation time: 10–15 minutes
Cooking time: 10–15 minutes

1. Peel the pumpkin, cut it in half, discard the seeds, then cut the flesh into small pieces.
2. Heat the oil in a pan and sauté the pumpkin and onion on a low heat until soft.
3. Add the stock and simmer the soup for 10 minutes
4. Pour the soup into a blender and purée briefly.
5. To serve, garnish each portion with chopped parsley.

PUMPKINS: NUTRIENT-RICH FOOD

Pumpkins and other winter squash are particularly rich in beta-carotene, which the body converts into Vitamin A and which has protective antioxidant properties. Pumpkins are also rich sources of Vitamin E, which is another antioxidant. The seeds of the plant are not only first-rate sources of iron and phosphorus, they are also brimming with potassium, magnesium and zinc. In some cultures, the seeds are prescribed to help expel worms, in conjunction with a suitable purgative, while there is evidence that pumpkin seeds can help to treat prostate and urinary problems.

MINESTRONE

(SERVES 4)

Ingredients
1 carrot
¼ celeriac (celery root)
1 celery stick (stalk)
½ cauliflower
1 large potato
1 tbsp vegetable oil
1.5 litres/2½ pints/6¼ cups Vegetable Stock (see page 206)
1 tsp dried basil
1 tsp dried oregano
freshly ground black pepper
grated fresh Parmesan cheese, to serve

Preparation time: 15 minutes
Cooking time: 15 minutes

1. Peel the carrot and celeriac (celery root) and cut into strips.
2. Wash the celery and cut into pieces.

3. Wash the cauliflower and separate into florets.
4. Peel the potato and dice into cubes.
5. Heat the oil in a large, non-stick pan and sauté the vegetables for 5 minutes.
6. Add the stock to the pan and bring to the boil, then reduce the heat and simmer the soup for 10 minutes.
7. Season to taste with basil, oregano and freshly ground pepper. For an authentic Italian touch, serve sprinkled with grated Parmesan cheese.

ARTICHOKE BISQUE

(SERVES 4)

Ingredients

3 large globe artichokes
1 tbsp lemon juice
2 tbsp olive oil
2 garlic cloves, peeled and chopped
1 litre/1¾ pints/4 cups water
1 tbsp butter
1 small onion, peeled and shredded
700 ml/1¼ pints/3 cups Vegetable Stock (see page 206)
freshly ground cayenne pepper
1 tbsp chopped fresh basil, to season
125 ml/4 fl oz/½ cup cream

Preparation time: 15–20 minutes
Cooking time: 50–55 minutes

1. Wash the artichokes and trim the stalks, leaving around 1 cm/½ inch. Break off the outermost leaves, then slice off the rest of the leaves, leaving those at the base around the 'choke' still attached. Set the leaves aside for later.
2. Combine the lemon juice, olive oil, garlic and water in a pan. Bring to the boil, add the artichoke bases, cover with a lid and cook for about 40–45 minutes, until tender enough to be pierced easily with a fork.
3. Remove the cooked bases, reserving 375 ml/13 fl oz/1⅔ cups of their cooking water. Add the artichoke leaves to the cooking water and simmer for 20 minutes. Drain the liquid, setting it aside for later. Let the leaves cool, then separate the edible pulp from them with a teaspoon.
4. Remove the 'choke' from the artichoke bases and cut off and discard the leaves around the edges. Chop the bases.
5. In a separate pan, melt the butter and cook the shredded onion until soft, then add the reserved artichoke liquid and the stock.
6. Add the pulp from the leaves and chopped bases. Heat the soup through and then purée.
7. Season with cayenne pepper and basil. Ladle the soup into heated bowls and serve hot with a swirl of cream.

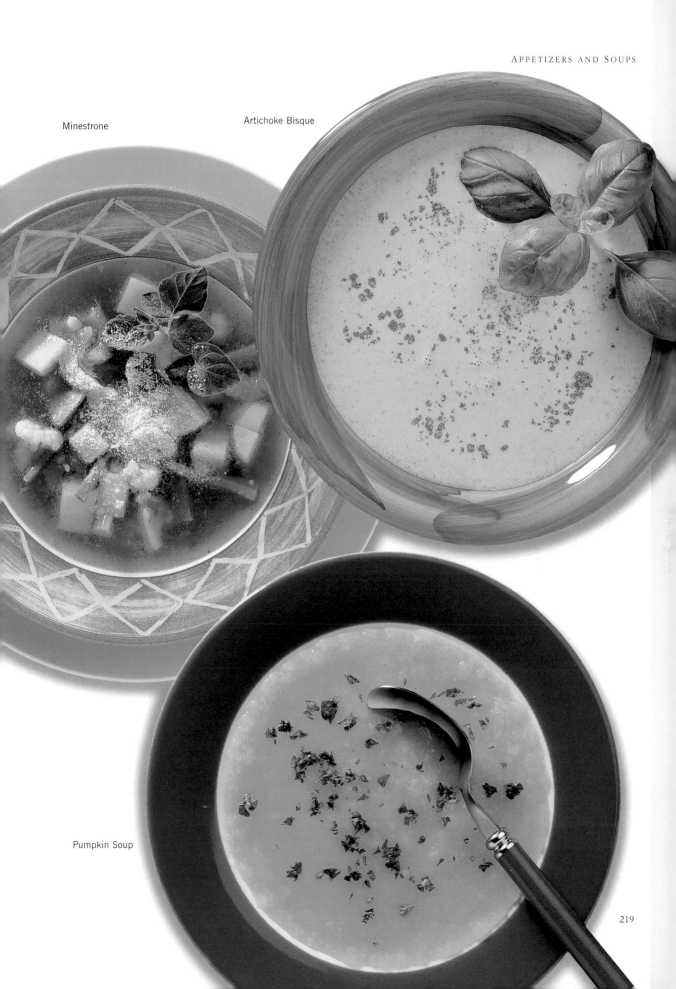

Minestrone

Artichoke Bisque

Pumpkin Soup

CRUDITES AND DIPS

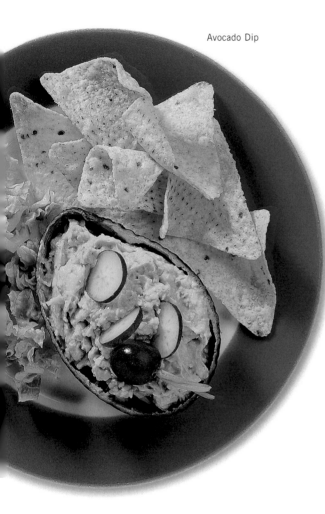

Avocado Dip

For a quick snack – or perhaps for an informal buffet – you can tempt yourself and your family and friends with a medley of raw vegetables: carrots, celery, cauliflower florets and sliced (bell) peppers, served with an attractive array of healthy dips. Eating raw vegetables like this is a significant part of any successful food-combining regime. Crudités are what the experts define as 'neutral' foods. This means that they mix happily with both proteins and starches. Of course, they are all delicious in their own right.

RAW VEGETABLES WITH DIPS

(SERVES 2)

Ingredients
1 cucumber
10 radishes
10 mushrooms
3 carrots
cherry tomatoes
Dips: Yogurt Dressing, Aioli, Cocktail Sauce, Istanbul Garlic Sauce (see pages 190–193)

Preparation time: 10 minutes

1. Peel the cucumber and cut it into strips about 7 cm/ 2¾ inches long for dipping.
2. Wash the radishes, cutting off any green parts, leaving around 2.5 cm/1 inch to make them easy to hold.
3. Wipe the mushrooms clean, blanch or steam them briefly, then cut them into strips.
4. Peel the carrots and cut into 7 cm/2¾ inch batons.
5. Wash the cherry tomatoes, pat them dry and insert a cocktail stick (toothpick) into each one.
6. Arrange the vegetables on a large serving platter. Serve with the dips.

AVOCADO DIP

(SERVES 4)

Ingredients
2 ripe avocados
2 tsp lemon juice
4 radishes
3 fresh basil leaves, finely shredded
shredded lettuce and tacos, to serve

Preparation time: 10 minutes

1. Cut the avocados in half, remove the stones (pits) and scoop out the flesh from the shells with a teaspoon. Reserve the shells.
2. Purée the flesh in a blender until smooth. Add a little lemon juice to prevent discoloration.
3. Wash the radishes, dry them and thinly slice.
4. Fill the hollow shells with the avocado purée and garnish with the radish slices.
5. Place the avocados on four small plates and garnish with the shredded basil leaves.
6. Serve with lettuce and warm Mexican tacos.

NO TIME FOR DIPS?

If you do not have time to make dips yourself, there is no need to despair. Practically all good supermarkets and food stores stock the classic varieties: you can find these in the chilled food section, or, if you are lucky, you can buy them fresh at the delicatessen counter. Here are four all-time favourites, complete with their respective nutritional values, based on an average serving.

Guacamole
Consisting of a mixture of avocado, lemon juice, tomatoes and salt, guacamole is rich in Vitamins E and C and also contains useful amounts of pantothenic acid. Another plus is the fact that it does not contain cholesterol.
Protein: 1.4 g
Carbohydrate: 2.2 g
Fat: 12.7 g

Hummus
Like taramasalata (see below), this tasty dip originated in the Near East, spreading from there to Greece and the Balkans. It is made from chickpeas (garbanzo beans), garlic, olive oil and lemon juice, with salt and pepper seasoning. It contains iron and thiamine and is protein-rich. Again, this healthy dip does not contain any cholesterol.
Protein: 7.6 g
Carbohydrate: 11.6 g
Fat: 12.6 g

Taramasalata
A richer dip than the others, as its relatively high fat content indicates, taramasalata consists of white breadcrumbs, smoked cod's roe, olive oil, lemon juice and pepper seasoning. It is a good source of Vitamin B_{12}. The high fat content is not so bad as it appears, since almost half is monounsaturated. However, taramasalata does contain some cholesterol.
Protein: 3.2 g
Carbohydrate: 4.1 g
Fat: 46.4 g

Salsa
This spicy dip, which consists of a mixture of tomato, onion, chilli peppers, garlic, olive oil, lemon juice and various spices, originated in the New World. Although it is low in protein, it is also low in calories.
Protein: 1 g
Carbohydrate: 7.2 g
Fat: 3.5 g

GUACAMOLE

(SERVES 4)

Ingredients
2 ripe avocados
3 tbsp lime juice
1 tomato, skinned, deseeded and chopped
1 shallot, peeled and finely chopped
freshly ground black pepper
2–5 drops Tabasco sauce

Preparation time: 10 minutes

1. Halve the avocados, remove the stones (pits), peel and chop the flesh into pieces.
2. Add the lime juice, tomato and shallot.
3. Purée until the sauce becomes smooth. Season with the pepper and Tabasco to taste.

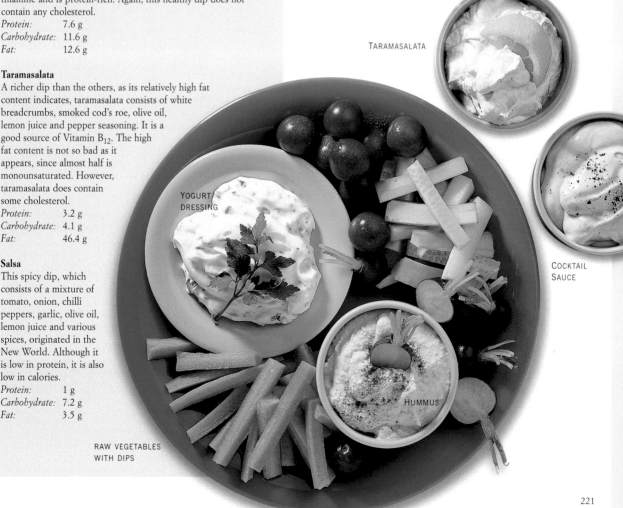

TARAMASALATA

COCKTAIL SAUCE

YOGURT DRESSING

HUMMUS

RAW VEGETABLES WITH DIPS

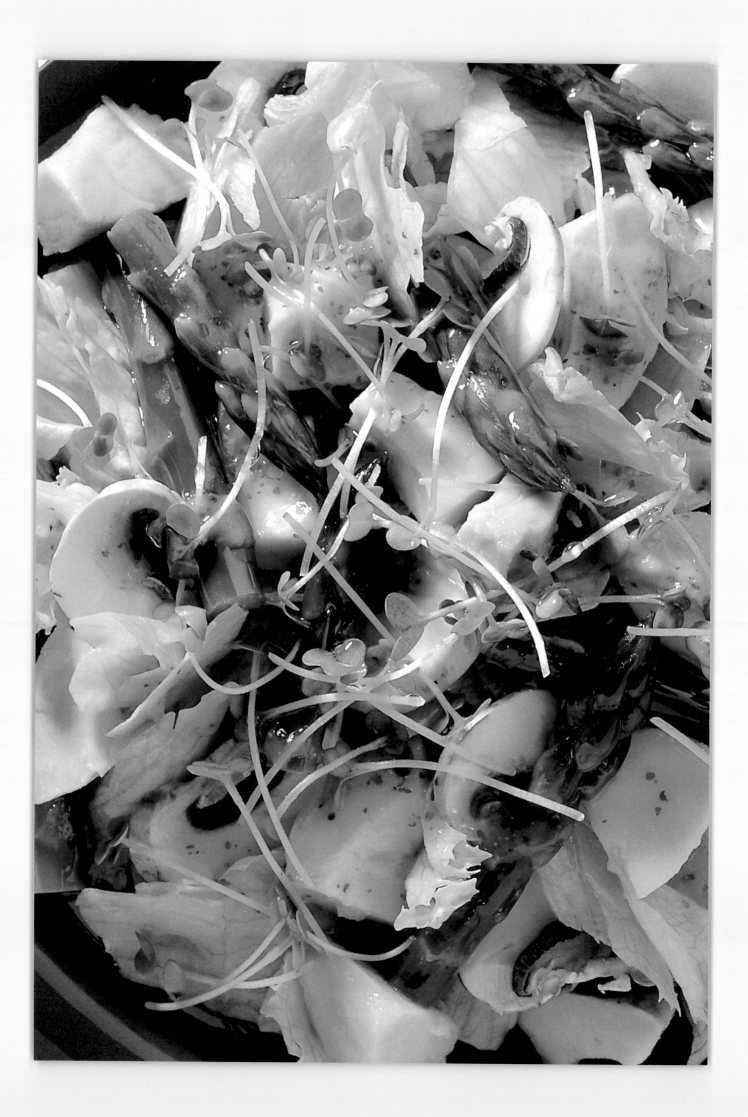

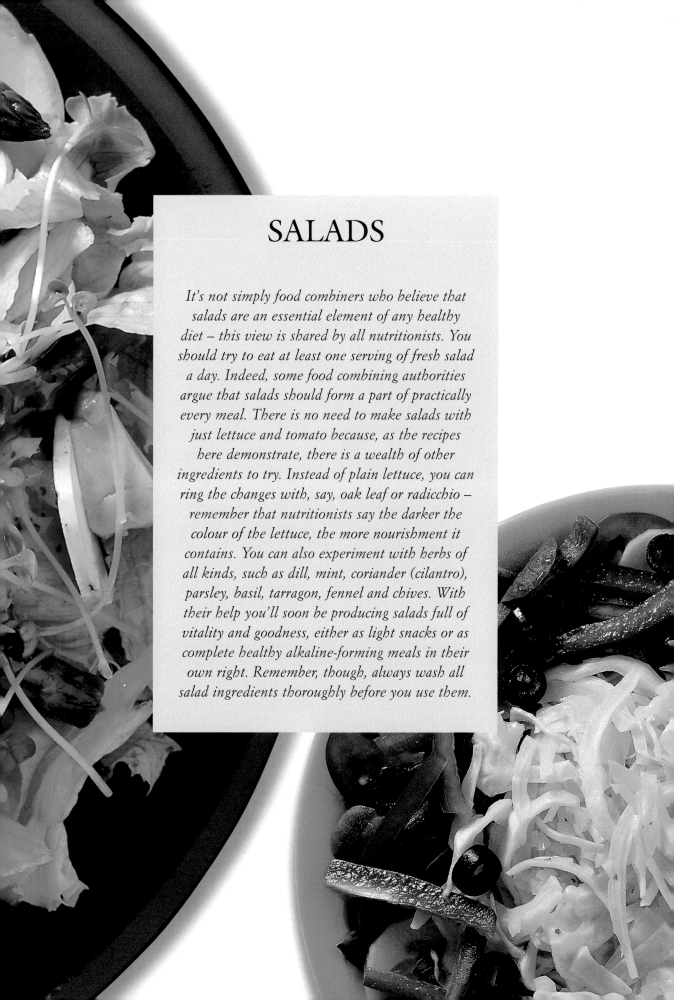

SALADS

It's not simply food combiners who believe that salads are an essential element of any healthy diet – this view is shared by all nutritionists. You should try to eat at least one serving of fresh salad a day. Indeed, some food combining authorities argue that salads should form a part of practically every meal. There is no need to make salads with just lettuce and tomato because, as the recipes here demonstrate, there is a wealth of other ingredients to try. Instead of plain lettuce, you can ring the changes with, say, oak leaf or radicchio – remember that nutritionists say the darker the colour of the lettuce, the more nourishment it contains. You can also experiment with herbs of all kinds, such as dill, mint, coriander (cilantro), parsley, basil, tarragon, fennel and chives. With their help you'll soon be producing salads full of vitality and goodness, either as light snacks or as complete healthy alkaline-forming meals in their own right. Remember, though, always wash all salad ingredients thoroughly before you use them.

LEAVES, LETTUCES AND TOMATOES

All salad leaves (greens) share the same nutritional benefits. They are low in calories (90 per cent water) and are useful sources of many nutrients, including beta-carotene and folate, and minerals such as calcium and iron. As far as food combining is concerned, their chief advantage is

that they are alkaline-forming, which makes them an essential part of any food combining plan or diet. Tomatoes provide potassium, Vitamins C and E, and also carotenoids, which reduce the risk of free-radical damage. Free radicals are highly reactive, unstable particles that damage cell structures and DNA in the body.

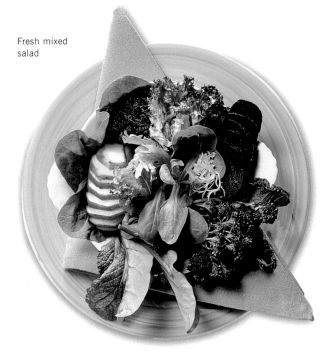

Fresh mixed salad

WATERCRESS, SPINACH, RADISHES AND CABBAGE

Particularly nutritious when eaten raw, spinach is rich in beta-carotene, folate and Vitamin C. Watercress, too, is an excellent beta-carotene and Vitamin C source and also contains iron, iodine, calcium and phosphorus. When it comes to the cabbage family, Chinese (cabbage) leaves are a good alternative to lettuce, while radishes are beneficial to the kidney and the gallbladder. Eat the tops as well as the roots, if they are fresh. Cabbage contains sulphur compounds which help to combat respiratory infections. It is also rich in iron, Vitamins A, C, E and K, Vitamin B complex, folic acid and beta-carotene.

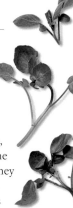

Watercress

TOMATOES

A member of the potato family, tomatoes are extremely good for you. Not only do they contain potassium, beta-carotene, and Vitamins C and E, according to some medical researchers there is evidence to suggest that their lycopene (the pigment that colours the skin as they ripen) reduces the chances of free radicals damaging the body and so helps to protect it against some forms of cancer.

Tomatoes are low in calories, too: a medium tomato contains only around 11 calories. They have one main drawback, however. They are a common trigger of allergies, associated with the development of mouth ulcers and eczema, for example. Eating green varieties can cause migraine.

As far as lettuce and salad leaves (greens) are concerned, the exact nutritional content varies from variety to variety. It also depends on the season and time of year, the freshness of the plant and, sometimes, on whether you are eating the outer or the inner leaves. On the whole, dark coloured lettuce is considered to be far more nourishing than paler varieties, and the dark outer leaves contain up to twice as much beta-carotene as the paler inner ones have. Most salad greens are also important sources of folate. In herbal medicine, lettuce leaves are used to cure insomnia – eating a large bowl of fresh leaves in the evening, herbalists say, will reduce nervous stress and help you sleep.

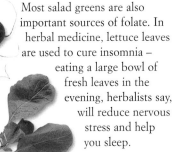

LEFT: Radishes

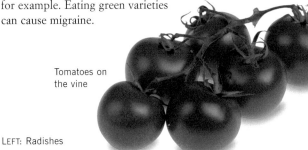

Tomatoes on the vine

SALAD LEAF VARIETIES

Ringing the changes is an excellent way of stopping salad from becoming boring. Here is a guide to some of the lettuces and other leaves you can try.

Butterhead (round) lettuce
Limp, light green lettuce, with a bland flavour.

Chicory (Belgian endive)
Pale, elongated, tapering leaves with a crisp texture and a somewhat bitter flavour.

Chinese leaf (Chinese cabbage)
A pale green leaf with crisp white ribs. It forms a cylinder-shaped head.

Cos (romaine) lettuce
Firm, long leaves that are full of flavour.

Curly lettuce
Firmer leaves than those of a butterhead (round) lettuce, with a slightly sharper taste.

Dandelion
A slightly bitter flavour that enlivens salads. The leaves contain up to one-and-a-half-times the amount of iron as the same quantity of spinach.

Frisée lettuce
Curly, ragged fronds of leaves, the outer ones being more bitter than the inner ones.

Iceberg lettuce
Round in shape with tightly packed, pale green leaves that have a crunchy texture, but tend to lack flavour.

Lamb's lettuce (mâche)
Small, velvety leaves with a delicate, nutty flavour.

Lollo Rosso
Distinguished by the reddish tinge around the frilly edges of its green leaves. Mild in flavour.

Oak-leaf lettuce
Leaves have a reddish tinge and are slightly bitter-tasting.

Radicchio
Firm, reddish-purple leaves that are crisp in texture and bitter to the taste buds. The plant's appearance resembles that of a small, red cabbage.

Rocket (arugula)
A dark green leaf, resembling that of a dandelion, which tastes peppery.

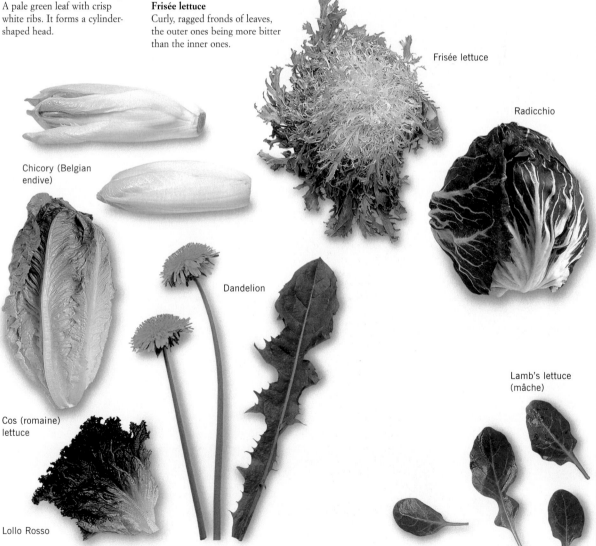

Frisée lettuce

Radicchio

Chicory (Belgian endive)

Dandelion

Cos (romaine) lettuce

Lamb's lettuce (mâche)

Lollo Rosso

Gardener's Salad

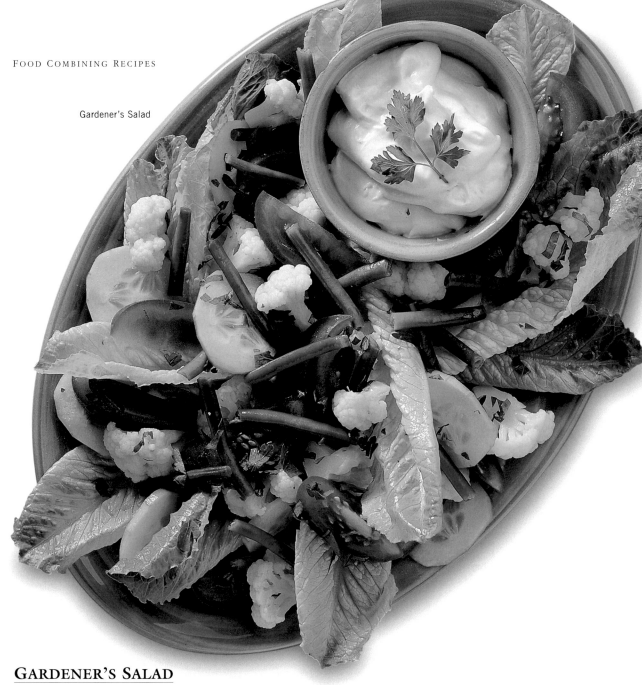

GARDENER'S SALAD

(SERVES 4)

Ingredients
½ head lettuce
1 cauliflower
200 g/7 oz/1⅓ cups green beans
2 ripe tomatoes
½ cucumber
1 tbsp finely chopped fresh parsley, to garnish
Salad Dressing or Mayonnaise (see pages 192–193), to serve

Preparation time: 10–15 minutes
Cooking time: 5–8 minutes

1. Wash and dry the lettuce.
2. Wash the cauliflower and separate into florets.

3. Steam or boil the cauliflower and set aside to cool.
4. Clean the green beans. Steam them until tender, then set aside to cool.
5. Wash the tomatoes and cut into thin wedges.
6. Peel and thinly slice the cucumber.
7. Arrange all of the ingredients on a large dish and sprinkle with chopped parsley.
8. Serve with a salad dressing or with mayonnaise.

FINE ASPARAGUS SALAD

(SERVES 4)

Ingredients
1 bundle green asparagus
1 bundle white asparagus
150 ml/5 fl oz/⅔ cup Mustard Sauce (see page 191)
cress, to garnish

Preparation time: 5–8 minutes
Cooking time: 10 minutes

1. Remove the fibrous parts of the green and white asparagus, then cut the trimmed stems into 2.5 cm/1inch long pieces. Set aside the tips.
2. Bring a large pan of water to the boil and cook the asparagus until tender. Add the tips for the last 3 minutes of the cooking time.
3. Drain the cooked asparagus on an asparagus dish or on kitchen paper (paper towels).
4. Put the asparagus on a dish and coat well with the mustard sauce. Garnish with the cress.

SWEETCORN (CORN) AND CHEESE SALAD

(SERVES 4)

Ingredients
150 g/5½ oz Gouda cheese
150 g/5½ oz canned or frozen sweetcorn (corn)
6 endive (chicory) leaves
½ red (bell) pepper
8 cherry tomatoes
salad dressing or Mayonnaise (see pages 192–193), to serve

Preparation time: 10–12 minutes

1. Remove the cheese rind and cut the cheese into cubes.
2. If using frozen sweetcorn (corn), cook briefly and set aside to cool. Place the sweetcorn (corn) and cheese cubes in a salad bowl.
3. Wash the endive (chicory) leaves and cut into strips.
4. Wash the red (bell) pepper, deseed and slice thinly.
5. Wash the tomatoes and cut in half.
6. Add all the vegetables to the cheese and sweetcorn (corn) mixture and toss until they are thoroughly mixed.
7. Serve with a salad dressing, or with mayonnaise.

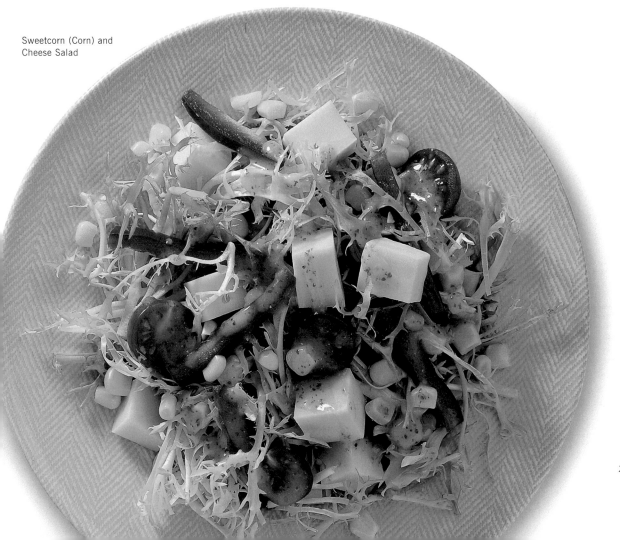

Sweetcorn (Corn) and
Cheese Salad

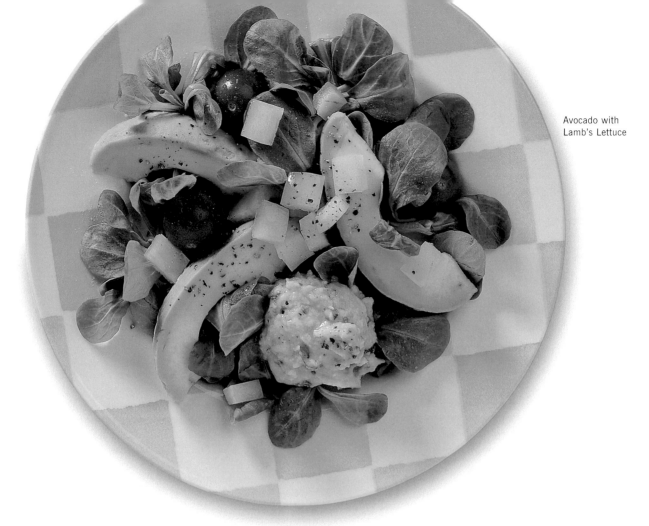

AVOCADO WITH LAMB'S LETTUCE (MÂCHE)

(SERVES 4)

Ingredients
300 g/10½ oz lamb's lettuce (mâche)
2 ripe avocados
juice of ½ lemon
freshly ground black pepper
1 tbsp chopped fresh basil
1 yellow (bell) pepper
12 cherry tomatoes

Preparation time: 10–15 minutes

1. Wash the lamb's lettuce (mâche), pat it dry, and divide it between four salad plates.
2. Peel the avocados and remove their stones (pits). Cut one of the avocados into slices, and sprinkle the sliced flesh with a little lemon juice to avoid any discoloration. Arrange the slices on the four salad plates.
3. Purée the other avocado with a little lemon juice. Season the purée with pepper and basil. Wash and deseed the yellow (bell) pepper and then dice it. Reserve for the garnish.
4. Divide the avocado purée between the plates. Garnish with cherry tomatoes and the cubes of yellow (bell) pepper.

POTATO SALAD

(SERVES 4)

Ingredients
600 g/1 lb 5 oz potatoes
2 shallots, peeled and finely chopped
5 tbsp Mayonnaise (see page 192)
1 tsp finely chopped fresh chives
1 tsp finely chopped fresh parsley

Preparation time: 10 minutes
Cooking time: 15–20 minutes

1. Scrub the potatoes thoroughly. Bring a pan of water to the boil and add the potatoes. Boil them in their skins until cooked. Allow to cool, then peel and slice them.
2. Add the shallots and mayonnaise to the potato slices and stir well to combine them.
3. Add most of the chives and parsley and mix in well. Reserve a little chopped chives and parsley to garnish.

FESTIVE RADICCHIO SALAD

(SERVES 2)

Ingredients
3 spears radicchio
100 g/3½ oz lamb's lettuce (mâche)
100 g/3½ oz frisée lettuce
6 radishes

For the dressing:
2 tbsp walnut oil
½ tbsp ground mustard seeds
1½ tbsp lemon juice
freshly ground cayenne pepper
10 shelled walnuts, to garnish

Preparation time: 10 minutes

1. Wash the radicchio, remove the bitter core, and chop finely. Place in a large salad bowl.
2. Wash the lamb's lettuce (mâche) and frisée lettuce and pat dry. Shred the frisée lettuce and add it to the radicchio with the lamb's lettuce (mâche).
3. Wash the radishes, remove any green parts, slice and mix with the salad.
4. To make the dressing, blend together the walnut oil, mustard seeds and lemon juice and season the mixture with the cayenne pepper.
5. Toss the salad in the dressing and garnish with walnuts.

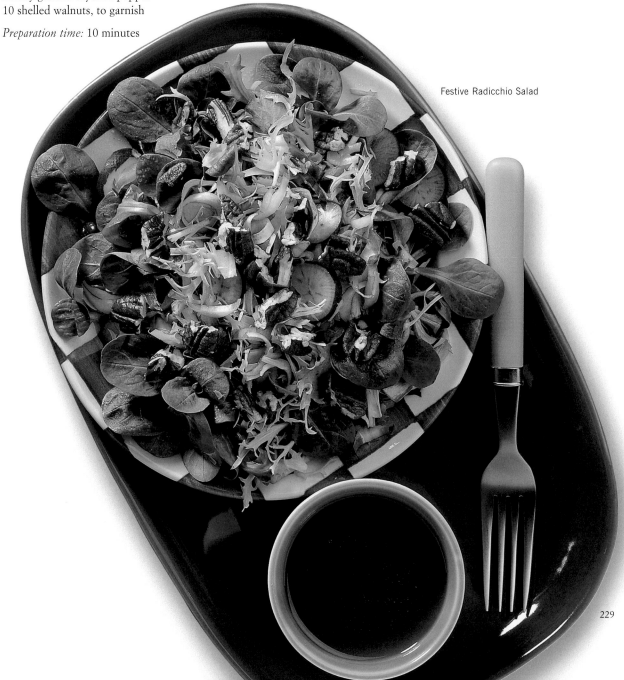

Festive Radicchio Salad

Red Cabbage Salad

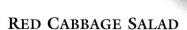

RED CABBAGE SALAD

(SERVES 2)

Ingredients
½ small red cabbage
1 shallot
1½ tbsp red wine vinegar
1 tsp mustard
4 tbsp olive oil
1 tbsp chopped fresh parsley

Preparation time: 10 minutes plus 2–3 hours chilling

1. Wash the red cabbage, dry, and slice finely using a bread-slicer or food processor. Put the cabbage in a bowl.
2. Peel the shallot and slice. Cover the shallot slices with vinegar, mustard and olive oil.
3. Pour this dressing on to the red cabbage and garnish with the chopped parsley.
4. Chill the red cabbage salad for a few hours – preferably overnight – before serving.

MIXED SALAD WITH ROASTED SESAME SEEDS

(SERVES 2)

Ingredients
400 g/14 oz mixed salad leaves (greens), such as lollo rosso and butterhead (round) lettuce, frisée lettuce, radicchio, and lamb's lettuce (mâche)
2 tbsp walnut oil
3 tbsp sesame seeds

Preparation time: 5–8 minutes
Cooking time: 2–3 minutes

1. Wash the salad leaves (greens), pat dry, and tear them into small pieces.
2. Put them into a large bowl and toss with the walnut oil.
3. Lightly roast the sesame seeds in a non-stick frying pan (skillet) and sprinkle on to the salad. (As alternatives to the sesame seeds, you could try pine nuts or sunflower seeds.)

SUPER SEEDS

Seeds of all descriptions are an excellent source of protein, Vitamin E and the B vitamins (with the exception of Vitamin B_{12}). They also provide the body with dietary fibre, which helps to regulate the bowels. Although they are high in calories, almost half their fat content consists of unsaturated fats. Seeds are usually sold cooked, to destroy any toxins, so any raw seeds are best toasted before serving. Salted seeds should be eaten only in moderation owing to their high sodium content. Try adding the following seeds to salads to add flavour and texture.

SESAME SEEDS
These come from the Middle East, where the classic dishes they play a part in making halva (a sweetmeat), and tahini (a spread). As well as Vitamin E, they contain calcium.

SUNFLOWER SEEDS
Another good source of Vitamin E, sunflower seeds are rich in linoleic acid, a substance which maintains healthy cells.

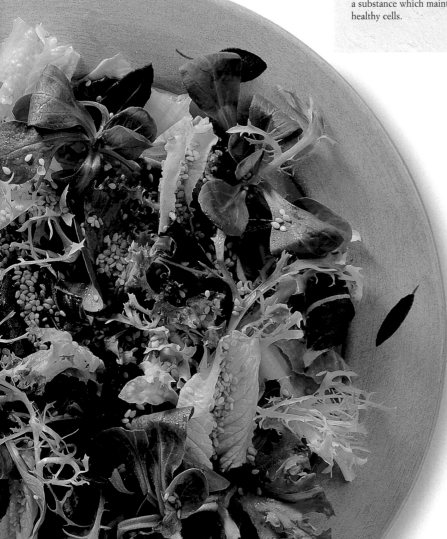

Mixed Salad with
Roasted Sesame Seeds

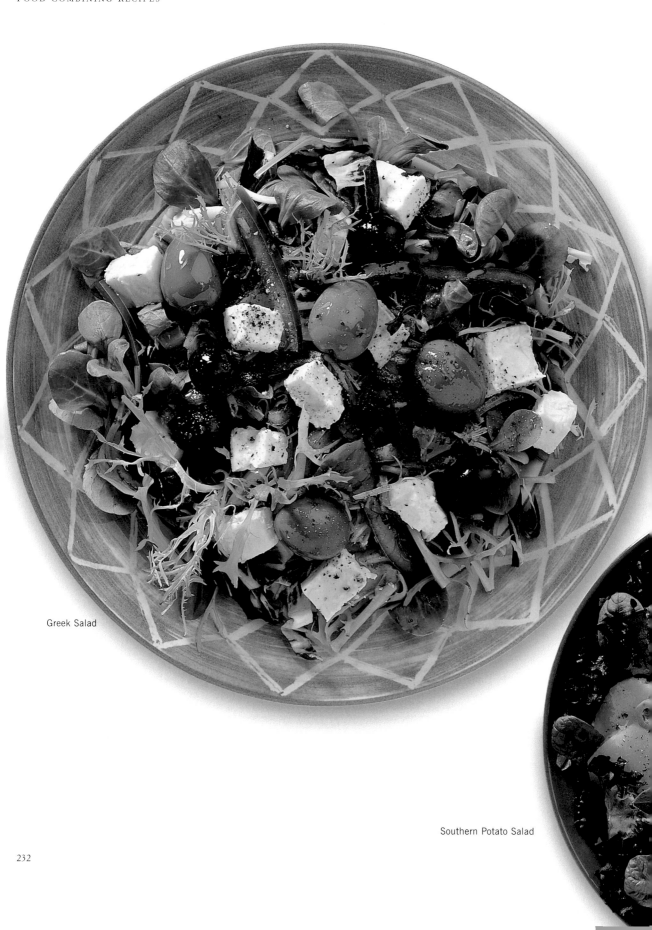

Greek Salad

Southern Potato Salad

GREEK SALAD

(SERVES 2)

Ingredients
150 g/5½ oz lamb's lettuce (mâche)
1 green (bell) pepper, to garnish
½ radicchio
4 leaves frisée lettuce
150 g/5½ oz feta cheese
4 stoned (pitted) black olives, to garnish
4 stoned (pitted) green olives, to garnish
3–4 tbsp Vinaigrette (see page 192)
freshly ground black pepper

Preparation time: 10 minutes

1. Wash and dry the lamb's lettuce (mâche) and put it in a large bowl.
2. Wash and deseed the green (bell) pepper and cut it into strips. Reserve it for the garnish.
3. Wash the radicchio and frisée lettuce, cut them into strips and add to the lettuce.
3. Break the feta cheese into cubes and sprinkle them over the salad leaves (greens).
3. Garnish the dish with the black and green olives and the strips of green (bell) pepper.
5. Drizzle the vinaigrette over the salad and season with black pepper before serving.

OLIVES AND OLIVE OIL

Olives have been valued for at least 5000 years in the Mediterranean region. In ancient Greece, for instance, the olive tree was sacred to the goddess Athena. Olives taste extremely bitter when eaten raw, so the practice grew of salting or pickling them and then marinating them in their own oil to make them palatable. This is one of the reasons why it used to be thought that olives were a high-calorie food, but this is, in fact, not the case. Not only are both green and black olives themselves low in calories, but the oil derived from them does not raise the level of cholesterol in the blood. Although olive oil has a high fat content, it consists of monounsaturated fatty acids, which, if anything, help to lower cholesterol levels, unlike the potentially harmful saturated variety of fats. (Medical studies have linked saturated fats with an increased risk of heart disease.) Olives are a good source of Vitamin E, a natural antioxidant, but they do have the drawback of being rich in sodium. For this reason, you should be careful how many you eat if you suffer from raised blood pressure.

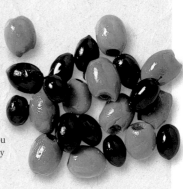

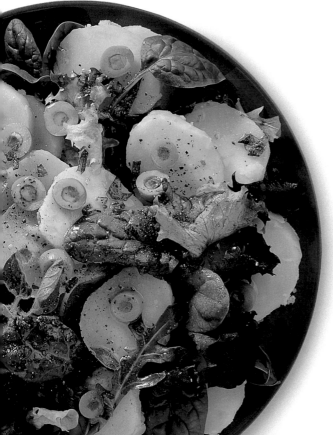

SOUTHERN POTATO SALAD

(SERVES 2)

Ingredients
500 g/1 lb potatoes
50–85 g/2–3 oz mixed salad leaves (greens)
6 green stuffed olives

For the dressing:
2 tbsp olive oil
1 tsp mustard
3 fresh oregano sprigs, finely chopped

Preparation time: 10–12 minutes
Cooking time: 15–20 minutes

1. Scrub the potatoes thoroughly. Plunge them into a pan of boiling water and cook them in their skins until tender. Set aside to cool, then peel and slice them.
2. Wash and dry the salad leaves (greens), arrange them in a bowl and put the potato slices on top.
3. Garnish the salad with the green olives, sliced thinly.
4. For the dressing, mix the olive oil with the mustard and the fresh oregano. Drizzle it over the potatoes and serve.

Asparagus and Avocado Salad

(SERVES 4)

Ingredients
500 g/1lb 2oz asparagus
4 lettuce leaves
100 g/3½ oz/scant 1½ cups mushrooms
1 ripe avocado
juice of ½ lemon

For the dressing:
1½ tbsp sherry vinegar
3 tbsp vegetable oil
1 tbsp ground mustard seeds
cress, to garnish

Preparation time: 10–15 minutes
Cooking time: 6–8 minutes

1. Cut the asparagus carefully into equal pieces. Cut off the tips and put to one side. Bring a pan of water to the boil and cook the asparagus (without the tips) for 6–8 minutes until tender, adding the tips for only the last 3 minutes of the cooking time. Remove the asparagus from the heat, let it cool, and then drain it. Arrange the pieces on a dish.
2. Wash the lettuce, pat dry and tear into small pieces.
3. Wipe the mushrooms clean and slice thinly. Add the lettuce and the mushrooms to the asparagus.
4. Peel the avocado, remove its stone (pit), cut the flesh into cubes, and sprinkle with lemon juice to avoid discoloration. Mix the cubes into the salad.
5. To make the dressing, combine the sherry vinegar, oil and ground mustard seeds. Drizzle the mixture over the salad and garnish with cress.

Southern Radicchio Salad

(SERVES 2)

Ingredients
1 yellow (bell) pepper
2 spears radicchio
5 stuffed green olives
2 tomatoes

For the dressing:
2 tbsp mustard
3 tbsp olive oil

To season:
1 tsp chopped fresh basil
freshly ground black pepper
paprika

Preparation time: 8–10 minutes

1. Wash the yellow (bell) pepper, deseed and cut into slices.
2. Wash the radicchio, pat dry, slice thinly and mix with the (bell) pepper slices in a large bowl.
3. Slice the olives and tomatoes and add both to the bowl.
4. Mix the mustard with the olive oil to make a dressing.
5. Drizzle the dressing over the salad and season with the chopped basil, black pepper and paprika.

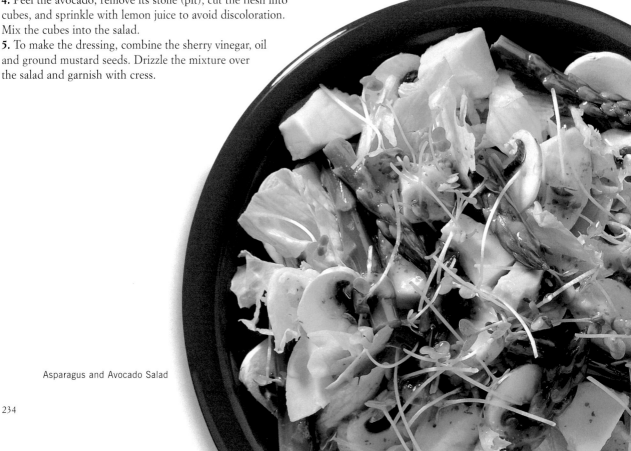

Asparagus and Avocado Salad

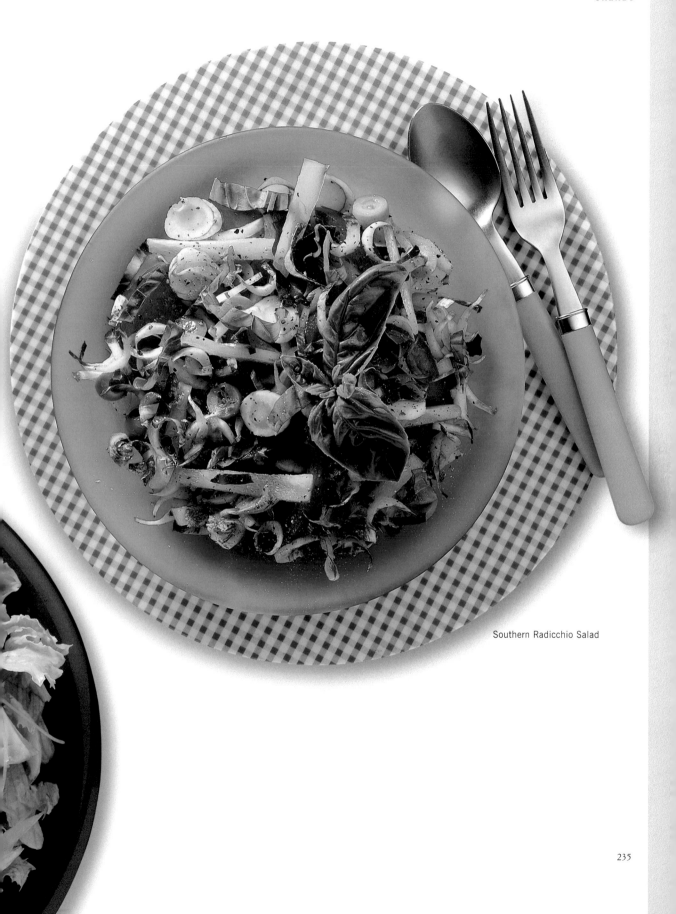

Southern Radicchio Salad

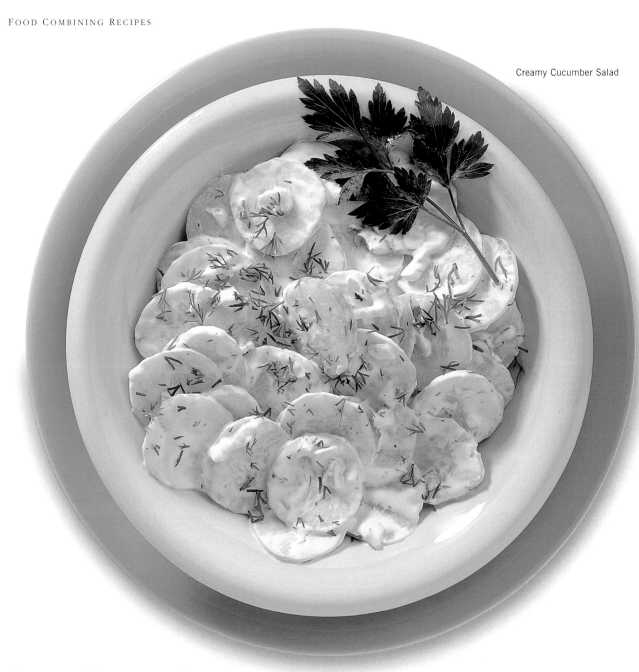

Creamy Cucumber Salad

CREAMY CUCUMBER SALAD

(SERVES 2)

Ingredients
1 cucumber
½ shallot
125 ml/4 fl oz/1/2 cup cream
1 tbsp Mayonnaise (see page 192)

To season:
1 tbsp chopped fresh parsley
1 tbsp chopped fresh dill
salt

Preparation time: 6–8 minutes

1. Peel the cucumber and slice thinly. Use a food processor if possible. Place in a bowl.
2. Peel the shallot, chop it finely and add it to the sliced cucumber in the bowl.
3. Add the cream and mayonnaise and mix the ingredients together well. Season the salad with the chopped parsley, dill, and, if necessary, salt.

RADICCHIO SALAD

(SERVES 4)

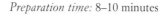

Ingredients
1 radicchio head
90 g/3¼ oz lamb's
lettuce (mâche)
1 avocado
juice of ½ lemon

For the dressing:
1 tsp mustard
3 tbsp natural (plain) yogurt
1 tbsp Mayonnaise (see page 192)
freshly ground black pepper
small handful chopped fresh mixed herbs, to garnish

Preparation time: 8–10 minutes

1. Wash the radicchio, tear the leaves into fine strips and place in a large bowl.
2. Wash the lamb's lettuce (mâche), pat dry, tear into strips and add to the radicchio leaves.
3. Cut the avocado in half, remove its stone (pit) and scoop out the flesh. Cut the flesh into pieces. Sprinkle with lemon juice, to avoid discoloration and mix into the salad.
4. To make the dressing, combine the mustard, yogurt and mayonnaise and season well with black pepper.
5. Combine the dressing with the salad and serve garnished with some chopped mixed herbs.

Radicchio Salad

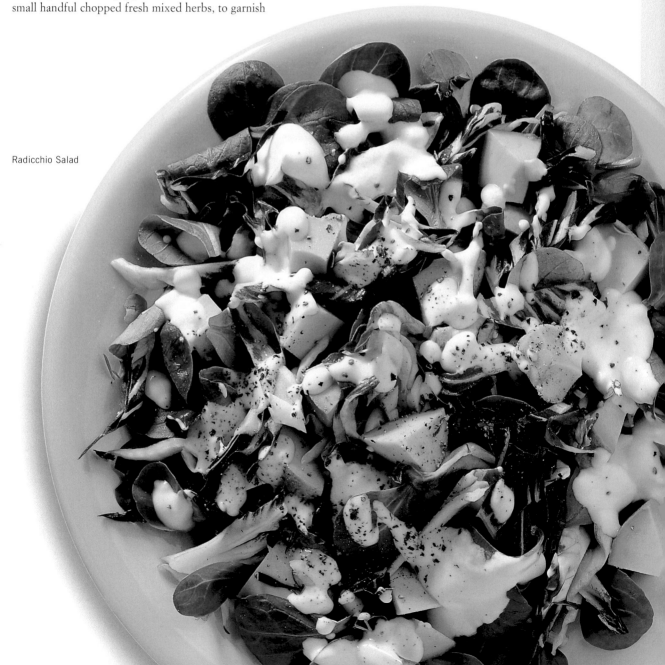

WHITE CABBAGE DRESSED FOR SUMMER

(SERVES 4)

Ingredients
¼ white cabbage
175 ml/6 fl oz/¾ cup Vinaigrette (see page 192)
200 g/7 oz lamb's lettuce (mâche)
12–15 black olives, stoned (pitted) and sliced
½ red (bell) pepper
½ green (bell) pepper
2 tomatoes
¼ cucumber

Preparation time: 8–10 minutes

1. Wash and dry the white cabbage. Shred and place in a large bowl. Add the vinaigrette, toss well and set aside for about 2 hours.
2. Wash the lamb's lettuce (mâche), pat dry and arrange it on a dish.
3. Wash and cut the tomatoes into slices. Wash the (bell) peppers, deseed them and slice. Peel and slice the cucumber.
4. To assemble, put the cabbage on top of the lamb's lettuce (mâche) and garnish with the sliced black olives and the (bell) pepper, tomato and cucumber slices.

CELERIAC (CELERY ROOT) SALAD

(SERVES 4)

Ingredients
1 celeriac (celery root)
3 tsp lemon juice
2 tbsp Mayonnaise (see page 192)
4 fresh chives, to garnish

Preparation time: 10–15 minutes

1. Peel the celeriac (celery root) and shred the flesh. Mix a little lemon juice into the shreds to prevent discoloration.
2. Add the mayonnaise and mix it into the shredded celeriac (celery root).
3. Shred the chives over the salad to garnish. (You can vary the recipe by using a combination of carrots and celeriac [celery root], or by using carrots alone.)

RADISH SALAD

(SERVES 4)

Ingredients
1 bunch radishes
½ cucumber
6 lettuce leaves
3 tbsp creamed horseradish

Preparation time 10 minutes

1. Remove the stalks from the radishes. Wash and slice the radishes, then put them in a bowl.
2. Peel the cucumber, slice and mix with the radishes.
3. Wash the lettuce, pat dry, tear into strips and add to the radishes and cucumber.
4. Add the creamed horseradish and blend well. Serve with a green salad (salad greens) or with bread.

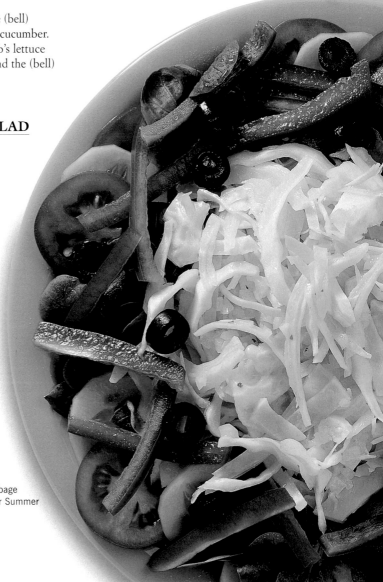

White Cabbage
Dressed for Summer

NEW ORLEANS COLESLAW

(SERVES 4)

Ingredients
¼ red cabbage
¼ white cabbage
3 carrots
3 spring onions (scallions)
½ yellow (bell) pepper

For the dressing:
4 tbsp sour cream
4 tbsp Mayonnaise (see page 192)
2 tbsp lemon juice
1 tbsp chopped fresh parsley
1 tbsp chopped celery leaves
1 tbsp shredded onion
freshly ground cayenne pepper

Preparation time: 15 minutes

1. Wash and dry the red and white cabbage quarters.
Cut them both into thin strips with a knife or a bread slicer,
or use a food processor.
2. Peel and shred the carrots.
3. Wash the spring onions (scallions), remove and discard the
roots and slice finely.
4. Wash the yellow (bell) pepper, deseed it and cut into strips.
Put all the vegetables in a bowl and mix them well.
5. For the dressing, combine the sour cream, mayonnaise and
lemon juice. Season the mixture with the chopped parsley,
celery leaves, shredded onion and cayenne pepper. Blend the
dressing thoroughly with the raw vegetables before serving.

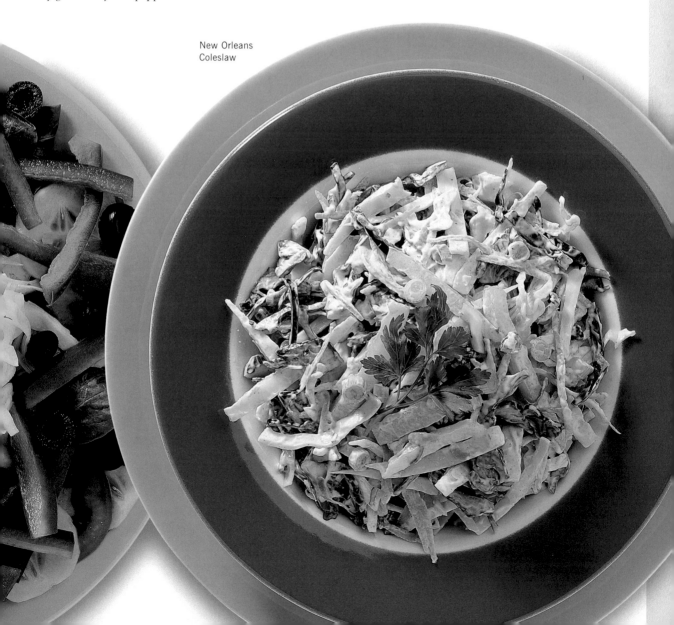

New Orleans
Coleslaw

SWEETCORN (CORN) SALAD

(SERVES 4)

Ingredients
250 g/9 oz/1½ cups cooked sweetcorn (corn)
2 young carrots
1 small courgette (zucchini)
12 cherry tomatoes
1 green (bell) pepper
½ red onion
100 g 3½ oz/scant 1 cup black olives
2 tsp chopped capers

For the dressing:
6 tbsp olive oil
3 tbsp white wine vinegar
1 tsp lime juice
1 tsp mustard
1 tbsp finely chopped fresh tarragon
freshly ground cayenne pepper, to season

Preparation time: 15 minutes

1. Drain any liquid from the sweetcorn (corn) and put the kernels into a large bowl.
2. Peel the carrots and courgette (zucchini) and cut them into small batons. Wash the tomatoes and cut in half.
3. Wash the green (bell) pepper, deseed and cut the flesh into thin strips.

(BELL) PEPPERS AND SPICY CHILLIES

The colour of sweet (bell) peppers depends on their degree of ripeness: they change from green to red and then to yellow, depending on how long they are left to ripen. All peppers are an excellent source of Vitamin C – weight for weight, a red (bell) pepper contains three times more of the vitamin than an orange – and they also contain beta-carotene and bioflavonoids. The heat in chilli peppers comes from the capsaicin they contain, which is particularly concentrated around the seeds and in the internal white ribs. This means that you need to take care when preparing chillies for cooking, because the capsaicin can irritate unprotected skin. Chillies, too, are a good source of Vitamin C, and their ability to make the eyes water and the nose run when you eat them can be put to good use in helping to relieve nasal congestion. The claim that chillies stimulate the stomach to secrete a mucus to protect its lining, however, is medically unproven. It is more likely that they irritate the digestive system, although there is scientific evidence to suggest that chillies can help to lower raised blood pressure and cholesterol levels. They are also thought to protect against blood clots.

4. Peel and thinly slice the onion. Put all the vegetables in the bowl. Add the black olives and chopped capers and mix well.
5. For the dressing, blend the olive oil with the wine vinegar, lime juice, mustard and fresh tarragon. Season with cayenne pepper and drizzle the dressing over the salad before serving.

SOUTHERN SALAD

(SERVES 2)

Ingredients
½ cucumber
2 tomatoes
½ onion
½ yellow (bell) pepper
½ red (bell) pepper
125 ml/4 fl oz/½ cup Vinaigrette (see page 192)
6 black olives

Preparation time: 10 minutes

1. Peel and slice the cucumber, then put in a salad bowl.
2. Wash the tomatoes, slice and add to the bowl.
3. Peel the onion, cut into rings and then add to the bowl.
4. Wash the yellow and red (bell) pepper halves, deseed and cut into strips. Mix with the cucumber, tomato and onion.
5. Drizzle the vinaigrette over the salad and chill in the refrigerator for 1 hour.
6. Garnish with the black olives before serving.

LEEK SALAD

(SERVES 4)

Ingredients
8 leeks
1 garlic clove

For the dressing:
1 tsp mustard
125 ml/4 fl oz/½ cup vegetable oil
4 tbsp white wine vinegar
1 tbsp fresh lemon juice
6 fresh chives, chopped

Preparation: 5–10 minutes plus 1–2 hours chilling
Cooking time: 15 minutes

1. Wash the leeks thoroughly and cut off and discard the roots and any green parts. Chop the white parts. Bring a pan of water to the boil, and add the leeks. Cook for 15 minutes with the garlic. Drain the leeks and arrange on a dish.
2. For the dressing, blend the mustard, oil, wine vinegar and lemon juice and pour the mixture over the leeks.
3. Garnish with the chopped chives. Chill for 1–2 hours.

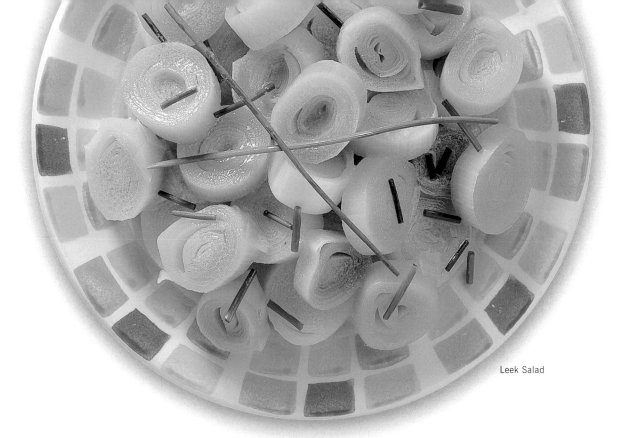

Leek Salad

Sweetcorn (Corn) Salad

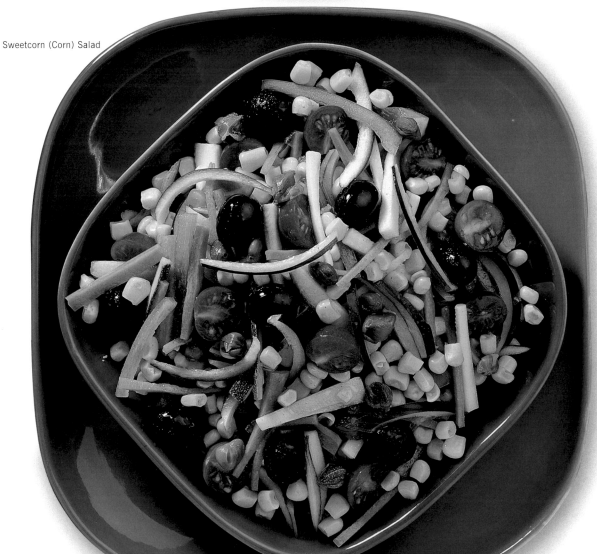

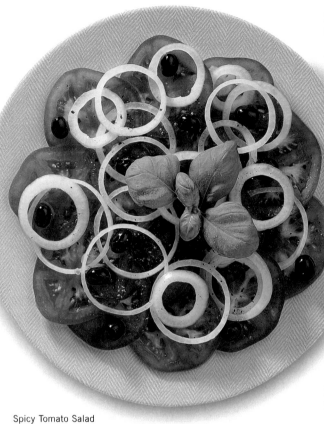

Spicy Tomato Salad

MIXED SALAD WITH TOMATO VINAIGRETTE

(SERVES 2)

Ingredients
½ cucumber
2 tomatoes
½ yellow (bell) pepper
3 Chinese cabbage or iceberg (romaine) lettuce leaves
3–4 tbsp Tomato Vinaigrette (see page 192)

Preparation time 10 minutes

1. Peel and slice the cucumber and arrange the slices in a shallow dish.
2. Wash the tomatoes, cut them into quarters and add them to the cucumber.
3. Wash the yellow (bell) pepper, deseed and cut the flesh into strips.
4. Wash the Chinese cabbage or lettuce leaves and cut into strips. Add the yellow (bell) pepper and cabbage or lettuce to the dish. Mix the salad vegetables well and drizzle the tomato vinaigrette over them.

SPICY TOMATO SALAD

(SERVES 2)

Ingredients
4 tomatoes
2 garlic cloves
1 onion
25 g/1 oz/¼ cup black olives
1 tbsp olive oil
1 tsp finely chopped fresh basil
1 tsp dried oregano
salt and freshly ground black pepper

Preparation time: 5–10 minutes

1. Wash and slice the tomatoes, then arrange them on a large dish.
2. Peel and finely slice the garlic and divide the slices among the tomatoes.
3. Peel the onion, cut into rings and add to the salad.
4. Garnish with the black olives.
5. Pour the olive oil over the salad and sprinkle with finely chopped fresh basil and dried oregano. Season with salt and pepper, if you like.

SPICY OYSTER MUSHROOM SALAD

(SERVES 4)

Ingredients
300 g/10½ oz/4¼ cups oyster mushrooms
1 tbsp butter
1 garlic clove, peeled and crushed
pinch chicken spices (a spicy mixture of herbs for chicken dishes)
pinch cayenne pepper
1 head of lettuce
10 cherry tomatoes
50 g/1¾ oz/scant ½ cup pecan nuts
16 fresh thyme sprigs, to garnish

Preparation time: 8–10 minutes
Cooking time: 4–5 minutes

1. Wipe the mushrooms clean. Melt the butter in a pan on a low heat, add the mushrooms and the garlic and sauté gently, stirring occasionally.
2. While the mushrooms and garlic are cooking, sprinkle the chicken spices and cayenne pepper over them. Continue cooking for 4–5 minutes more, until the mushrooms have turned golden brown.
3. Wash the lettuce and pat dry. Tear the leaves into strips and place in a bowl. Add the mushrooms, tomatoes and pecan nuts and toss well to mix thoroughly. Garnish with the thyme sprigs.

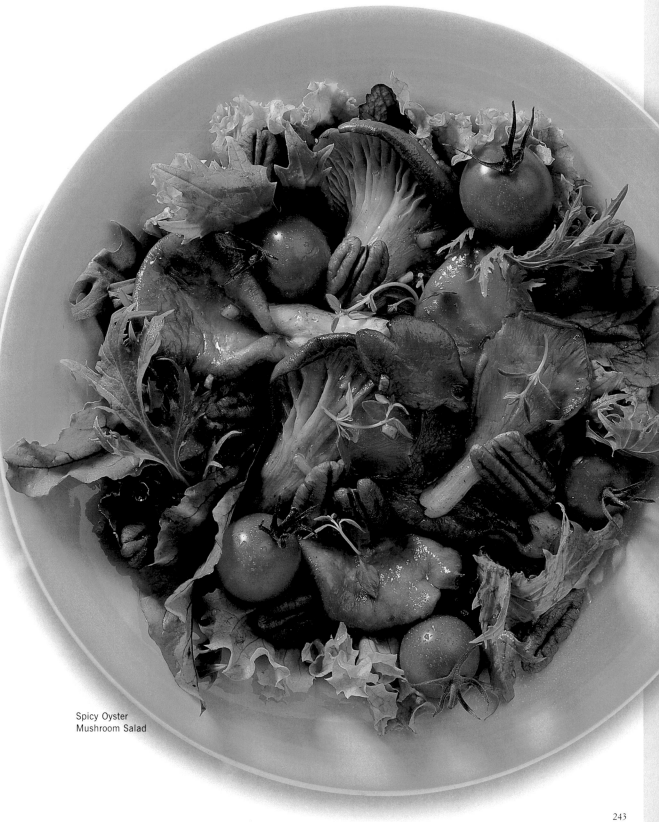

Spicy Oyster
Mushroom Salad

Mushroom Salad

(SERVES 4)

Ingredients
250 g/9 oz/3⅔ cups mushrooms
juice of ½ lemon
½ onion
1 bunch fresh chervil
6 fresh chives
1 garlic clove, peeled and crushed
125 ml/4 fl oz/½ cup Vinaigrette (see page 192)

Preparation time: 10 minutes plus 1 hour chilling

1. Wipe the mushrooms clean, remove the lower part of the stalks (stems), slice and sprinkle the lemon juice over them.
2. Peel and finely chop the onion and then add it to the mushroom slices.
3. Wash and chop the chervil and chives. Combine them with the mushrooms and onion and arrange the mixture on a dish.
4. Mix the crushed garlic into the vinaigrette. Stir with a fork and pour the dressing over the mushroom salad. Chill for 1 hour before serving.

Fennel Salad

(SERVES 2)

Ingredients
2 bulbs fennel complete with feathery fronds
½ red lettuce

For the dressing:
125 ml/4 fl oz/½ cup olive oil
4 tbsp wine vinegar
pinch each dried basil, oregano and paprika
green stuffed olives, to garnish

Preparation time: 10–15 minutes

1. Wash the fennel bulbs. Remove any feathery fronds and save them for the garnish. Roughly shred or finely slice the bulbs and place in a dish.
2. Wash the lettuce, tear the leaves into strips and add them to the fennel.
3. To make the dressing, combine the olive oil and wine vinegar, then season to taste with basil, oregano and paprika. Pour the dressing over the fennel salad and toss well.
4. Garnish with the feathery fronds from the fennel and the green stuffed olives.

Avocado and Spinach Salad

(SERVES 2)

Ingredients
200 g/7 oz young spinach leaves
1 avocado
1 tsp lemon juice
½ cucumber
10 cherry tomatoes
1 tbsp toasted sunflower seeds

Preparation time 10–15 minutes

1. Wash the spinach leaves and tear them into rough strips. Divide them among two plates – each plate should take a good handful of leaves.
2. Halve the avocado, remove the stone (pit) and peel both halves. Cut the flesh into slices and sprinkle with a little lemon juice to prevent discoloration.
3. Wash and slice the cucumber.
4. To assemble the salad, top the spinach with the avocado, cherry tomatoes and cucumber and garnish with the toasted sunflower seeds.

SPINACH: FACT AND FABLE

Contrary to popular belief, spinach is not a particularly rich source of iron for the body. The misconception came about through a mistake by an early food analyst, who, while working out the vegetable's iron content, misplaced the decimal point, so ending up with a figure ten times greater than it should have been. Nevertheless, there is no doubt that spinach is extremely good for you: it is a concentrated source of carotenoids, including beta-carotene, Vitamin C, potassium and folate. The drawback is the high amount of oxalic acid the vegetable contains, which may interfere with the body's ability to absorb iron and calcium from the vegetable. Your body will absorb more of the former if you eat spinach in combination with a food that is high in Vitamin C.

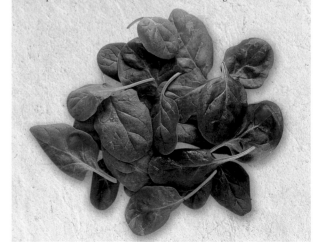

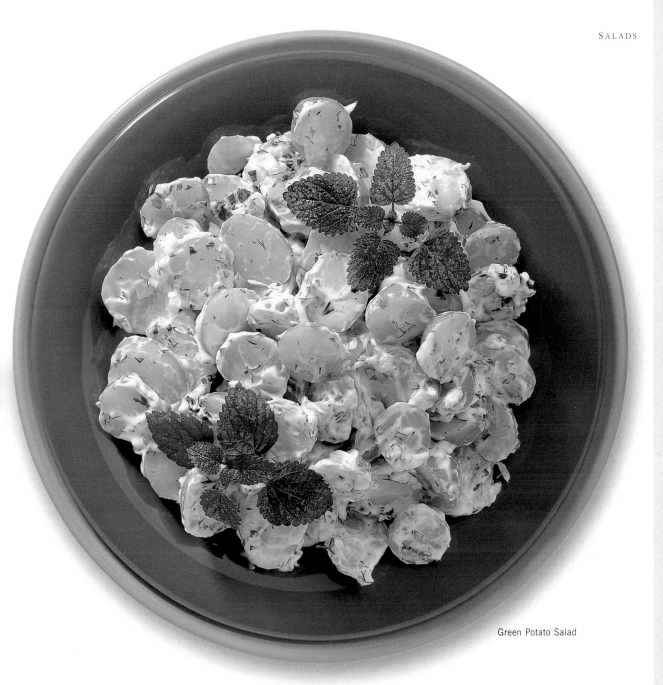

Green Potato Salad

GREEN POTATO SALAD

(SERVES 4)

Ingredients
1 kg/2 lb 4 oz new potatoes
1 shallot, peeled and chopped
1 bunch fresh dill
1 bunch fresh parsley
5 fresh sage leaves
1 fresh lemon balm sprig
2 tbsp Mayonnaise (see page 192)
1 tbsp sour cream

Preparation time: 8–10 minutes
Cooking time: 15–20 minutes

1. Scrub the potatoes thoroughly. Bring a pan of water to the boil and cook the potatoes in their skins until tender. Remove from the heat, drain, set aside to cool, then slice them.
2. Put the potato slices in a bowl with the chopped shallot.
3. Wash and dry the herbs, including the leaves from the lemon balm sprig, and chop finely.
4. Blend the mayonnaise with the sour cream and mix with the chopped herbs. Add this mixture to the potato slices and stir together well.

245

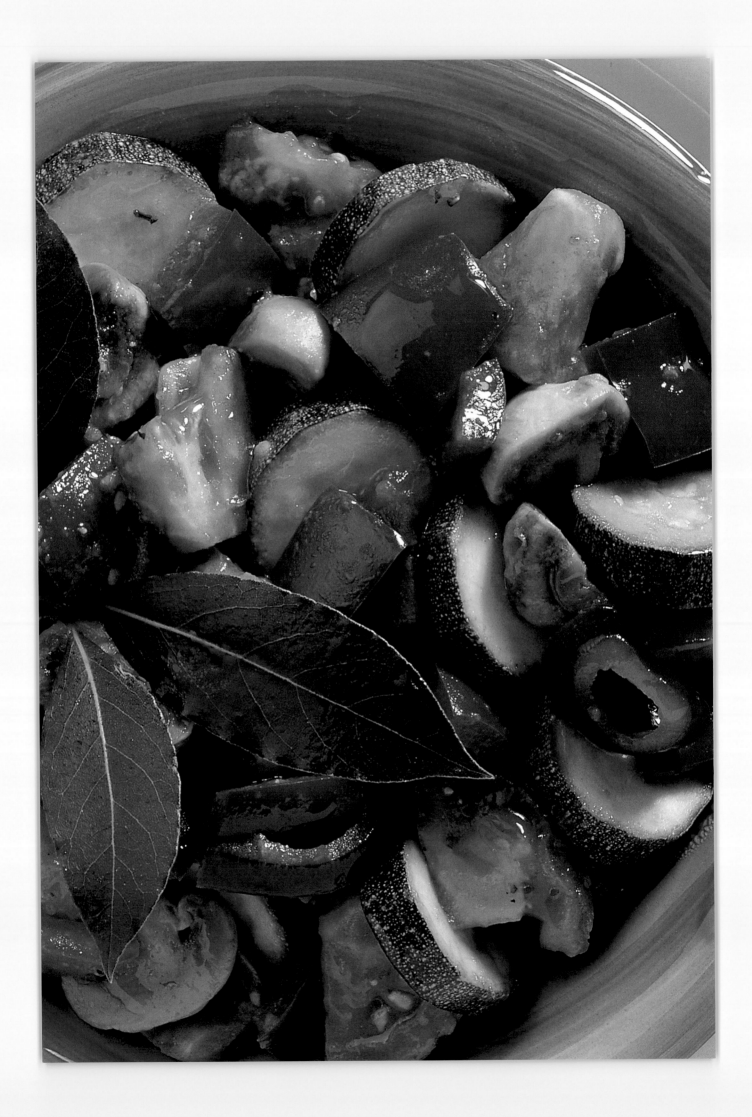

VEGETABLES

Experts at the World Health Organization state categorically that we should all eat at least five portions of vegetables and fruit a day. You would certainly not find a food combining authority who would disagree with this notion, especially since there is a long list of vegetables that will happily mix with either proteins or starches, so making them an essential element in any food combining plan. Vegetables are packed full of the vital fibre, vitamins and minerals we all need to maintain good health. They also provide other substances, such as bioflavonoids and enzymes, which play a vital role in the healthy functioning of the body. Eating a wide variety is the best way of being sure of a healthy intake of all these various nutrients. It is also important to cook vegetables correctly. Vitamins, in particular, can be destroyed by boiling vegetables, which allows valuable nutrients to leach away into the cooking water. For these reasons, vegetables are better eaten lightly steamed, roasted or baked.

VEGETABLES, FOOD COMBINING AND HEALTH

With the exception of sauerkraut, vegetables containing lactic acid and tomatoes, all vegetables may be combined with virtually any type of food. Because of their powerful alkaline effect, they are good for the body's all-important acid-base balance. As far as fighting off illness is concerned, *various scientific studies around the world have demonstrated that people who follow a diet rich in vegetables and fruit seem to run a lower risk of contracting life-threatening diseases, such as cancer. This is thought to be linked to protective substances in plants known as phytochemicals.*

PHYTOCHEMICALS: NATURE'S POWERFUL HEALERS

Scientists believe that, as well as containing beneficial nutrients of all kinds, vegetables also contain powerful non-nutritional compounds known as 'phytochemicals'. It is these compounds, they believe, that may play an important part in protecting the body against the risk of contracting cancer and possibly other life-threatening disorders, such as diabetes, coronary heart disease, circulatory

LEFT: Vegetables are thought to play an important role in preventing many diseases.

problems, high blood pressure and osteoporosis, a degenerative disorder of the bones. Phytochemicals known as carotenoids (plant pigments) have antioxidant properties, which means that they are powerful weapons against free radicals, particles which have the potential to damage the body's cells and DNA. All vegetables have their share of phytochemicals, although the cruciferous varieties – cabbage, cauliflower, broccoli, sprouts, kale and turnips – appear to be particularly rich in these compounds. Vegetables with the greatest amounts of carotenoids are watercress, broccoli, spinach, yellow-fleshed squashes, carrots, pumpkins and red (bell) peppers.

Other valuable phytochemicals include allicin compounds, which are present in garlic, onions, chives and leeks; indoles, contained in cruciferous vegetables; isothiocyanates, the main sources for which are sprouts, cabbage and broccoli; bioflavonoids, found in fruits, such as grapefruit, lemons, blackcurrants and cherries; and coumaric acid, found in tomatoes, green (bell) peppers and carrots.

THE IMPORTANCE OF VEGETABLES

Food combiners rank foods in order of their importance to the body, starting with fruits, then all salad and leafy green vegetable foods, followed by root vegetables, then grains and proteins. So clearly it is important to eat plenty of vegetables.

Whatever food combining regime you are following, you should remember that it is better to spread your food intake evenly throughout the day, if at all possible. Nutritional research has demonstrated that people who divide up their food intake like this seem to manage to take in a greater variety of the essential nutrients and to eat less fatty foodstuffs into the bargain. If you are prone to snacking, remember that, if you choose plenty of vegetables – raw vegetable sticks for instance – snacking becomes a healthy option, rather than a potential disaster area.

PREVENTING NUTRIENT LOSS

All vegetables contain varying quantities of different nutrients, so eating a wide selection of fresh food is the best way of being sure of a healthy nutrient intake. As far as what you should eat and when to eat it is concerned, the simplest advice is to look for what is in season and, if practical, favour foods that are locally grown. The further vegetables have to be transported, the more their nutrient levels can become depleted – some start to lose nutrients as soon as they are picked – which is why, paradoxically enough, frozen vegetables can, at least in theory, be more nutritious than fresh ones. In any event, frozen varieties are usually better for you than their canned equivalents.

You should try to store vegetables somewhere cool – (bell) peppers, courgettes (zucchini) and tomatoes should be kept at around 10°C/50°F to keep them as fresh as possible. For most other vegetables, the optimum storage temperature is 0°C/32°F, apart from potatoes, which should not be stored at temperatures below 4°C/40°F.

Courgettes (zucchini)

248

WHAT'S FRESHEST WHEN?

SEASON	LOOK FOR

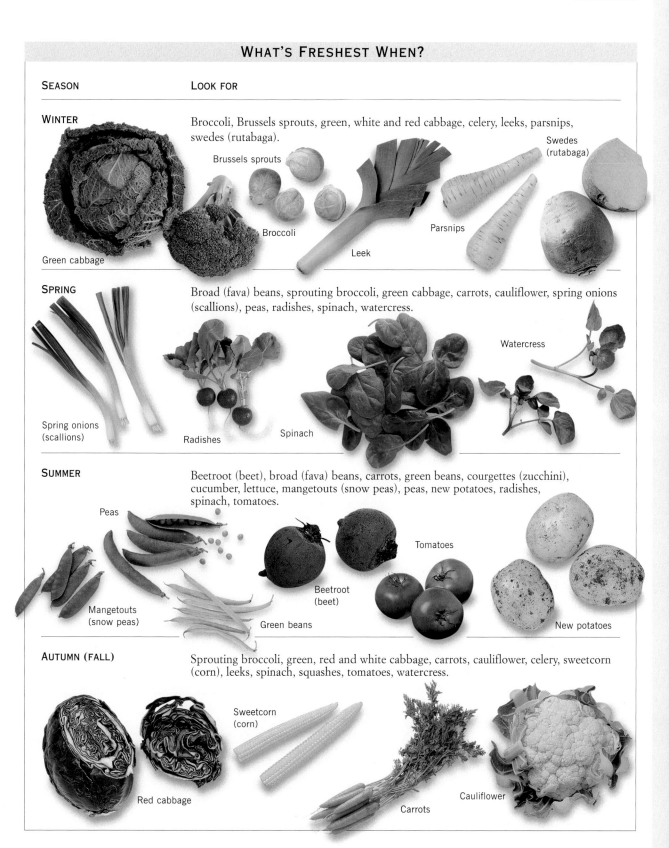

WINTER

Broccoli, Brussels sprouts, green, white and red cabbage, celery, leeks, parsnips, swedes (rutabaga).

Brussels sprouts

Swedes (rutabaga)

Broccoli

Parsnips

Leek

Green cabbage

SPRING

Broad (fava) beans, sprouting broccoli, green cabbage, carrots, cauliflower, spring onions (scallions), peas, radishes, spinach, watercress.

Watercress

Spring onions (scallions)

Radishes

Spinach

SUMMER

Beetroot (beet), broad (fava) beans, carrots, green beans, courgettes (zucchini), cucumber, lettuce, mangetouts (snow peas), peas, new potatoes, radishes, spinach, tomatoes.

Peas

Tomatoes

Beetroot (beet)

Mangetouts (snow peas)

Green beans

New potatoes

AUTUMN (FALL)

Sprouting broccoli, green, red and white cabbage, carrots, cauliflower, celery, sweetcorn (corn), leeks, spinach, squashes, tomatoes, watercress.

Sweetcorn (corn)

Red cabbage

Cauliflower

Carrots

STEAMED VEGETABLES

(SERVES 4)

Ingredients
1 head of broccoli
½ small cauliflower
4 carrots

For the sauce:
1 tbsp butter
1 tbsp flour
175 ml/6 fl oz/¾ cup vegetable stock (see page 206)
4 tbsp cream
pinch each ground nutmeg, freshly ground black pepper
and paprika

Preparation time: 15–20 minutes
Cooking time: 10 minutes

1. Wash the broccoli, peel the stems and cut them into pieces. Separate the rest into florets.
2. Separate the cauliflower into florets and wash thoroughly.
3. Peel and slice the carrots or cut into small batons.
4. Steam all the vegetables for 10 minutes until tender.
5. To make the sauce, heat the butter in a pan on a low heat until melted. Add the flour, a little at a time, stirring constantly. When the flour has been absorbed by the butter, gradually stir in the stock. Simmer until the sauce has thickened and then add the cream.
6. Season the sauce with the nutmeg, pepper and paprika.
7. Cover the warm vegetables with the sauce and serve with new potatoes.

CHINESE CABBAGE AU GRATIN

(SERVES 4)

Ingredients
1 Chinese cabbage
½ tsp stock granules or bouillon powder
200 g/7 oz/2¾ cups mushrooms
1 tbsp butter
100 g/3½ oz/scant 1 cup grated Gruyère (Swiss) or
Emmenthal cheese

Preparation time: 5 minutes
Cooking time: 10–12 minutes

1. Cut the Chinese cabbage into four pieces and wash thoroughly. Bring a pan of water to the boil. Add the Chinese cabbage and the stock granules or bouillon powder and simmer for 8 minutes. Drain the pieces and put into a greased, flameproof dish.

2. Meanwhile wipe the mushrooms clean, then slice them. Melt the butter in a pan on a low heat and gently cook the mushrooms for several minutes.
3. Spread the mushrooms over the Chinese cabbage and sprinkle liberally with the grated cheese.
4. Put the dish under the grill (broiler) and cook for a few minutes until the cheese starts to bubble. Serve with a salad.

STUFFED (BELL) PEPPERS

(SERVES 4)

Ingredients
4 large red or yellow (bell) peppers
300 g/10½ oz/1½ cups long grain rice
1 onion
1 small green (bell) pepper
150 g/5½ oz/2¼ cups mushrooms
1 tbsp vegetable oil
pinch each paprika, curry powder and freshly ground
black pepper
lettuce leaves to serve

Preparation time: 20 minutes
Cooking time: 30–35 minutes

1. Preheat the oven to 200°C/400°F/gas 6.
2. Wash the red or yellow (bell) peppers, cut off the tops, remove the seeds, then blanch or steam them for 2–3 minutes. Turn off the heat, lift them out of the pan, then turn them upside down to drain.
3. Cook the rice, following the instructions on the packet.
4. While the rice is cooking, peel and finely chop the onion.
5. Wash the green (bell) pepper, deseed it and cut the flesh into fine strips.
6. Wipe the mushrooms clean and slice them.
7. When the rice is almost ready, heat the oil in a pan and sauté the onion for 2–3 minutes. Add the green (bell) pepper and mushrooms. Drain the rice, add it to the onion and season with paprika, curry powder and black pepper.
8. Fill the red or yellow bell peppers with the rice mixture and place them in a casserole. Cover and cook the (bell) peppers in the preheated oven for 15 minutes.
9. Serve with fresh lettuce.

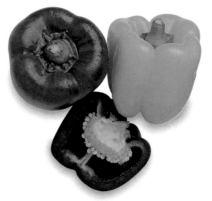

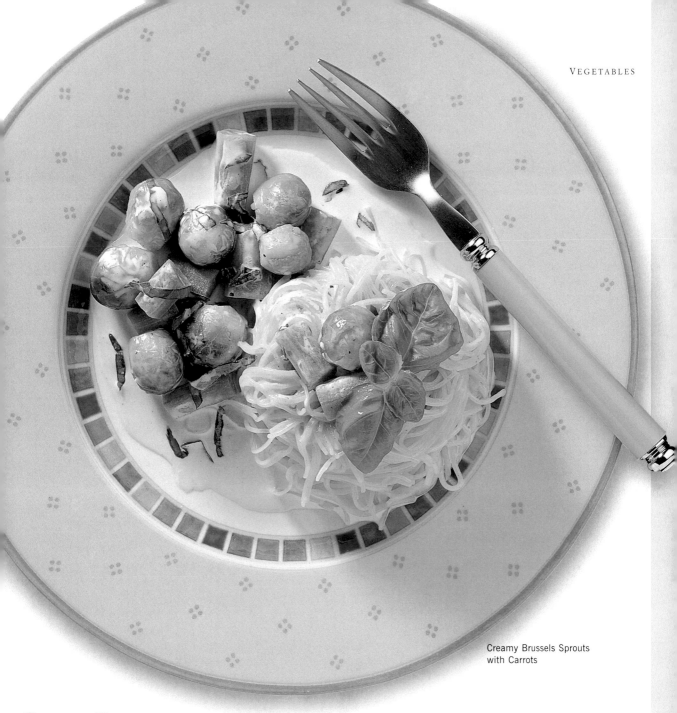

Creamy Brussels Sprouts
with Carrots

CREAMY BRUSSELS SPROUTS WITH CARROTS

(SERVES 4)

Ingredients
800 g/1 lb 12 oz Brussels sprouts
6 young carrots

For the sauce:
125 ml/4 fl oz/½ cup cream
4 fresh basil leaves, finely chopped, plus 1 whole basil
leaf to garnish
pinch each ground black pepper and paprika, to season

Preparation time: 10–15 minutes
Cooking time: 10–15 minutes

1. Clean the sprouts.
2. Peel the carrots and cut them into batons. Steam
the carrots and the sprouts for 8–10 minutes until they are
both tender.
3. In a separate small pan, heat the cream gently, but do not
boil, and add the chopped basil leaves.
4. Season the sauce with pepper and paprika and pour it over
the vegetables. Garnish with the whole basil leaf. Serve with
pasta or potatoes.

251

RATATOUILLE

(SERVES 4)

Ingredients
1 courgette (zucchini)
250 g/9 oz/3⅔ cups mushrooms
1 red (bell) pepper
1 large onion
2 garlic cloves
5 or 6 beefsteak (beef) tomatoes
1 tbsp olive oil
2 bay leaves
½ tbsp stock granules or bouillon powder

Preparation time: 15–20 minutes
Cooking time: 50 minutes

1. Wash the courgette (zucchini) and cut into slices.
2. Wipe the mushrooms clean, remove the lower part of the stalks (stems), then cut the caps in half.
3. Wash the red (bell) pepper, remove the seeds and cut the flesh into strips.
4. Peel the onion and cut into rings.
5. Peel the garlic and cut the cloves in half.
6. Skin the tomatoes (plunge them briefly into just boiled water to make this easier) and cut into chunky pieces, discarding the cores.
7. Heat the olive oil in a pan on a medium heat and sauté the onion rings for 2–3 minutes. Add the rest of the vegetables and mushrooms. Add the bay leaves and stock granules or bouillon powder, then simmer on a low heat for 50 minutes.

STEAMED CAULIFLOWER WITH HERB SAUCE

(SERVES 4)

Ingredients
1 large cauliflower

For the sauce:
1 tbsp butter
1 tbsp flour
250 ml/9 fl oz/generous 1 cup vegetable stock (see page 206)
4 tbsp cream, whipped
pinch ground nutmeg
freshly ground black pepper
1 tbsp chopped fresh parsley
2 fresh basil leaves, finely shredded

Preparation time: 8–10 minutes
Cooking time: 10 minutes

1. Wash the cauliflower thoroughly, separate into florets and steam until tender for 10 minutes.
2. To make the sauce, melt the butter in a pan on a low heat. Add the flour and stir briskly.
3. When the butter has absorbed the flour completely, gradually add the stock, stirring constantly. Remove the sauce from the heat and stir in the cream. Season with nutmeg, pepper, parsley and basil.
4. Serve with boiled or steamed potatoes.

Ratatouille

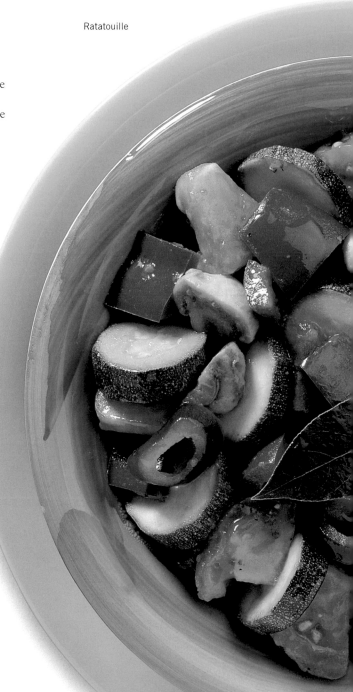

VEGETABLE STRIPS WITH CORIANDER SAUCE

(SERVES 4)

Ingredients
100 g/3½ oz carrots, peeled
100 g/3½ oz kohlrabi
100 g/3½ oz courgettes (zucchini)

For the sauce:
1 tbsp butter
1 spring onion (scallion)
2 tsp ground coriander
250 ml/9 fl oz/generous 1 cup cream

Preparation time: 8–10 minutes
Cooking time: 4–6 minutes

1. Wash the carrots, kohlrabi and courgettes (zucchini). Use a vegetable peeler to cut them into ribbons. Only use the outer part of the courgette (zucchini) flesh, not the seeds.
2. Blanch or steam the vegetable ribbons for 2–3 minutes.
3. Meanwhile, to make the sauce, heat the butter in a pan on a low heat. Shred the spring onion (scallion) and sauté in the butter for 2–3 minutes until soft.
4. Add the coriander and cream to the spring onion (scallion) and blend together. Pour the sauce over the vegetable ribbons and serve immediately.

MIXED STIR-FRIED VEGETABLES

(SERVES 4)

Ingredients
1 onion
1 garlic clove
1 red (bell) pepper
½ Chinese cabbage
200 g/7 oz/2¼ cups closed cup mushrooms
200 g/7 oz broccoli
    2 tbsp vegetable oil
    2 tbsp soy sauce
    1 tsp ground ginger
    ½ tsp paprika
    freshly ground black pepper

Preparation time: 10–15 minutes
Cooking time: 5 minutes

1. Peel the onion, cut in half, then slice into rings.
2. Peel the garlic clove and cut into four pieces.
3. Wash and deseed the (bell) pepper and cut into strips.
4. Wash the Chinese cabbage, pat dry and cut into strips.
5. Wipe the mushrooms clean and cut them in half.
6. Wash the broccoli, separate the florets from the stems, then cut the stems into small pieces.
7. Heat the oil in a wok or large frying pan (skillet) and stir-fry the onion for 1 minute. Add the garlic and (bell) pepper strips and stir-fry for 2 minutes. Add the broccoli and stir-fry for 1 minute. Add the Chinese cabbage and the mushrooms and stir-fry for 1 minute more.
8. Season the vegetables with soy sauce, ginger, paprika and pepper. Serve with boiled rice.
Note: omit the soy sauce if you have high blood pressure.

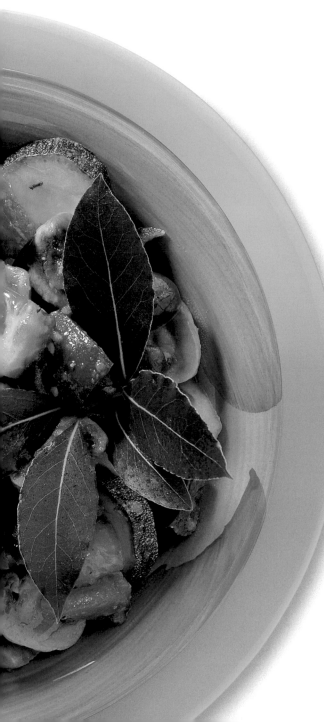

STEAMED CARROTS WITH COURGETTES (ZUCCHINI) AND SAGE

(SERVES 4)

Ingredients
1 bunch of new carrots
1 courgette (zucchini)

For the sauce:
1 small onion
1 tbsp butter
2–3 fresh sage leaves, finely chopped
125 ml/4 fl oz/½ cup cream

Preparation time: 20 minutes
Cooking time: 15 minutes

1. Remove the green leafy parts from the carrots and discard them, then wash the carrots thoroughly.
2. Wash the courgette (zucchini) and cut into slices or dice into cubes. Steam the carrots and courgette (zucchini) for 5–10 minutes, until tender.
3. To make the sauce, peel and finely chop the onion. Melt the butter in a pan and sauté the onion until soft. Add the sage and the cream. Pour the cream sauce over the hot vegetables and serve with potatoes.

BROCCOLI WITH LEEK CREAM SAUCE

(SERVES 4)

Ingredients
500 g/1 lb 2 oz broccoli
1 leek
1 tbsp butter
125 ml/4 fl oz/½ cup cream
pinch curry powder
freshly ground black pepper

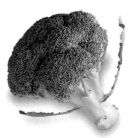

Preparation time: 10 minutes
Cooking time: 15 minutes

1. Wash the broccoli, chop the stems, separate out the florets and steam until tender.
2. Remove any green parts from the leek, cut off the roots, and cut the rest into rings.
3. Melt the butter in a pan. Cook the leek rings gently for 5 minutes until soft.
4. In a separate pan, heat the cream gently, but do not boil. Add the leeks and season to taste with curry powder and black pepper.
5. Serve the steamed broccoli with the leek cream sauce and potatoes or pasta.

BRUSSELS SPROUTS AND CHERRY TOMATOES IN HERB BUTTER

(SERVES 2)

Ingredients
300 g/10½ oz Brussels sprouts
200 g/7 oz cherry tomatoes
1–2 tbsp butter
1 tbsp finely chopped fresh herbs, such as parsley, tarragon, chives or sage

Preparation time: 10 minutes
Cooking time: 8–12 minutes

1. Clean the sprouts, then steam for 5–8 minutes until tender.
2. Wash and dry the tomatoes.
3. Leave the butter in a warm place to soften. In a small bowl mix the butter with the finely chopped herbs.
4. Heat the herb butter in a pan on a low heat. Sauté the sprouts and the tomatoes for 3–4 minutes.
5. Serve with a green salad (salad greens).

CARROTS: BETTER COOKED THAN RAW

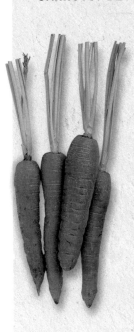

The orange pigment in carrots makes them an excellent source of the cancer-protective phytochemical beta-carotene, a carotenoid which the body converts into Vitamin A. Despite popular belief, they are better eaten cooked, rather than raw because the tough cell walls of the uncooked vegetable hinder the body's ability to manufacture Vitamin A. Cooking breaks down the cell walls, making absorption easier and does not affect beta-carotene levels. The belief that carrots can help you to see in the poor light is correct – Vitamin A helps your eyes to adjust from light to darkness. Carrots do have one drawback, however – unless they are grown organically, their skin often contains high levels of pesticides, so if you are unable to buy organic, make sure that you peel them before use.

STUFFED CABBAGE ROLLS WITH SPICED RICE

(SERVES 4)

Ingredients
100 g/3½ oz/½ cup long grain rice
1 small onion
½ red (bell) pepper
1 tbsp butter
1 tsp curry powder
1 Savoy cabbage

Preparation time: 20 minutes
Cooking time: 15–20 minutes

1. Cook the rice, following the instructions on the packet, drain and set aside to cool.

2. Peel and chop the onion.
3. Wash and deseed the pepper and chop into fine strips.
4. Melt the butter in a pan on a low heat, add the onion and red (bell) pepper and sauté until soft. Add the cooked rice and curry powder, mix well and cook for a 1–2 minutes before removing from the heat.
5. Meanwhile remove the outermost leaves from the cabbage. Cut out the thick central stalk, then wash them and cook in boiling water for 4–5 minutes. Drain and pat dry.
6. Put a spoonful of rice mixture in the middle of each leaf and roll up. Secure with a skewer or cocktail stick (toothpick).
7. Serve the rolls with the rest of the spiced rice mixture.

Stuffed Cabbage Rolls with Spicy Rice

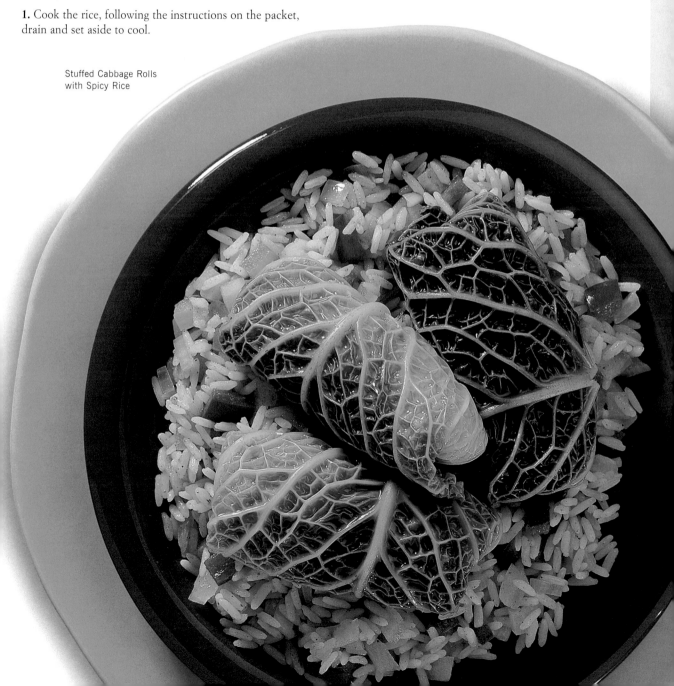

STUFFED MUSHROOMS WITH LEEK

(SERVES 2)

Ingredients
12 large mushrooms
1 leek
1 tbsp butter
3 fresh chives
4 tablespoons cream, whipped
freshly ground cayenne pepper, to season
paprika, to season

Preparation time: 15 minutes
Cooking time: 10 minutes

1. Wipe the mushrooms clean. Cut off the stalks (stems) and chop finely. Reserve the mushroom caps.
2. Clean and wash the leek, trimming off any roots and discarding any green parts. Slice into rings.
3. Wash the chives, pat dry and shred.
4. Heat the butter in a pan on a low heat and sauté the leeks and mushroom stalks (stems) for 5 minutes until soft. Add the chives and the cream and mix well. Season with cayenne pepper and paprika.
5. Fill the mushroom caps with the leek mixture and cook under a preheated medium grill (broiler) until brown.
6. Serve with pasta.

STUFFED FENNEL

(SERVES 2–3)

Ingredients
4 large fennel bulbs
½ red (bell) pepper
1 tbsp butter
1 shallot, peeled and finely chopped
1 garlic clove, peeled and crushed
100 g/3½ oz/scant 1 cup grated cheese

Preparation time: 30 minutes plus 30 minutes cooling
Cooking time: 35 minutes

1. Wash the fennel, removing the feathery fronds and any brown spots. Steam the bulbs whole for 30 minutes until tender. Remove from the heat and set aside to cool.
2. Using a teaspoon, scoop out the flesh, leaving the outer parts intact. Chop the flesh.
3. Wash, quarter and deseed the red (bell) pepper, and roughly chop into strips.
4. Melt the butter in a pan on a medium heat. Cook the (bell) pepper, shallot, fennel and crushed garlic for 4–5 minutes.
5. Fill the fennel bulbs with the vegetable mixture and sprinkle some grated cheese on top. Cook under a preheated hot grill (broiler) for 5 minutes until the cheese has melted.

OVEN-BAKED AUBERGINE (EGGPLANT) AND TOMATOES

(SERVES 4)

Ingredients
3 aubergines (eggplant)
8 beefsteak (beef) tomatoes
1–2 tbsp olive oil
4 fresh oregano sprigs, chopped
12 fresh basil leaves, chopped plus 8 whole leaves to garnish

Preparation time: 15 minutes
Cooking time: 55–60 minutes

1. Wash the aubergines (eggplant), slice, sprinkle with salt and drain for an hour. Rinse them well.
2. Preheat the oven to 200°C/400°F/gas 6.
3. Wash the tomatoes and cut into rings.
4. Heat the olive oil in a pan on a medium heat. When the oil is very hot, add the aubergine (eggplant) slices and sauté in batches until lightly browned.
5. Arrange the aubergine (eggplant) and tomato slices alternately in an ovenproof dish.
6. Sprinkle with the chopped oregano and basil and bake in the oven for 40 minutes. Garnish with the basil leaves before serving.

THREE VEGETABLES IN CHEESE SAUCE

(SERVES 4)

Ingredients
1 small cauliflower
300 g/10½ oz broccoli
4 carrots
1 tbsp chopped fresh parsley

For the cheese sauce:
2 tbsp butter
25 g/1 oz/¼ cup flour
300 ml/10 fl oz/1¼ cups milk
55 g/2 oz/½ cup grated cheese

Preparation time: 5–10 minutes
Cooking time: 10–15 minutes

1. Wash the cauliflower and broccoli. Separate into florets.
2. Peel the carrots and cut into batons.
3. Steam all the vegetables for 10 minutes until tender.
4. To make the cheese sauce, melt the butter in a pan on a low heat. Stir in the flour and cook, stirring constantly for 1 minute. Gradually stir in the milk and bring to the boil, stirring constantly. Remove the pan from the heat, stir in the cheese and pour the sauce over the steamed vegetables.

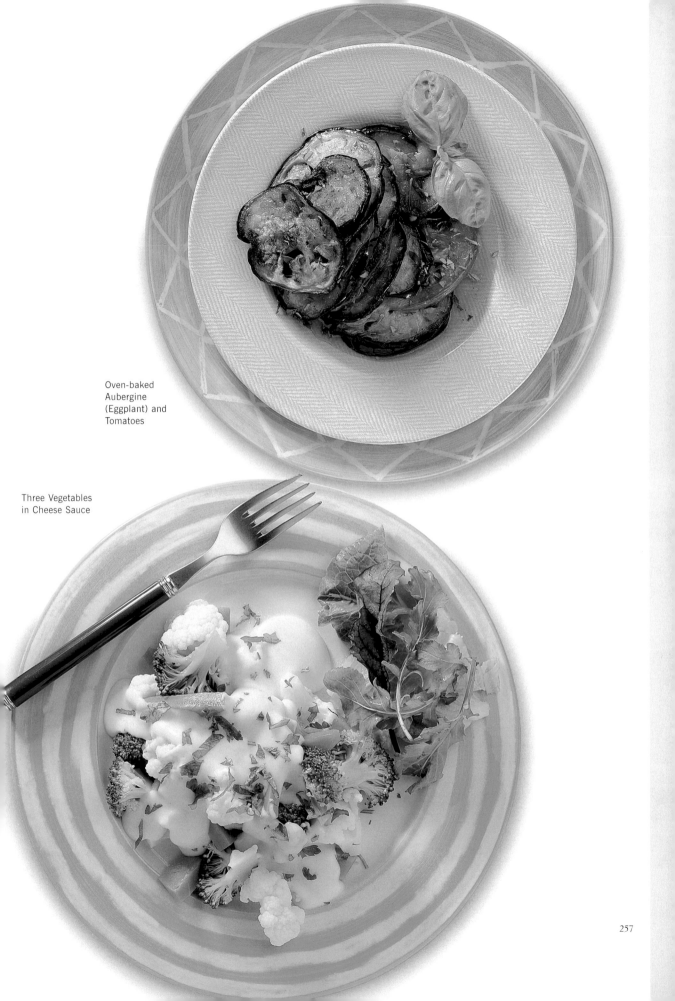

Oven-baked
Aubergine
(Eggplant) and
Tomatoes

Three Vegetables
in Cheese Sauce

257

STUFFED AUBERGINES (EGGPLANT)

(SERVES 4)

Ingredients
4 small aubergines (eggplant)
1 shallot
½ red (bell) pepper
2 tomatoes
1 tbsp olive oil
1 garlic clove, peeled and crushed
2 fresh basil leaves, chopped
3 mozzarella cheeses

Preparation time: 15 minutes
Cooking time: 50 minutes

1. Preheat the oven to 180°C/350°F/gas 4.
2. Wash the aubergines (eggplant), cut them in half and scoop out the flesh. Cut the flesh and reserve the shells.
3. Peel the shallot and chop finely.
4. Wash and deseed the (bell) pepper and cut into fine strips.
5. Skin the tomatoes (score them and plunge them into just boiling water for 2 minutes to help ease off the skins) and cut them into chunks.
6. Heat the olive oil in a pan on a low heat. Sauté the shallot, aubergine (eggplant) flesh, red (bell) pepper and tomatoes for 5 minutes. Add the garlic and cook for 2–3 minutes more.
7. Remove from the heat and add the chopped basil.
8. Fill the aubergine (eggplant) halves with the vegetable mixture and place in a greased ovenproof dish. Slice the mozzarella cheese with an egg slicer, if possible, and arrange the slices over the aubergines (eggplant). Bake for 40 minutes, or until the cheese is golden and bubbling.

AUBERGINES (EGGPLANT): EASTERN EXOTICS

A native of India, the aubergine (eggplant) features prominently in Asian, Middle Eastern and Mediterranean cuisine. It reached Europe in the Middle Ages, when Arab traders introduced it into Spain. Although in Africa and south-east Asia the vegetable was revered for its healing powers, Europeans took a different view. For centuries, they believed that eating aubergines (eggplant) could lead to leprosy and cancer and could drive people insane.

If baked, the vegetable is low in calories, but, if fried, aubergines (eggplant) will soak up substantial amounts of fat during cooking. The tastiest specimens are young and firm with shiny smooth skins and fresh green caps and stems.

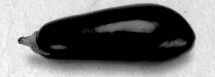

KOHLRABI AU GRATIN

(SERVES 4)

Ingredients
4 kohlrabi
1 small onion
200 g/7 oz/2¼ cups mushrooms
1 tbsp butter
1 garlic clove, peeled and crushed
freshly ground black pepper
1 tsp stock granules or bouillon powder
90 g/3¼ oz/scant 1 cup grated low-fat cheese or
90 g/3¼ oz/scant ½ cup Quark
125 ml/4 fl oz/½ cup cream

Preparation time: 15 minutes
Cooking time: 6–8 minutes

1. Peel the kohlrabi and dice into cubes.
2. Peel the onion and chop finely.
3. Wipe the mushrooms clean and slice thinly.
4. Melt the butter in a pan on a medium heat and sauté the onion, kohlrabi and mushrooms for 4–5 minutes until soft.
5. Add the crushed garlic to the pan and season the mixture with pepper and the stock granules or bouillon powder. Cook for 2–3 minutes more.
6. Combine the cheese or Quark and cream in a dish. Add the vegetable mixture and mix together.
7. Serve hot with a mixed salad.

MIXED ASPARAGUS WITH CREAM SAUCE

(SERVES 2 TO 3)

Ingredients
2 bundles asparagus, green and white
2 fresh parsley sprigs
2 tbsp butter
125 ml/4 fl oz/½ cup cream, whipped
freshly ground cayenne pepper

Preparation time: 8–10 minutes
Cooking time: 10 minutes

1. Wash the asparagus. Cut the stems into equal pieces and discard the fibrous stalks. Cut off the tips and reserve.
2. Steam the asparagus for 10 minutes, adding the tips 3 minutes before the end of the cooking time.
3. Wash the parsley, pat dry and chop finely.
4. Melt the butter in a pan on a low heat. Stir in the cream and season with cayenne pepper. Pour the cream sauce over the steamed asparagus and garnish with the chopped parsley.

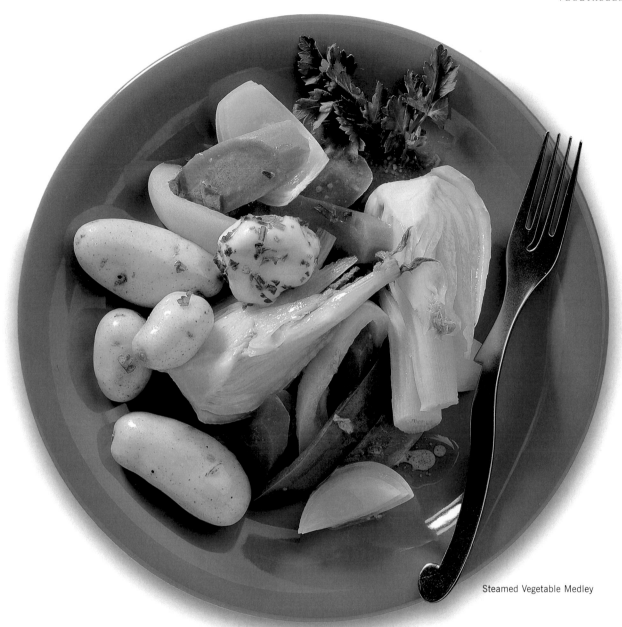

Steamed Vegetable Medley

STEAMED VEGETABLE MEDLEY

(SERVES 2)

Ingredients
2 fennel bulbs
½ red (bell) pepper
½ yellow (bell) pepper
1 onion
3 carrots
1 bay leaf
1 tbsp stock granules or bouillon powder
2–3 tbsp softened butter
50 g/1¼ oz/scant 1 cup finely chopped fresh herbs

Preparation time: 10–15 minutes
Cooking time: 8–10 minutes

1. Wash and trim the fennel, then cut into quarters.
2. Wash and deseed the (bell) peppers, then cut into chunks.
3. Peel the onion and carrots and chop into large pieces.
4. Put the fennel, (bell) peppers, onion and carrots into a steaming basket. Add the bay leaf to the water and steam the vegetables until tender.
5. Combine the butter with the chopped herbs. Arrange the steamed vegetables on a dish and spread with the herb butter.
6. Serve with potatoes.

ENDIVE (CHICORY) IN PASTRY

(SERVES 4)

Ingredients
1 large head of endive (chicory)
1 tbsp butter
125 ml/4 fl oz/½ cup Sour Cream Dressing (see page 193)
1 garlic clove, peeled and crushed
1 tbsp stock granules or bouillon powder
pinch nutmeg
4 puff pastry cases

Preparation time: 5–10 minutes
Cooking time: 12–18 minutes

Preheat the oven to 180°C/350°F/gas 4.
1. Wash the endive (chicory). Melt the butter in a pan on a low heat and cook the endive (chicory) until just wilted.
2. Remove from the heat and stir in the sour cream dressing.
3. Season with the crushed garlic, stock granules or bouillon powder and nutmeg. Fill the puff pastry cases with the endive (chicory) mixture and heat through in a hot oven.

FRIED VEGETABLES

(SERVES 4)

Ingredients
1 shallot
½ red (bell) pepper
200 g/7 oz broccoli
90 g/3¼ oz/1⅓ cups mushrooms
2 tbsp butter

To season:
freshly ground black pepper
pinch paprika
pinch curry powder

Preparation time: 5–10 minutes
Cooking time: 12–18 minutes

1. Peel and finely chop the shallot.
2. Wash and deseed the (bell) pepper, and cut into fine strips.
3. Wash the broccoli. Steam whole, then drain well and cut into pieces.
4. Wipe the mushrooms clean and slice thinly.
5. Melt the butter in a pan on a medium heat. Add all the vegetables and sauté for 10 minutes. Season with pepper, paprika and curry powder. Serve with mashed potato or rice.

POTATO AU GRATIN

(SERVES 2)

Ingredients
500 g/1 lb 2 oz potatoes
1 garlic clove
125 ml/4 fl oz/½ cup cream
freshly ground black pepper
100 g/3½ oz/1¼ cups breadcrumbs

Preparation time: 10–15 minutes
Cooking time: 15–20 minutes

1. Peel the potatoes and slice them thinly – use a food processor if possible. Steam the potato slices until just cooked. Do not overcook.
2. Grease a shallow, flameproof dish and rub it with a cut garlic clove. Arrange the potato slices in the dish.
3. Pour the cream over the sliced potatoes. Season with pepper and sprinkle with the breadcrumbs.
3. Cook the potatoes under a hot grill (broiler) for 5 minutes or until a brown crust forms on them.

ALL ABOUT POTATOES

One of the most enduring food myths is the belief that potatoes are bad for you because they are fattening. They are not bad for you – they are packed with nutrients. Potatoes provide complex carbohydrates, which are needed for long-lasting energy, fibre, Vitamin C, Vitamin B6, potassium and other minerals. The potato's skin contains much of the nutrients, so it is best to leave it on. It is also a good idea to eat potatoes baked or boiled, rather than fried, because fat added during cooking increases calorie content substantially. The Vitamin C content starts to drop almost as soon as potatoes are lifted from the soil, so the fresher the potatoes you eat the better. Because potatoes are treated with chemicals, try to buy organically grown ones whenever possible, while any potato that has sprouted or has green patches on it should be discarded. (The green patches contain alkaloids, which can be poisonous.)

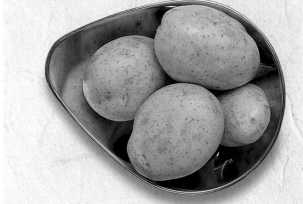

Potato Skins
with Sour Cream

(SERVES 2)

Ingredients
4 large new potatoes
55 g/2oz/¼ cup butter
handful fresh mixed herbs, chopped
150 ml/5fl oz/⅔ cup sour cream
handful chopped fresh chives

Preparation time: 5–10 minutes
Cooking time: 25–30 minutes

1. Preheat the oven to 230°C/450°F/gas 8.
2. Scrub the potatoes well, cook them whole in boiling water until soft, then drain them.
3. Cut the potatoes lengthways into four quarters. Remove most of the flesh with a sharp knife, taking care to leave a layer of flesh on the potato skin.
4. Arrange the skins on a greased baking (cookie) sheet. Melt the butter and coat the skins with it. Sprinkle with herbs and bake in the oven for 15–20 minutes, or until crisp.
5. Serve the potato skins lukewarm or warm with sour cream, chopped chives and a salad.

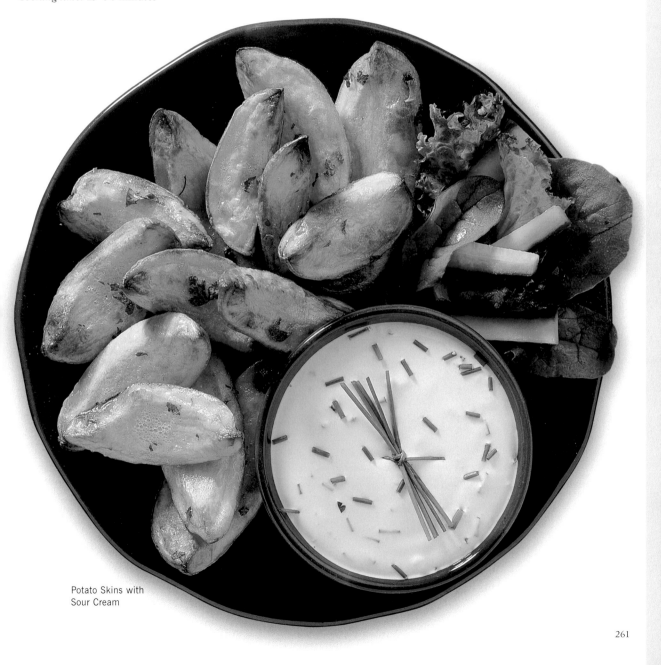

Potato Skins with
Sour Cream

WINTER WARMING POTATOES

(SERVES 4)

Ingredients
1 kg/2 lb 4 oz potatoes
1 onion
1 tbsp butter
1 bay leaf
freshly ground black pepper
stock granules or bouillon powder

Preparation time: 5–10 minutes
Cooking time: 15–20 minutes

1. Peel the potatoes and dice into cubes.
2. Peel the onion and chop into thin rings.
3. Melt the butter in a large pan and gently cook the potatoes and onions over a low heat for 15–20 minutes. Add the bay leaf and season with pepper and the stock granules.

POTATO RÖSTI

(SERVES 4)

Ingredients
4 large potatoes
1 tbsp butter
salt
freshly ground black pepper

Preparation time: 8–10 minutes
Cooking time: 10–12 minutes

1. Peel the potatoes and use a food processor to shred them roughly. Squeeze out the shredded potato on to a clean dish towel or put in a colander to drain. Divide the mixture into eight spoonfuls.
2. Melt the butter in a pan on a medium heat. When it is very hot, add the potatoes and press down and shape them with a fork, creating 8 small cakes. You may have to do this in batches. Season with salt and pepper. Cook for 5 minutes until the undersides of the cakes turn golden brown, then turn them over and cook the other sides until they are the same colour. Serve immediately.

Potato Rösti

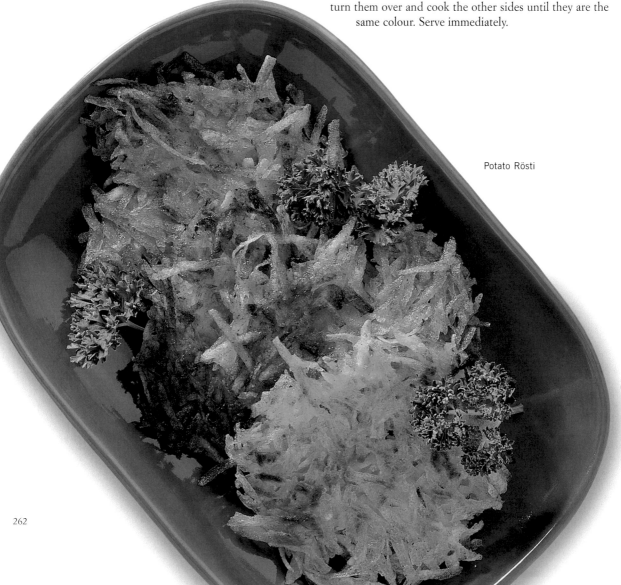

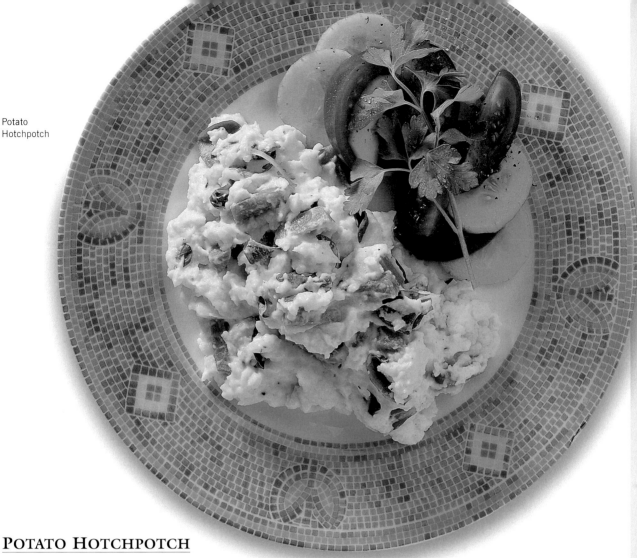

Potato
Hotchpotch

POTATO HOTCHPOTCH

(SERVES 4)

Ingredients
1 kg/2 lb 4 oz potatoes
125 ml/4 fl oz/½ cup cream
125 ml/4 fl oz/½ cup Vegetable Stock (see page 206)
2 tbsp butter
pinch each nutmeg and mace, to season
freshly ground black pepper, to season
selection of prepared vegetables such as carrots, cauliflower and spinach, raw or cooked

Preparation time: 10–15 minutes
Cooking time: 5–10 minutes

1. Peel the potatoes and chop into cubes. Cook the potatoes in boiling water for 5–10 minutes until soft, then drain.
2. Using a masher or blender, mash the potatoes, adding the cream, vegetable stock and butter. Season the mash with nutmeg, mace and black pepper.
3. Combine the mashed potato with the prepared boiled, steamed or raw vegetables.
4. Serve the hotchpotch with a refreshing salad.

POTATO-CELERIAC (CELERY ROOT) PUREE

(SERVES 4)

Ingredients
500 g/1 lb 2 oz potatoes
300 g/10½oz peeled celeriac (celery root)
butter
4 tbsp cream
nutmeg
freshly ground black pepper

Preparation time: 10 minutes
Cooking time: 15 minutes

1. Peel and dice the potatoes and celeriac (celery root) and steam them for 15 minutes until tender.
2. Put the potatoes and celeriac (celery root) in a food processor, add the butter and cream and process to a smooth purée. Season with nutmeg and black pepper.

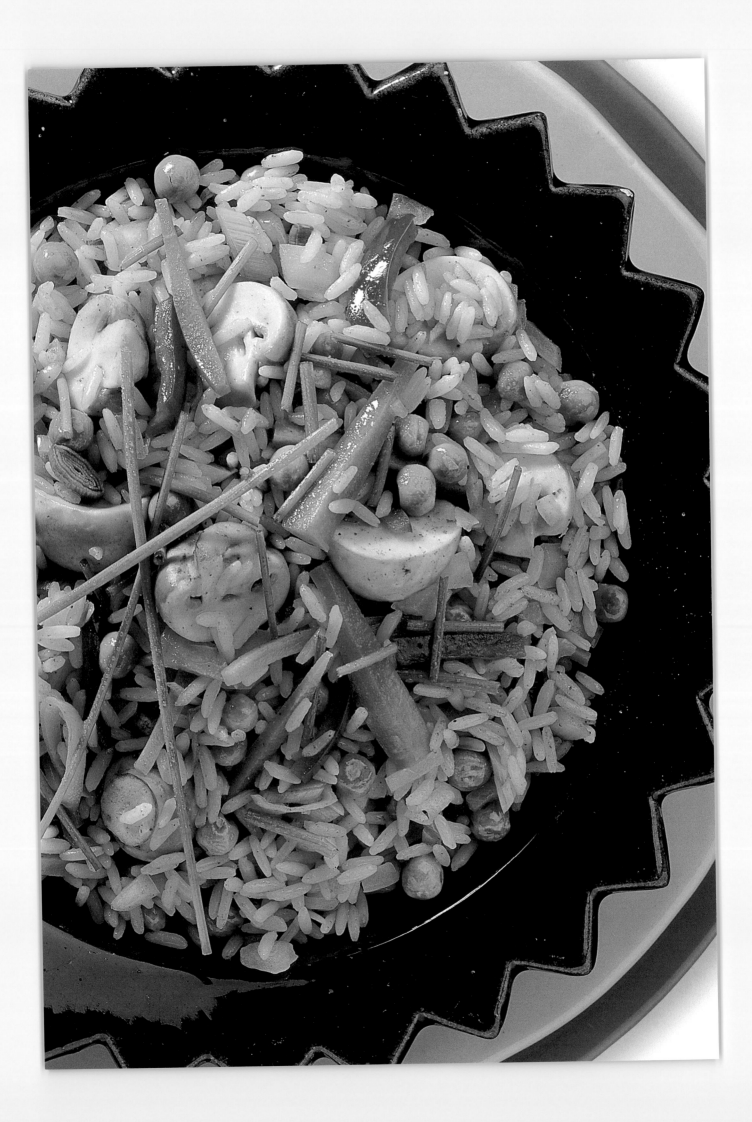

PASTA AND RICE DISHES

Once it was thought best to avoid pasta because it was considered to be extremely fattening. Nowadays, the health bonuses of the complex carbohydrates pasta contains, together with protein, are universally recognized. The body breaks down these carbohydrates to build up its reserves of energy-providing glycogen. The unhealthy culprit, in all probability, is the rich sauce with which pasta is all-too-frequently served. If you are eating healthily, you should cut back on or avoid sauces that feature cream, butter or cheese heavily among their ingredients. In fact, all dairy products are high in fat, two-thirds of which is saturated. Rice, for its part, is a good source of starch and of gluten-free carbohydrate. Most of its nutrients are contained in the bran and the germ, so brown rice varieties are more nutritious on the whole than white ones. Eating too much white rice can lead to a lack of thiamine in the body, while too much brown rice can result in iron and calcium deficiencies developing.

PASTA PERFECTION

One of the staple foods in the much vaunted Mediterranean diet, pasta is undoubtedly good for you. Indeed, the fact that so much pasta is eaten in Italy and other parts of southern Europe has been scientifically linked to the low levels of heart disease found in those areas. The starch and fibre in rice make it similarly beneficial, keeping blood sugar levels steady and helping to maintain the healthy functioning of the digestive system. It is also a useful, safe source of carbohydrates for anyone who has a wheat allergy.

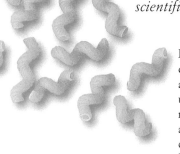

Pasta is literally a paste or dough made with flour, oil and sometimes eggs, and is used fresh or dry. Its chief nutritional virtue is its abundance of complex carbohydrates. The body breaks these down to build up its reserves of glycogen, the essential energy-providing substance. This is one of the reasons that pasta frequently features as a favourite energy-giving food among athletes and other sportspeople as part of their training plans. Of course, another reason for its popularity is that pasta dishes are easy to make and delicious to eat. Food combining experts agree that pasta should be kept egg-free – the protein from eggs does not combine well with the starchy pasta flour. In food combining terms, pasta is regarded as acid-forming.

PASTA FLOURS

When it comes to which sort of pasta to buy, you should take into account the type of flour that has been used to make it. Wholewheat pasta – which is made from 100 per cent wholewheat or whole durum wheat flour – is more nutritious than white pasta, which is made with refined flour that has had its wheatgerm and bran content removed during the milling process. White pasta retains starch and some fibre, but wholewheat pasta is a much better source of fibre and thiamine – the B vitamin the body requires to convert complex carbohydrates into glycogen. Wholewheat pasta also contains five per cent more protein than pasta made with white flour. It takes only 2–3 minutes longer to cook than the white variety and has a slightly coarser texture.

A NOTE ON ACCOMPANIMENTS

In Italy, it would be unthinkable to contemplate eating pasta without sauce or vegetables. Food combiners advise eating sauces in moderation, however, as they can interfere with the digestion if combined with cereal products too liberally, since their content is usually acidic. To maintain the body's acid-base balance, the ideal accompaniment for spaghetti and any other form of pasta is vegetables, cooked or (preferably) raw.

VERSATILE RICE

Rice is the staple food of half the world. It is packed with useful starches, and contains B vitamins, calcium and iron – although the more refined it is, the fewer nutrients it contains. The many different types of rice now available make it a versatile food – it can be used to make risotto, or in stir-fries and stuffed vegetables, and for sweet desserts. For optimum nutrition, it is best to eat brown or wild rice. Brown rice, in particular, is an excellent source of dietary fibre, although the phytic acid it contains can hinder the body's absorption of iron and calcium if it is eaten in large quantities. All rice has the added health bonus of being easily digestible and is an ideal gluten-free food for those who suffer from gluten intolerance. The starch it contains provides the body with a slow, steady flow of energy by keeping the blood sugar levels steady.

> **The quantities in the pasta recipes that follow are all based on using dried pasta. If you use fresh pasta for any of the recipes, you will need twice the weight.**

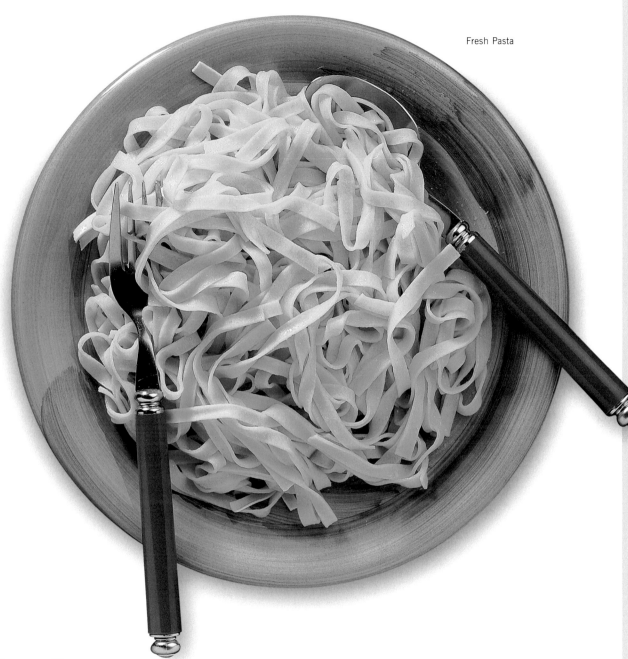

Fresh Pasta

FRESH PASTA

(SERVES 2)

Ingredients
200 g/7oz/generous 1⅔ cups whole durum wheat flour
2 eggs
1 tbsp oil

Preparation time: 10–12 minutes plus 30 minutes resting
Cooking time: 4–5 minutes

1. Put the flour in a bowl, and make a well in the middle. Break the eggs into the flour.
2. Add the oil and knead into a dough for 5 minutes until elastic in consistency. Knead the dough into a ball, then cover and set aside for 30 minutes.
3. Divide the dough into manageable pieces and roll with a rolling pin or use a pasta machine. Cut the dough into strips, slices, or other shapes.
4. Bring a large pan of water to the boil. Add the pasta and cook for 4–5 minutes until *al dente* (cooked, but not soft). Drain and then serve.

Fine Spaghetti with Mixed Vegetables

(SERVES 4)

Ingredients
400 g/14 oz/5¼ cups sugar snap peas
12 baby corn cobs
300 g/10½ oz/4¼ cups mushrooms
3 spring onions (scallions)
2 tbsp butter
salt and freshly ground cayenne pepper
300 g/10½ oz fine spaghetti
300 ml/10 fl oz/1¼ cups Creamy Red (Bell) Pepper Sauce
(see page 191)

Preparation time: 5–10 minutes
Cooking time: 10 minutes

1. Wash the sugar snap peas and remove their fibrous threads. Wash the baby corn cobs.
2. Wipe the mushrooms clean. Remove and discard the lower parts of the stalks (stems). Slice the rest.
3. Remove and discard the roots and any withered green parts from the spring onions (scallions). Cut the remainder into strips, then slice them.
4. Melt the butter in a pan on a low heat and sauté the mushrooms, baby corn and sugar snap peas for 5–10 minutes until soft. Season with salt and cayenne pepper.
5. Meanwhile, cook the spaghetti according to the instructions on the packet and drain. Divide equally among four warmed plates. Add a few spoonfuls of mixed vegetables to each plate. Serve with the creamy red (bell) pepper sauce.

Three-coloured Pasta with Leek Sauce

(SERVES 4)

Ingredients
3 leeks
200 g/7 oz/2¼ cups mushrooms
500–600 g/1 lb 2 oz–1 lb 5 oz three-coloured pasta
1 tbsp butter
pinch curry powder
freshly ground black pepper
½ tsp stock granules or bouillon powder
350 ml/12 fl oz/1½ cups cream

Preparation time: 5–10 minutes
Cooking time: 10 minutes

1. Cut off the roots and any green parts from the leeks. Cut the leeks in half, wash thoroughly, then cut into rings.
2. Wipe the mushrooms clean. Remove and discard the lower parts of the stalks (stems), then slice the remainder.

3. Cook the three-coloured pasta, following the instructions on the packet, until it is *al dente* (cooked, but not soft), then drain and place into a bowl.
4. Meanwhile, heat the butter in a pan on a medium heat and cook the leeks and the mushrooms until soft. Season with curry powder, pepper and stock granules or bouillon powder.
5. Stir in the cream, then pour the sauce over the pasta. Toss well and serve with a salad.

Cold Pasta Salad

(SERVES 1)

Ingredients
100 g/4 oz/1 cup mixed pasta
1 head broccoli
3–4 iceberg (romaine) lettuce
1 bunch watercress
2 carrots
2 tbsp Mayonnaise (see page 192)

Preparation time: 5–10 minutes plus chilling time
Cooking time: 10 minutes

1. Cook the pasta until it is *al dente* (cooked but not soft). Drain and set aside to cool.
2. Wash the broccoli and separate into florets. Steam the florets and set them aside to cool.
3. Wash the lettuce leaves, pat dry and cut into strips.
4. Wash the watercress, pat dry and add to the pasta with the lettuce strips and the broccoli florets.
5. Roughly shred the carrots and mix with the pasta.
6. Add the mayonnaise and mix together thoroughly to coat all of the ingredients.

Pasta with Herbs

(SERVES 4)

Ingredients
500 g/1lb pasta
4 tbsp olive oil
2 tbsp chopped fresh basil or parsley

Preparation time: 1–2 minutes plus chilling time
Cooking time: 10 minutes

1. Cook the pasta until it is *al dente* (cooked, but not soft), then drain and place in a dish.
2. Heat the oil and pour it over the pasta.
3. Sprinkle with the chopped basil or parsley.

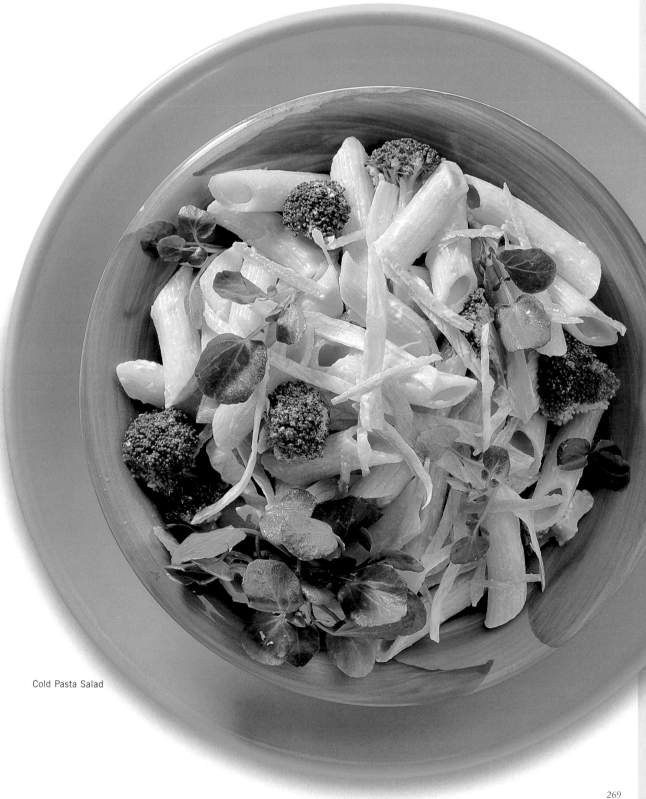

Cold Pasta Salad

VEGETARIAN LASAGNE

(SERVES 4)

Ingredients
450 g/1 lb broccoli
½ tsp stock granules or bouillon powder
salt and freshly ground black pepper
1 frisée lettuce
2 tbsp butter
200 g/7 oz/2¾ cups mushrooms
250 ml/8 fl oz/1 cup cream
500 g/1 lb 2 oz lasagne
3 tbsp breadcrumbs

Preparation time: 20–25 minutes
Cooking time: 15–20 minutes

1. Wash the broccoli, then cut off and reserve the stalks. Divide the head into florets, cut the stalks into pieces and steam for 6–8 minutes until tender. Drain, purée the cooked broccoli, and season with stock granules or bouillon powder, salt and pepper.

2. Wash and shred the the frisée lettuce. Melt a little of the butter in a pan on a low heat and sauté the frisée lettuce for 1–2 minutes until wilted. Season to taste.

3. Wipe the mushrooms clean, slice and cook in a separate pan for 2–3 minutes using the remaining butter.

Vegetarian Lasagne

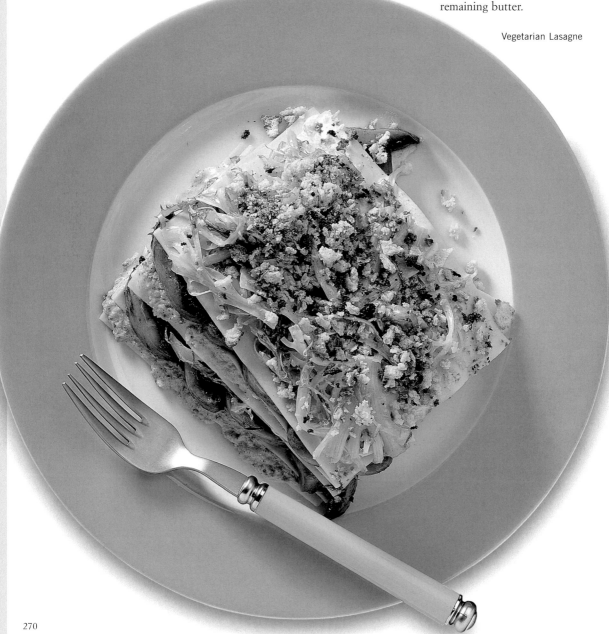

4. Stir half the cream into the broccoli purée and the other half into the frisée lettuce.
5. Cook the lasagne following the instructions on the packet.
6. Grease a square, flameproof dish and cover the base with some of the cooked lasagne strips. Pour a layer of broccoli sauce over the lasagne. Then top with another layer of lasagne, followed by the mushrooms, another layer of lasagne then the frisée mixture. Continue doing this until the sauces, lasagne and mushrooms have been used up. Make sure that you use frisée for the final layer.
7. Sprinkle with breadcrumbs and cook under a medium grill (broiler) for 10–20 minutes.

REFRESHING PASTA SALAD

(SERVES 1)

Ingredients
100 g/3½ oz/scant 1 cup butterfly pasta
1 carrot
1 carton cress
2 tbsp chopped beansprouts
2 tbsp Herb Mayonnaise (see page 192)

Preparation time: 5 minutes
Cooking time: 10 minutes

1. Cook the pasta according to the instructions on the packet until *al dente* (cooked, but not soft). Drain and set aside to cool.
2. Peel the carrot, shred it and add to the cooled pasta.
4. Wash the cress and combine with the pasta. Add the beansprouts and mix well.
5. Stir in the herb mayonnaise and combine well.

PASTA WITH STEAMED VEGETABLES

(SERVES 4)

Ingredients
1 small courgette (zucchini)
3 new carrots
300 g/10½ oz fresh peas
3 spring onions (scallions)
400 g/14 oz pasta

For the sauce:
½ onion
1 tbsp butter
250 ml/8 fl oz/1 cup cream
pinch saffron threads
salt freshly ground black pepper
6–10 fresh thyme sprigs, to garnish

Preparation time: 15–20 minutes
Cooking time: 10 minutes

1. Wash the courgette (zucchini) and the carrots and cut them into equal-size small pieces.
2. Remove the fresh peas from their pods, discard any fibrous threads, then wash them.
3. Remove the roots and any withered parts from the spring onions (scallions). Wash well, then cut each green part into two pieces and the white parts into four.
4. Put all the vegetables into a steamer and cook them gently for 3–5 minutes.
5. Meanwhile, cook the pasta according to the instructions on the packet until it is *al dente* (cooked, but not soft). Drain.
6. To make the sauce, peel and finely chop the onion. Melt the butter in a pan on a low heat and sauté the onion for 5 minutes until soft.
7. Add the cream and saffron threads to the onion. Season with salt and pepper if required.
8. Pour the cream sauce over the vegetables. Serve the pasta and the vegetables in two separate bowls, garnished with sprigs of thyme.

TAGLIATELLE WITH OYSTER MUSHROOMS

(SERVES 4)

Ingredients
1 kg/2 lb 4 oz/14½ cups oyster mushrooms
1 shallot
1 tbsp butter
1 tbsp olive oil
2 garlic cloves, peeled and crushed
freshly ground cayenne pepper
400–500 g/14 oz–1 lb 2 oz) tagliatelle
250 ml/8 fl oz/1 cup cream
6 fresh basil leaves, to garnish

Preparation time: 10 minutes
Cooking time: 10 minutes

1. Wipe the mushrooms clean. Remove the lower parts of the stalks (stems) and slice the remainder.
2. Peel and finely chop the shallot.
3. Heat the butter and olive oil in a pan over a low heat. Add the mushrooms and the shallot and cook until soft. Season with garlic and a little cayenne pepper and continue cooking for 1–2 minutes more.
4. Meanwhile, cook the pasta according to the instructions on the packet until it is *al dente* (cooked, but not soft). Drain and combine with the mushroom mixture in a large bowl. Stir in the cream and mix well.
5. Garnish with basil leaves.

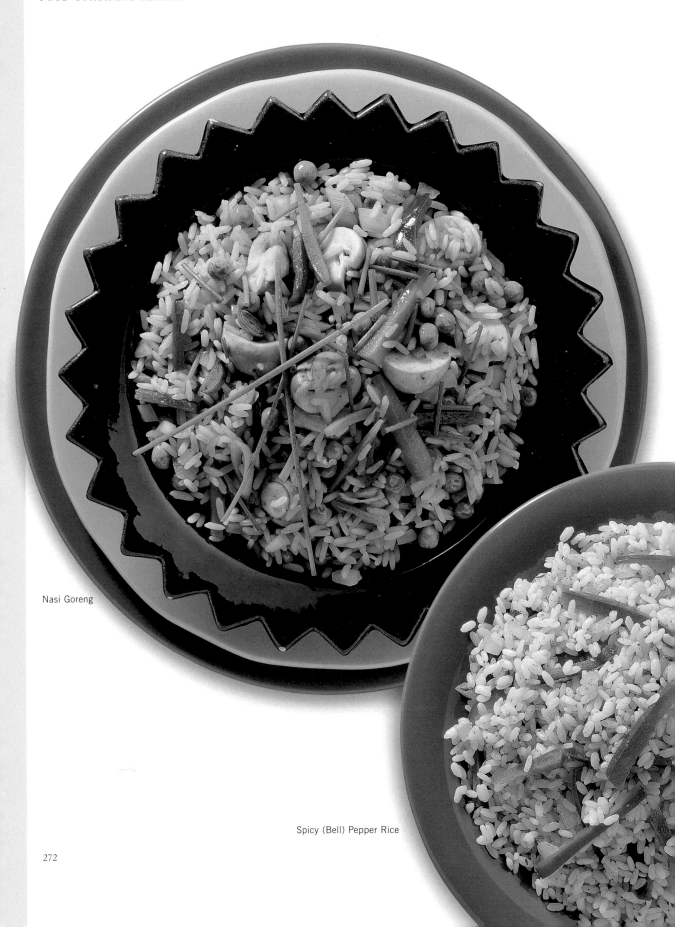

Nasi Goreng

Spicy (Bell) Pepper Rice

NASI GORENG

(SERVES 4)

Ingredients
300 g/10½ oz/1½ cups long grain rice
1 small onion
1 garlic clove
1 large carrot
1 leek
½ red (bell) pepper
200 g/7 oz fresh peas
150 g/5½ oz/2¼ cups baby button (white) mushrooms
1 tbsp vegetable oil
1 tbsp soy sauce
½ tsp paprika
¼ tsp curry powder
¼ tsp ground ginger
6–8 fresh chives, chopped, to garnish

Preparation time: 25–30 minutes
Cooking time: 15–20 minutes

1. Start cooking the rice, following the instructions on the packet. The vegetables can be prepared while it is cooking.
2. Peel and slice the onion and peel and crush the garlic.
3. Peel the carrot and cut it into fine strips.
4. Wash the leek and red (bell) pepper. Remove and discard the leek roots and deseed the (bell) pepper. Cut both into fine strips or rings.
5. Boil the peas for 5 minutes until tender.
6. Wipe the mushrooms clean and cut in half.
7. When the rice is almost ready, heat the oil in a wok or deep frying pan (skillet). When the oil is very hot, add all the vegetables and stir-fry rapidly for 5 minutes.
8. Place the stir-fried vegetables in a bowl and season with soy sauce. Drain the cooked rice and mix it in. Season with paprika, curry powder and ginger. Garnish the dish with chopped chives before serving.

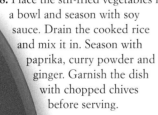

SPICY (BELL) PEPPER RICE

(SERVES 4)

Ingredients
200 g/7 oz/1 cup long grain rice
1 red (bell) pepper
1 green (bell) pepper
½ tbsp vegetable oil
½ onion, peeled and chopped
1 garlic clove, peeled and crushed
2 drops Tabasco sauce
½ tsp curry powder

Preparation time: 5–10 minutes
Cooking time: 15–20 minutes

1. Cook the rice, following the instructions on the packet, then drain.
2. Wash and deseed both (bell) peppers and cut the flesh into fine strips.
3. Heat the oil in a pan and cook the onion, garlic and (bell) peppers until soft.
4. Add the cooked rice. Mix together thoroughly, adding the Tabasco and the curry powder as you do so. Serve on its own or with a side dish.

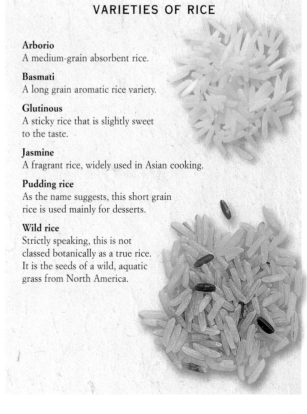

VARIETIES OF RICE

Arborio
A medium-grain absorbent rice.

Basmati
A long grain aromatic rice variety.

Glutinous
A sticky rice that is slightly sweet to the taste.

Jasmine
A fragrant rice, widely used in Asian cooking.

Pudding rice
As the name suggests, this short grain rice is used mainly for desserts.

Wild rice
Strictly speaking, this is not classed botanically as a true rice. It is the seeds of a wild, aquatic grass from North America.

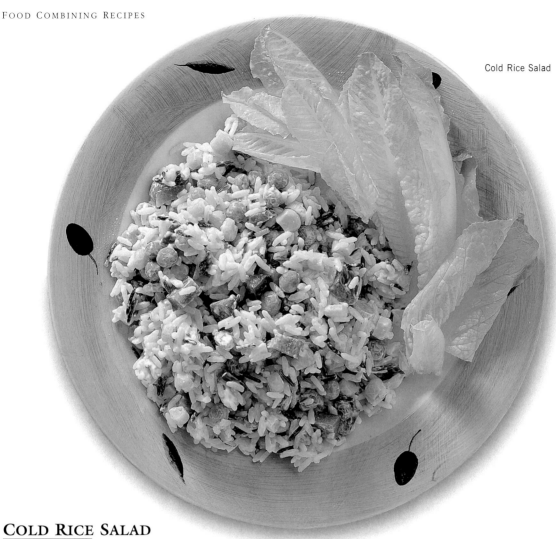

Cold Rice Salad

COLD RICE SALAD
(SERVES 4)

Ingredients
150 g/5½ oz/¾ cup long grain rice
½ red (bell) pepper
1 spring onion (scallion)
3 tbsp freshly cooked peas
3 tbsp cooked sweetcorn (corn)
3 tbsp Mayonnaise (see page 192)

Preparation time: 5–10 minutes
Cooking time: 20–30 minutes

1. Cook the rice, following the instructions given on the packet, then drain.
2. Wash and deseed the (bell) pepper and dice it finely.
3. Peel the spring onion (scallion), removing the roots and green parts, then chop the rest finely. Blend with the rice and (bell) pepper.
4. Mix the peas and the sweetcorn (corn) with the rice salad. Add the mayonnaise and blend well.
5. Serve with a green salad (salad greens).

MIXED RICE
(SERVES 4)

Ingredients
150 g/5½ oz/¾ cup long grain rice
50 g/1¼ oz/¼ cup wild rice
1 shallot
1 tbsp butter
pinch paprika
freshly ground black pepper
6 fresh chives, chopped

1. Cook both types of rice separately according to the instructions given on the packets. (You can recognize wild rice by its long, slim, black grains.) Drain.
2. Peel the shallot and shred it. Melt the butter in a pan on a low heat and cook the shallot for 2–3 minutes until soft.
3. Add the rice and the wild rice to the pan, mix well and season with paprika and pepper.
4. Garnish with the chopped chives and serve the rice as a side dish.

RISOTTO WITH MUSHROOMS

(SERVES 4)

Ingredients
250 g/9 oz/2¼ cups Arborio (risotto) rice
1 shallot
1 garlic clove
1 kg/2 lb 4 oz/14½ cups mixed mushrooms (such as oyster mushrooms, chanterelles, Parisian mushrooms, morels, ceps)
2 tbsp butter
freshly ground black pepper
250 ml/8 fl oz/1 cup cream
1 tbsp chopped fresh basil and oregano, to season

Preparation time: 5–10 minutes
Cooking time: 20–25 minutes

1. Cook the rice, following the instructions given on the packet, then drain.
2. Peel and finely chop the shallot and the garlic.
3. Wipe the mushrooms clean, slice the large ones and leave the smaller ones whole.
4. Melt the butter in a large pan on a low heat. Sauté the mushrooms, shallot and crushed garlic for 5 minutes until soft. Season with pepper.
5. Mix the cooked rice with the mushrooms and add the cream. Season the risotto with the basil and oregano.

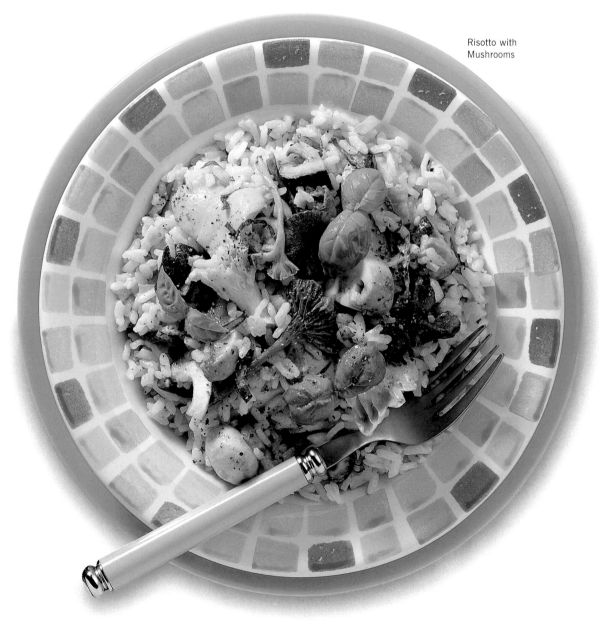

Risotto with
Mushrooms

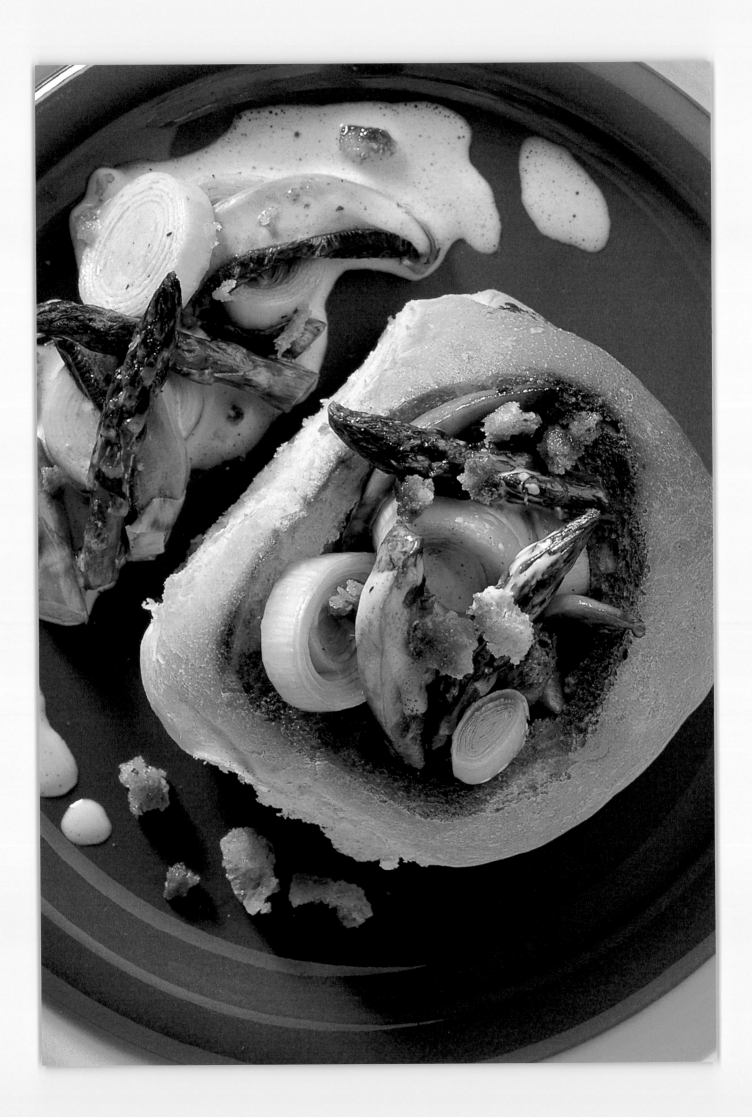

BREAD

Almost all grains and cereal products are acid-forming starches, which combine well with any kind of vegetables, salads, seeds and herbs. They do not mix well with proteins, however. Bread is healthy and full of flavour. Its high fibre content makes it a useful nutritional weapon in helping to prevent and treat intestinal disorders, although, according to food combining authorities, it is important not to eat too much of it too often.

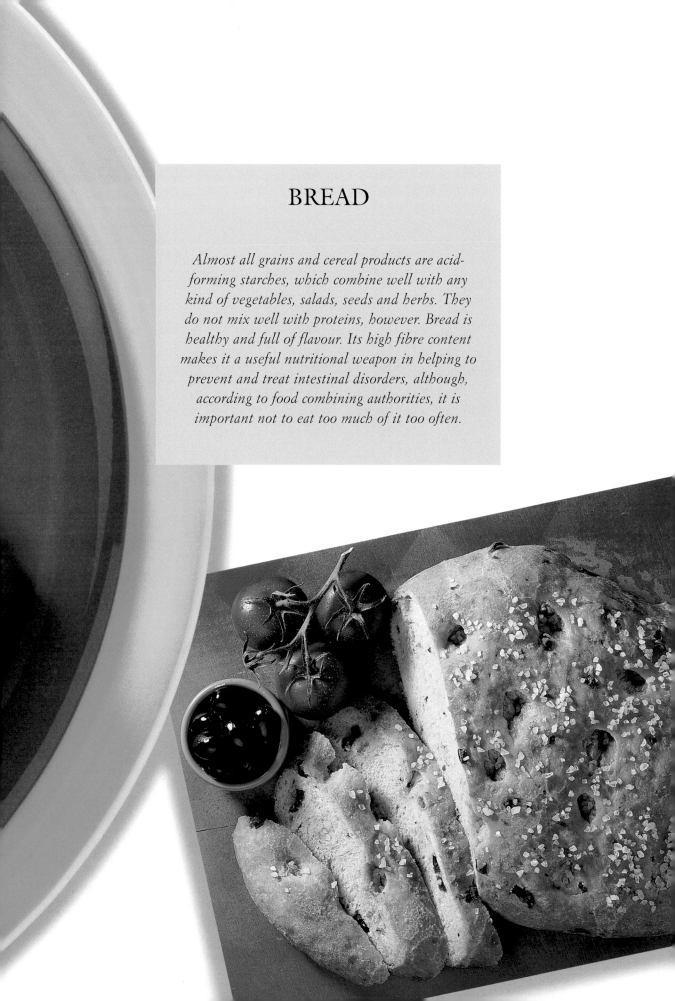

BREAD AND BREAD-MAKING

In recent years, bread's image has been transformed. It used to be considered fattening, stodgy and generally unappealing. Now, by contrast, it is recognized as an important part of a healthy diet, and the actual breads we prefer are now healthier and more varied. From bagels and brioche to pumpernickel and tortilla, there is a bread to catch everyone's fancy. Remember, though, that brioche should be only an occasional treat because it contains more fat, protein and calories than almost any other bread variety.

A wide variety of healthy breads is now available.

Conventional nutritionists and food combining experts tend to differ about how much and what types of bread we should eat and how often. The viewpoint of the former is that, particularly because of its high-fibre content, bread can help to prevent digestive problems and other disorders. It is rich in iron and vitamins, especially the B-complex group, and is also a valuable source of calcium, which is essential for the building of strong bones and teeth. Wholemeal (whole-wheat) varieties, in particular, are packed with natural goodness and fibre.

Although bread is undeniably nutritious, food combining authorities have a different view of its overall value to health. The starch in bread, they say, is slow to break down into its constituent sugars, which is exacerbated if too much bread is eaten: excessive quantities of starch disrupt the body's acid-base balance, which can lead to digestive difficulties. Added to this, some breads come heavily laced with extra yeast and extra gluten (one of the proteins in wheat flours); both are common food allergens. There is also the question of the other additives found in most mass-produced bread. These include fat, preservatives, salt, emulsifiers and, in the case of some white breads, flour bleaches. The salt, which is added for flavour and to strengthen the gluten, is certainly a nutritional drawback. A typical mass-manufactured white loaf can contain as much as 350 mg a slice.

The picture is not so gloomy as this might suggest, however. Combining starchy and fatty foods, such as bread and butter, is favourable to digestion, provided that the fat's overall degree of acidity is not too high. Healthier alternatives to standard mass-manufactured bread include yeast-free soda bread, rye bread or pumpernickel (black rye). Remember, too, that the denser the texture of the bread, the better it is for you. It will help to satisfy your appetite, provide improved levels of nourishment and can help to reduce the chance of developing cravings that can lead to binge-eating.

FOOD VALUES PER 100 G/3½ OZ

WHITE BREAD
Fibre: 1.5 g
Carbohydrate: 49.3 g
Protein: 8.4 g
Fat: 1.9 g
Calories: 235
Vitamins and minerals: the flour from which white bread is made is fortified artificially with calcium, niacin, iron and thiamine by its manufacturers. So white bread contains twice as much calcium as wholemeal (whole-wheat) bread.

WHOLEMEAL (WHOLE-WHEAT) BREAD
Fibre: 5.8 g
Carbohydrate: 41.6 g
Protein: 9.2 g
Fat: 2.5 g
Calories: 215
Vitamins and minerals: wholemeal (whole-wheat) bread has three times more zinc and 40 per cent more iron than white bread, with a higher phosphorus, magnesium and manganese content and more B vitamins than white or brown bread. Contains Vitamin E.
Wholemeal (whole-wheat) bread

BROWN BREAD
Fibre: 3.5 g
Carbohydrate: 44.3 g
Protein: 8.5 g
Fat: 2.0 g
Calories: 218
Vitamins and minerals: brown bread contains the same amount of calcium as white bread; other nutrient levels are slightly lower than wholemeal (whole-wheat) bread.

RYE BREAD
Fibre: 4.4 g
Carbohydrate: 45.8 g
Protein: 8.3 g
Fat: 1.7 g
Calories: 219
Vitamins and minerals: Rye bread has significant Vitamin E levels.

BREAD FACTS

* The flour used to make white bread is often bleached. The bread itself contains water, yeast and various additives, preservatives and emulsifiers.
* Brown bread's colour derives not only from the brown part of the wheatgrain that it used to make the flour for it – manufacturers also add colouring, such as caramel.

BREAD DIRECTORY

Among the breads most widely available are:

Bagel
By origin, an eastern European Jewish roll with a hole through its centre. The dough is boiled and then baked, often sprinkled with seeds.

Brioche
Light, yeast-leavened roll or loaf, originating from France, made from white flour enriched with butter and eggs.

Ciabatta
Italian bread made from white or brown flour, bound with olive oil and often flavoured with herbs.

Croissant
Rich, flaky French roll that takes its name from its crescent shape. It has a high fat content, especially when it is made with butter.

Focaccia
Italian yeasted dough bread baked as a large disc, flavoured with olive oil, rock or sea salt, herbs and garlic.

Matzo
Traditional Jewish unleavened bread similar to a cracker.

Pitta
Middle Eastern flat bread, sometimes split to form a pocket

Pumpernickel
Heavy, dark brown rye bread originating from Germany, with a slightly sour, but rich flavour.

Rye breads
Popular in Scandinavia, Germany and Russia. Their low gluten content makes them heavier and denser than other breads.

Tortilla
Originally from Mexico, tortillas are round unleavened breads, made by mixing corn or wheat flour with salt and water, flattening the dough, and baking on a hot griddle.

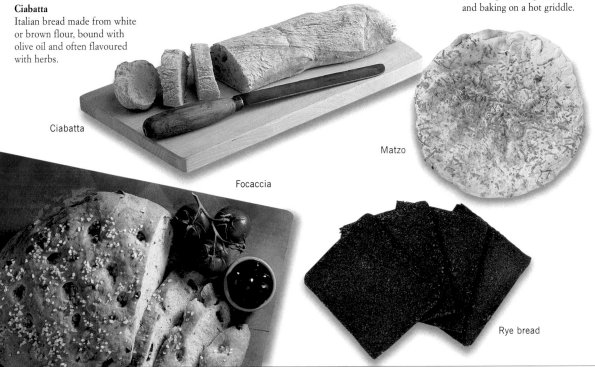

Ciabatta

Focaccia

Matzo

Rye bread

* Wholemeal (whole-wheat) bread is made with wholegrain flour or white flour with added wheatgerm and bran.
* Wheatgerm bread is made with brown or white flour, to which processed wheatgerm has been added.
* The added fibre in high-fibre white bread comes from non-wheat sources, such as rice, bran or soy.

BAKING BREAD AT HOME

Making your own bread lets you increase its fibre and nutritional content and to vary its flavours. To add calcium to your bread, for instance, replace some of the water in a standard recipe with skimmed (skim) milk or yogurt. Adding one or two tablespoons of skimmed milk powder (non-fat dry milk). For increased flavour, try using puréed fruit or babyfood fruit in place of some of the water. Not only does the fruit purée provide a different taste, it adds nutritional value and fibre, and helps to reduce the fat content when used in place of some of the fat in a conventional recipe. To add more fibre, use oats or other whole grains as substitutes for some of the regular flour. You can reduce the amount of sodium in the bread by cutting down the salt to 1 teaspoon for every 350 g/12 oz/3 cups of flour, but do not cut it out completely because yeast works better with some salt.

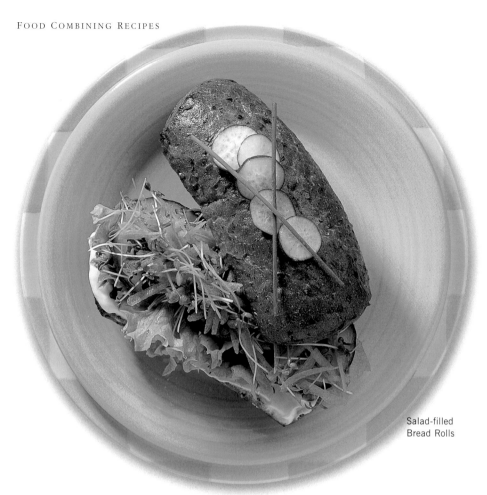

Salad-filled
Bread Rolls

SALAD-FILLED BREAD ROLLS

(SERVES 1)

Ingredients
2 bread rolls
2 tbsp Mayonnaise (see page 192)
4 lettuce leaves
¼ cucumber
2 tbsp shredded carrots
1 small handful of cress
6 radishes
chopped fresh chives, to garnish

Preparation time: 10–15 minutes

1. Cut the bread rolls in half and spread with the mayonnaise.
2. Wash the lettuce leaves, pat dry and tear into manageable pieces. Divide among the bread rolls.
3. Peel the cucumber, slice thinly and arrange on top of the open bread rolls with the shredded carrots and the cress.
4. Wash the radishes, remove and discard any green parts and slice. Use the slices to garnish the bread rolls. Sprinkle some finely chopped chives on the top.

AVOCADO BREAD ROLLS

(SERVES 1)

Ingredients
4 lettuce leaves
4 radishes
¼ cucumber
1 avocado
1 tbsp lemon juice
½ tbsp curry powder
2 bread rolls
1 small handful cress, to garnish

Preparation time: 10–15 minutes

1. Wash the lettuce, pat dry and tear into strips.
2. Wash the radishes, remove and discard the stalks and any green parts and slice. Peel and thinly slice the cucumber.
3. Peel the avocado, cut in half, remove the stone (pit) and purée the flesh. Add lemon juice to prevent discoloration and season with the curry powder.
4. Cut the bread rolls in half and spread them thickly with the avocado purée. Pile on the lettuce, radishes and cucumber slices and garnish with cress.

MUSHROOM TOASTS

(SERVES 4)

Ingredients
200 g/7 oz/2¼ cups mushrooms
1 tbsp butter
125 ml/4 fl oz/½ cup Cream Sauce (see page 193)
pinch nutmeg
pinch paprika
pinch stock granules or bouillon powder
freshly ground black pepper
1 tsp cornflour (cornstarch), optional
4 thick slices bread
2 tbsp breadcrumbs
carrot batons, cucumber slices, cherry tomatoes, to serve

Preparation time: 10 minutes
Cooking time: 10 minutes

1. Wipe the mushrooms clean and slice.
2. Melt the butter in a pan over a low heat and sauté the mushrooms for a few minutes.
3. Stir the cream sauce into the mushrooms. Season with nutmeg, paprika, stock granules or bouillon powder and pepper. Add some cornflour (cornstarch) paste (cornflour [cornstarch] mixed with water) to the sauce to thicken if necessary.
4. Meanwhile, toast the bread.
5. Spread a thick layer of the mushroom sauce over the toast and sprinkle with the breadcrumbs.
6. Place the mushroom toasts under a hot grill (broiler) and brown the surface. Arrange on plates decorated with raw salad vegetables.

STUFFED BREAD ROLLS

(SERVES 1)

Ingredients
2 round bread rolls
2 frisée lettuce leaves
100 g/3½ oz red cabbage
½–1 tbsp Herb Mayonnaise (see page 193)
2 tsp softened butter

Preparation time: 10 minutes
Cooking time: 5–10 minutes

1. Slice off the top of each bread roll, scoop out the contents and dice the soft bread into cubes.
2. Wash the frisée lettuce, pat dry, tear into fine strips and place into a mixing bowl.
3. Shred the red cabbage and add to the lettuce, followed by the herb mayonnaise. Mix well.
4. Heat the butter in a small frying pan (skillet). Sauté the bread cubes until golden brown and then add to the mixture.
5. Fill the rolls with the mixture and serve.

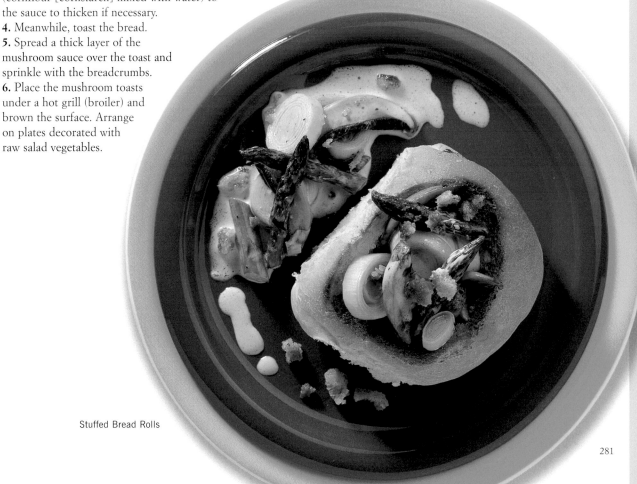

Stuffed Bread Rolls

TOAST WITH GARLIC MUSHROOMS

(SERVES 4)

Ingredients
75g/2¾ oz/6 tbsp butter
2 garlic cloves, crushed
350g/12 oz/4 cups mixed mushrooms, such as open-cap,
button, oyster and shiitake, sliced
8 slices French bread
1 tbsp chopped parsley
salt and pepper

Preparation time: 10 minutes
Cooking time: 10 minutes

1. Melt the butter in a frying pan (skillet). Add the crushed
garlic and cook for 30 seconds, stirring well.
2. Add the mushrooms to the butter and cook for about 5
minutes, stirring occasionally.
3. Toast the French bread slices under a preheated medium
grill (boiler) for 2–3 minutes, turning them once.
4. Transfer the pieces of toast to a serving plate.
5. Sprinkle the parsley into the mushrooms, mixing well, and
season with salt and pepper to taste.
6. Spoon the mushroom mixture over the toast and serve hot.

OYSTER MUSHROOM ROLLS

(SERVES 1–2)

Ingredients
200 g/7 oz/2¾ cups oyster mushrooms
1 tbsp butter
1 garlic clove, peeled and crushed
2 lettuce leaves
1 tbsp Mayonnaise (see page 192)
1 tbsp whipped cream
1–2 tsp chopped fresh herbs
salt and freshly ground black pepper
2 round bread rolls

Preparation time: 5 minutes
Cooking time: 4–5 minutes

1. Wipe the mushrooms clean and slice them.
2. Melt the butter in a pan over a low heat. Sauté the
mushrooms for 3–4 minutes. Add the crushed garlic and cook
for 1 minute more. Wash and dry the lettuce leaves.
3. Mix the mayonnaise with the cream and herbs and season
with salt and pepper.
4. Cut the bread rolls in half. Arrange lettuce and mushrooms
on each half and top with a spoonful of herb sauce.

STUFFED BREAD ROLLS WITH LEEK RAGOÛT

(SERVES 4)

Ingredients
1 leek
150 g/5½ oz/2¼ cups mushrooms
6 cooked asparagus spears
2 tbsp butter
125 ml/4 fl oz/½ cup whipped cream
freshly ground black pepper
pinch stock granules or bouillon powder
4 round crusty bread rolls
selection of raw vegetables, to serve

Preparation time: 15–20 minutes
Cooking time: 6–8 minutes

1. Clean the leek, discarding any root or green parts,
and cut into rings.
2. Wipe clean the mushrooms and slice.
3. Cut the asparagus into small even pieces.
4. Heat half the butter in a pan and sauté the leek rings and
mushroom slices for several minutes until tender. Add the
asparagus pieces and cook for 2–3 minutes more.
5. Remove the ragoût from the heat, stir in the cream and
season with pepper and stock granules or bouillon powder.
6. Slice off the top of each bread roll, scoop out the contents
of the rolls and cut into cubes. In a second pan, melt the
remaining butter. Sauté the cubes until golden brown to
make croûtons.
7. Fill the toasted rolls with the leek ragoût, sprinkle them
with the croûtons, and serve them with raw vegetables and
any remaining sauce.

WHAT IS GLUTEN INTOLERANCE?

According to the American Dietetic Association, one in 300
Americans is intolerant or sensitive to gluten, a protein that is
found in wheat, barley and rye. The results can include weight
loss, loss of appetite, abdominal cramps and, in children, poor
growth. Another consequence of gluten intolerance is poor
vitamin and mineral absorption from food. Treating gluten
intolerance means avoiding any foods that contain wheat, rye and
barley. Maize (corn), rice, soy, tapioca and potato flour are all
good alternatives to gluten-containing grains. If you
think you are suffering from the condition, you
should check with a doctor before making
any dietary changes. If you are diagnosed
as gluten intolerant, a dietician can help
you to develop an appropriate eating plan.

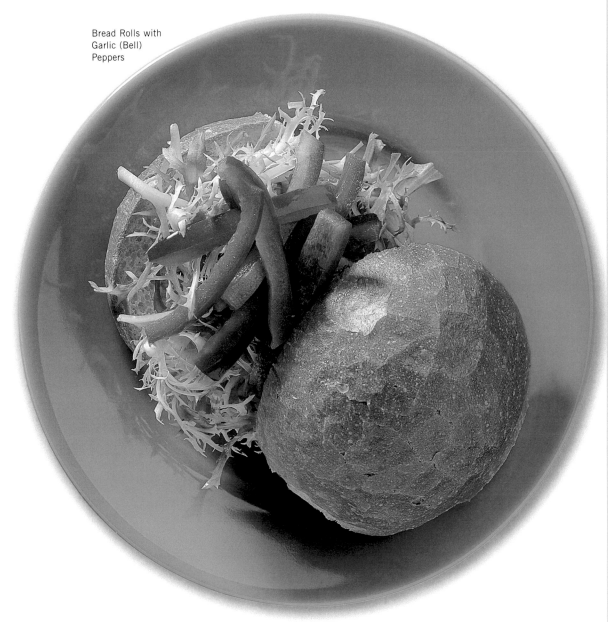

Bread Rolls with
Garlic (Bell)
Peppers

BREAD ROLLS WITH
GARLIC (BELL) PEPPERS

(SERVES 1–2)

Ingredients
2 bread rolls
1 red (bell) pepper
1 tbsp vegetable oil
1 garlic clove, peeled and crushed
2 frisée lettuce leaves

Preparation time: 5 minutes
Cooking time: 5 minutes

1. Cut the bread rolls in half.
2. Wash and deseed the (bell) pepper and cut into fine strips.
3. Heat the oil in a pan on a low heat and sauté the (bell) pepper strips with the crushed garlic until soft.
4. Tear the lettuce leaves into small pieces, then arrange them on the bread rolls with the (bell) pepper strips.

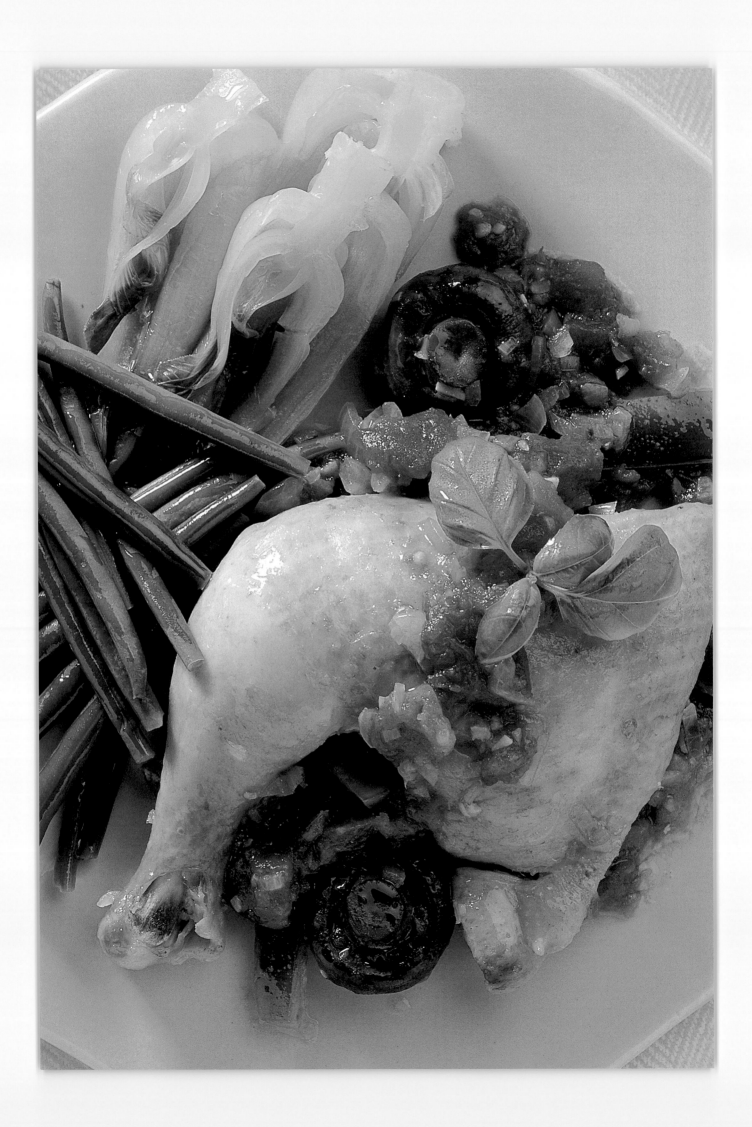

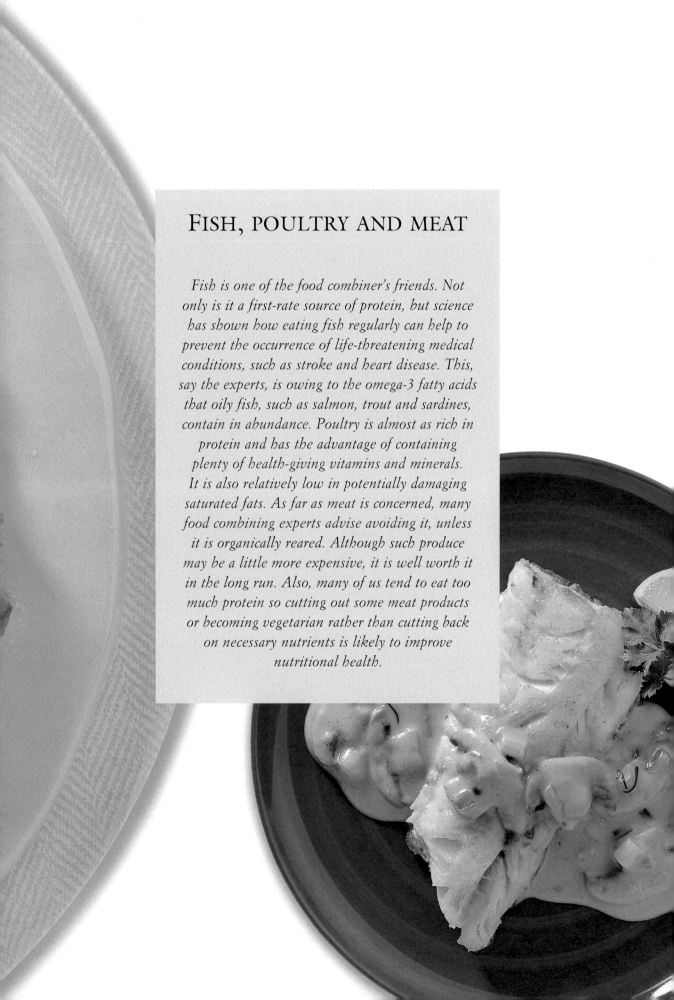

FISH, POULTRY AND MEAT

Fish is one of the food combiner's friends. Not only is it a first-rate source of protein, but science has shown how eating fish regularly can help to prevent the occurrence of life-threatening medical conditions, such as stroke and heart disease. This, say the experts, is owing to the omega-3 fatty acids that oily fish, such as salmon, trout and sardines, contain in abundance. Poultry is almost as rich in protein and has the advantage of containing plenty of health-giving vitamins and minerals. It is also relatively low in potentially damaging saturated fats. As far as meat is concerned, many food combining experts advise avoiding it, unless it is organically reared. Although such produce may be a little more expensive, it is well worth it in the long run. Also, many of us tend to eat too much protein so cutting out some meat products or becoming vegetarian rather than cutting back on necessary nutrients is likely to improve nutritional health.

FISH

The nutritional benefits of fish have long been recognized – scientific studies have proved that people who eat oily fish at least once a week are less likely to suffer from stroke or heart disease. This is largely owing to the omega-3

Sardines

fatty acids that oily fish, such as herring and mackerel, contain, which help to protect against heart and circulatory problems. As far as food combining is concerned, fish mixes well with non-starchy vegetables, salads, seeds and herbs, but not with starchy vegetables, grains and cereals.

Omega-3 fatty acids are not the only benefits fish contains, however. A single 100 g/3½ oz serving of fish a day will supply the body with between a third and a half of its daily protein requirements, while most fish are also rich in Vitamin B12 and iodine. The former plays an important part in keeping the nervous system healthy, while the thyroid gland needs iodine in order to function effectively. The Vitamin D that oily fish contains is also highly beneficial. For example, it is essential for skin and bone health.

WHITE FISH

White fish, such as cod, haddock, skate, sole and whiting, are all popular favourites. In fact, worldwide stocks of cod are dangerously low which, according to leading environmentalists, is the result of overfishing. Cod and haddock both store their fat reserves in their livers: cod liver oil is particularly rich in Vitamins A and D. The flesh of both fish is high in Vitamin B_{12}.

Cod steak

Flat fish, such as sole, plaice and flounder, all have a similar nutritional composition. They are low in fat and rich in protein in Vitamin B_{12}. When it comes to cooking flat fish, grilling (broiling) is healthier than frying, which can quadruple the calorific content. This is because flat fish absorb more oil when they are fried than their round fish equivalents.

OILY FISH AND CARTILAGINOUS FISH

Eating fresh tuna is always preferable to eating the canned variety. The fresh fish is rich in Vitamin D, Vitamin B12 and omega-3 fatty acids. Although canned tuna retains the same high vitamin content, the amount of fatty acids it contains is lowered during the canning process, when much of the fish oil the tuna contains is removed. Mackerel is similarly rich in fatty acids and also has a high Vitamin D and selenium content. The amount of fat mackerel contains

varies with the season – it is lowest in the summer after spawning and highest in the winter. Herring is equally rich in omega-3 fatty acids, as are salmon and trout, while sardines are a useful source of protein, calcium, iron and zinc, plus the other nutrients associated with all oily fish.

Cartilaginous fish is the term used to describe fish such as dogfish, shark, skate and ray. The flesh is firm and generally low in fat, while the livers are large and oily.

PRESERVING AND COOKING

Over the years, many ways of preserving fish have been devised, chief among them being smoking, pickling and salting. Smoking fish does not destroy its Vitamin D content, nor the beneficial omega-3 fatty acids. Pickling and salting are far less preferable. The high salt content of pickled herrings, for instance, can contribute to raised blood pressure, while the histamine and tyramine they contain can also trigger migraine attacks in susceptible individuals. Salted and smoked cod and haddock have an enhanced sodium content, which means that people at risk from high blood pressure should avoid them.

Oily fish, such as herring and mackerel, should be cooked and eaten fresh, because they spoil rapidly, while fish such as cod should always be cooked to make sure that any parasitic worms and their eggs are killed. The healthiest ways of cooking all fish are to steam, grill (broil) or bake them.

Plaice (right) and herring (below)

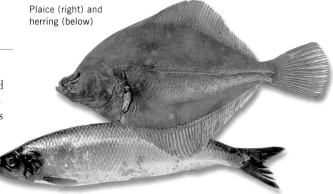

FOOD VALUES PER 100 G/3½ OZ

WHITE FISH
(cod, haddock, plaice, flounder, sole, whiting)

Protein: 19–23 g
Iron: 0.4–1 mg
Fat: 0.6–2 g
Calories: 96–104

OILY FISH
(herring, mackerel, salmon, sardines, trout)

Protein: 20–26 g
Iron: 0.4–2 g
Fat: 5–17 g
Calories: 135–240
Vitamins and Minerals: Good source of Vitamin B_{12} and omega-3 fatty acids.

SMOKED FISH
(mackerel, salmon, herring)

Protein: 19–25 g
Iron: 0.6–1.6 mg
Fat: 3–4.5 g
Calories: 142–354

OYSTERS
(raw)

Protein: 10.8 g
Fat: 1.3 g
Sodium: 510 mg.
Vitamins and Minerals: Good source of Vitamin B_{12}, Vitamin E, niacin, thiamin, riboflavin, zinc, copper, iron, potassium, selenium, iodine.

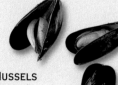

MUSSELS
(steamed)

Protein: 16.7 g
Fat: 2.7 g
Sodium: 360 mg
Vitamins and Minerals: Good source of Vitamin B_{12}, Vitamin E, riboflavin, folate, iron, iodine, selenium.

SCALLOPS
(steamed)

Protein: 23.2 g
Fat: 1.4 g
Sodium: 180 mg
Vitamins and Minerals: Good sources of Vitamin B_{12} and niacin, selenium, potassium and zinc.

LOBSTER
(boiled)

Protein: 22.1 g
Fat: 1.6 g
Sodium: 330 mg
Vitamins and Minerals: Good source of Vitamin B_{12} and niacin, selenium and zinc.

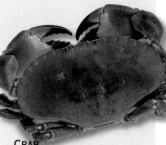

CRAB
(boiled)

Protein: 9.5 g
Fat: 5.5 g
Sodium: 420 mg
Vitamins and Minerals: Good source of Vitamin B_6, riboflavin, pantothenic acid, potassium, zinc, magnesium.

PRAWNS (SHRIMP)
(boiled)

Protein: 23.8 g
Fat: 2.4 g
Sodium: 3840 mg
Vitamins and Minerals: Good source of Vitamin B_{12} and niacin, iodine, selenium and calcium.

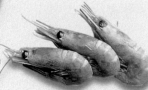

WHY FISH OILS ARE IMPORTANT

Modern medicine now regards an adequate intake of essential fatty acids (EFAs) as an important part of keeping healthy. These fats, notably the omega-3 and omega-6 varieties, are involved in so many bodily processes that scientists now believe that they can help us to overcome illness.

Recent studies and clinical trials have found that regular ingestion of essential fatty acids has had significant benefit in the reduction in the risk of heart disease and the symptoms of arthritis.The omega-3 fatty acids reduce triglyceride levels in the blood (the triglycerides are fats that build up in the arteries and obstruct the circulation). It has also been shown that omega-3 fatty acids reduce 'platelet aggregation' helping to prevent blood clots from forming. Fish oils can be taken as a food supplement in capsule or liquid form. The fish body oils are the ones that are rich in omega-3 fatty acids, while fish liver oils – from cod, halibut and shark – contain high amounts of Vitamins A and D. Cod liver oil has a concentrated supply of nutrients and is used to treat medical conditions such as eye disease caused by Vitamin A deficiency, and rickets, a bone disease triggered by a lack of Vitamin D. Other food supplements that contain essential fatty acids include flaxseed oil, which can be used as a dressing for salads or in soups, and evening primrose oil.

FRUITS OF THE SEA

High in protein but low in fat, many varieties of shellfish are also excellent sources of other important nutrients. Most shellfish contain abundant supplies of Vitamin B_{12}, which the body needs to form red blood cells and to keep the nervous system healthy, and zinc, which plays an important part in protein production, proper functioning of the reproductive organs and in the healing of wounds. Other vitamins and minerals include Vitamins B_1 and B_2, niacin, selenium, calcium, magnesium and iodine. In common with oily fish, shellfish also possess small amounts of essential fatty acids. In short, they are a powerful health-enhancing food.

However, all shellfish are highly perishable and prone to bacterial contamination. They should be eaten on the day of purchase or stored in the refrigerator at a temperature of 0–5°C/32–41°F, but only for a day or two. Shellfish are also more likely to trigger allergic reactions than other types of fish. The safest shellfish are those that have been farmed commercially in clean waters.

SCALLOPS

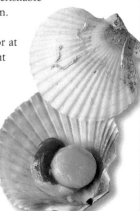

ROAST TUNA WITH OVEN-BAKED RATATOUILLE

(SERVES 4)

Ingredients
1 medium onion
2 garlic cloves
2 tbsp lemon juice
6 tbsp olive oil
salt and freshly ground black pepper
4 tuna steaks
2 (bell) peppers, 1 red, 1 yellow
4 courgettes (zucchini)
1 aubergine (eggplant)
2 tbsp tomato purée (paste)
1 kg/2 lb 4 oz canned chopped plum tomatoes
2 tbsp chopped fresh parsley

Preparation time: 10–15 minutes
Cooking time: 1 hour

1. Preheat the oven to 200°C/400°F/gas 6.
2. To make the marinade, peel and finely chop the onion, peel and crush one of the cloves of garlic and place them both in a mixing bowl. Add the lemon juice and 2 tablespoons of the olive oil, mix together well and season to taste. Put the tuna steaks into a dish, pour the marinade over them, cover and set aside to absorb the flavours.
3. Meanwhile, crush the second clove of garlic. Wash and deseed the (bell) peppers, then quarter and dice them. Quarter the courgettes (zucchini) lengthways and dice the slices. Slice the aubergine (eggplant) lengthways and dice.
4. Heat the remaining oil in a flameproof casserole, add the (bell) peppers and courgettes (zucchini) and sauté until they start to soften. Then add the aubergine (eggplant), followed by the garlic and a tablespoon of the tomato purée (paste). Stir well.
5. Add the plum tomatoes to the casserole, along with half the can juice, mix thoroughly, cover, and transfer to the preheated oven. Bake for 45 minutes, stirring frequently and adding more of the tomato can juice if the ratatouille begins to dry out. Remove from the oven.
6. Line a roasting tin (pan) with foil. Moisten the foil slightly with a little oil to make sure that the marinated tuna does not stick to it, then add the fish.
7. Roast for 8–10 minutes, or until the fish is just cooked and flakes easily with the point of a knife. Serve the steaks garnished with chopped parsley and accompanied by the ratatouille, which can be eaten either cold or hot.

TROUT AND ALMOND BAKE

(SERVES 4)

Ingredients
4 trout
juice of 2 lemons
4 tbsp flaked (sliced) almonds

Preparation time: 15–20 minutes
Cooking time: 12 minutes

1. Preheat the oven to 230°C/450°F/gas 8.
2. Gut the trout, if this has not already been done, and wash well. Pat dry and brush the insides with the lemon juice.
3. Spread out the almonds on a plate. Toss the trout in the almonds, so that both sides of each fish are covered lightly with the flakes (slices).
4. Line a baking (cookie) sheet with greaseproof (waxed) paper. Place the trout on the sheet and bake for 6 minutes each side, or until cooked through.
5. Transfer to serving plates and serve immediately with a green salad (salad greens).

HADDOCK FILLET WITH MUSHROOM SAUCE

(SERVES 2)

Ingredients
bunch spring onions (scallions)
400 g/14 oz/5⅔ cups mushrooms
6 tbsp olive oil
1 tsp lemon juice
300 ml/5 fl oz/⅔ cup Vegetable Stock (see page 206)
3 tbsp single (light) cream
small pinch saffron powder
1 tbsp cornflour (cornstarch)
2 haddock fillets
lemon wedges, to garnish

Preparation time: 8–10 minutes
Cooking time: 10–12 minutes

1. Trim the spring onions (scallions) and wash them well. Chop coarsely.
2. Wipe the mushrooms and slice thinly.
3. Heat 2 tablespoons of the oil in a frying pan (skillet), add the spring onions (scallions) and the mushrooms and cook over a low heat for 5 minutes.
4. Sprinkle the mixture with the lemon juice and add the vegetable stock. Simmer for 1 minute.

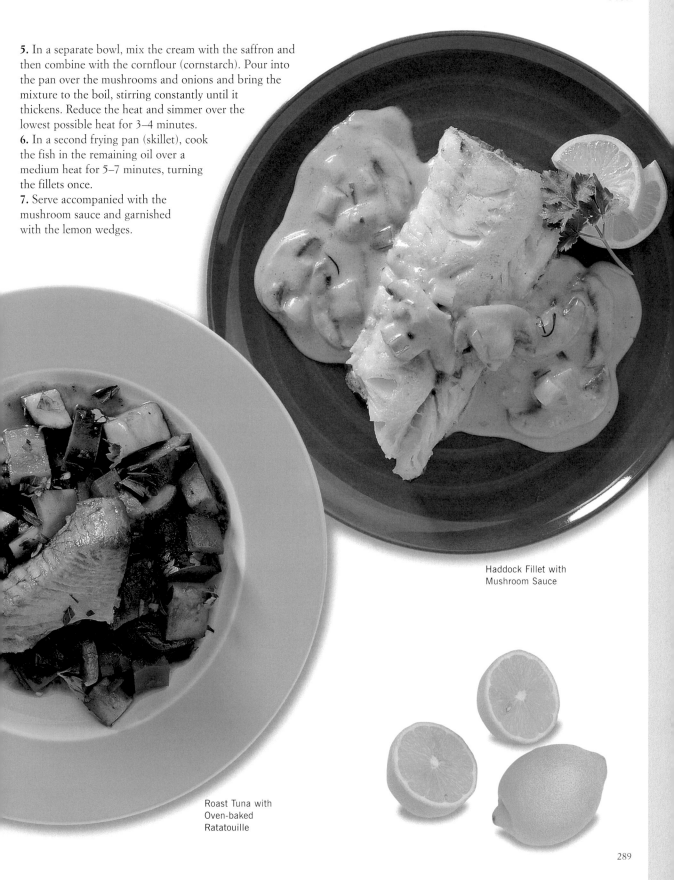

5. In a separate bowl, mix the cream with the saffron and then combine with the cornflour (cornstarch). Pour into the pan over the mushrooms and onions and bring the mixture to the boil, stirring constantly until it thickens. Reduce the heat and simmer over the lowest possible heat for 3–4 minutes.

6. In a second frying pan (skillet), cook the fish in the remaining oil over a medium heat for 5–7 minutes, turning the fillets once.

7. Serve accompanied with the mushroom sauce and garnished with the lemon wedges.

Haddock Fillet with
Mushroom Sauce

Roast Tuna with
Oven-baked
Ratatouille

ROAST COD WITH A SALAD OF MIXED LEAVES (GREENS)

(SERVES 4)

Ingredients
mixed salad leaves (greens) of your choice
3–4 tbsp Vinaigrette (see page 192)
½ cucumber
2–3 tsp finely chopped fresh mixed herbs
1 tbsp finely chopped capers
4 cod fillets
salt and freshly ground black pepper
2 tsp lemon juice
4 tbsp olive oil

Preparation time: 10 minutes
Cooking time: 10–14 minutes

1. Preheat the oven to 230°C/450°F/gas 8.
2. Tear the mixed salad leaves (greens) and place in a large mixing bowl. Dress with the vinaigrette, season to taste and mix to coat all the leaves thoroughly.
3. Peel, deseed and dice the cucumber. Add to the salad. Sprinkle with the herbs and toss. Arrange on four side plates and sprinkle the capers over each portion.
4. Season both sides of the cod with salt, freshly ground black pepper and lemon juice.
5. Heat the oil in a non-stick, ovenproof pan. Add the cod and cook, skin side down, for 3–4 minutes. Turn the fish over and place the pan in the oven for 5–7 minutes, or until the cod is fully cooked.
6. Just before serving, crisp the skin of the cod briefly under a hot grill (broiler). Serve immediately, with the salad.

PROVENÇAL COD

(SERVES 2)

Ingredients
2 cod fillets
500 g/1 lb 2 oz tomatoes
½ green (bell) pepper
½ red (bell) pepper
4 shallots
½ tbsp olive oil
2 tsp dried Provençal herbs

Preparation time: 10–15 minutes
Cooking time: 20–25 minutes

1. Dice the fish into cubes.
2. Plunge the tomatoes into just boiled water for 2 minutes, then remove the skins, quarter, deseed and dice.
3. Deseed the (bell) peppers and slice into thin strips.
4. Peel and dice the shallots.
5. Heat the oil in a pan over a low heat and sauté the diced shallots for 2–3 minutes until they soften. Add the sliced (bell) peppers, followed by the chopped tomatoes and the Provençal herbs. Bring to the boil.
5. Add the fish, cover the pan and simmer for about 20 minutes. Serve hot accompanied by a mixed green salad (salad greens).

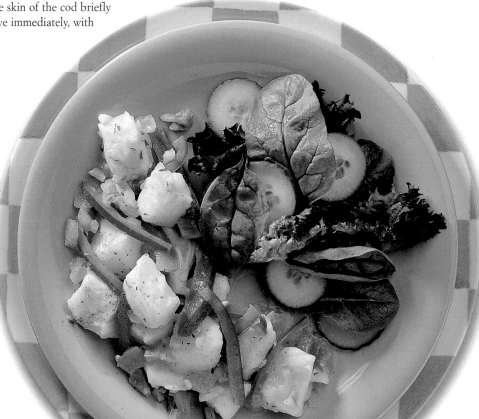

Provençal Cod

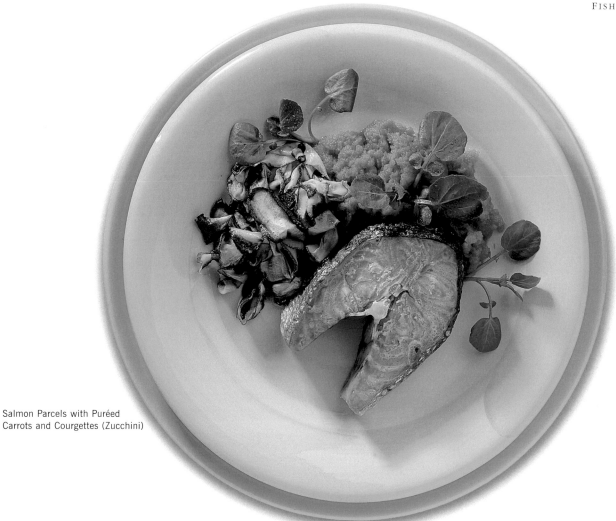

Salmon Parcels with Puréed
Carrots and Courgettes (Zucchini)

SALMON PARCELS WITH
PURÉED CARROTS AND
COURGETTES (ZUCCHINI)

(SERVES 4)

Ingredients

4 salmon steaks
2½ tbsp olive oil
salt and freshly ground black pepper
4 fresh tarragon sprigs
4 tbsp dry white wine
4 carrots
8 courgettes (zucchini)
4 watercress sprigs, to garnish

Preparation time: 10–15 minutes
Cooking time: 20–25 minutes

1. Preheat the oven to 190°C/375°F/gas 5.
2. Place each salmon steak on a square double-thickness of
greaseproof (waxed) paper, season with salt and pepper and
use half the oil to coat liberally. Place a sprig of tarragon
on each steak and spoon the white wine them.
3. Fold the paper into parcels, seal the edges, place on a
baking (cookie) sheet, and bake for 20 minutes, or until the
fish is cooked.
4. Meanwhile, trim and dice the carrots. Slice the courgettes
(zucchini) into long thin strips.
5. Bring a large pan of water to the boil. Add the carrots and
cook them until tender. Drain and purée them. Set aside and
keep warm.
6. Heat the remaining oil in a frying pan (skillet). Add the
courgettes (zucchini) and sauté the slices until they are soft
and just turning brown. Drain, set aside and keep warm.
7. When the fish is cooked, drain off any liquid from the
parcels, remove the fish and arrange on warm plates,
accompanied by the carrot purée and courgettes (zucchini).
Garnish each plate with a sprig of watercress and serve.

POULTRY AND GAME

There's no disguising the fact that poultry is good for you: organically reared chickens, ducks, turkeys and geese all provide an excellent source of protein, and they also contain most of the B vitamins and minerals the body requires. One drawback, though, is that the skin surrounding *the meat is high in fat, and another is that there is a risk of food-poisoning if poultry – especially chicken, which carries salmonella bacteria – is not cooked properly. Like fish, white meat combines well with non-starchy vegetables, salads, seeds and herbs.*

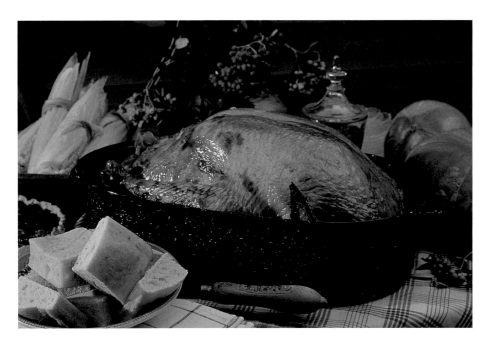

LEFT: Poultry of all kinds is a good source of many vital nutrients. Choose organic birds, which are not only healthier than those raised intensively, but are also much more flavoursome.

Poultry is a first-rate source of healthy nutrients – an average serving of turkey, for instance, is rich in protein and contains 93 per cent of the recommended daily niacin intake. Even the fat that poultry contains is not a major worry, since it is relatively low in saturated fats and, in any event, it is found mostly in the skin, which can be removed easily either before or after cooking.

If you are following a low-cholesterol or low-calorie diet, skinless turkey and chicken breast portions are the best choice. Bear in mind that, as far as chicken and turkey are concerned, eating dark meat as well as light is the healthiest option. The dark meat of chicken contains twice as much iron and zinc than the light meat does, and a portion of the dark meat from a roasted turkey will provide almost half of the required daily zinc intake. Duck and geese are rich sources of nutrients: duck contains three times as much iron as chicken, while an average serving of goose contains more than half of the daily recommended iron intake for men and a third of that recommended for women.

ORGANIC IS BEST

If you have the opportunity, organically reared or at least free-range chickens and turkeys are a far better buy than the factory-farmed varieties. Most factory-farmed birds are kept in crowded conditions and they have to be routinely treated with drugs to prevent the spread of disease. Organic and free-range birds, by contrast, have the freedom to run and scratch for food in conditions that are usually far less cramped.

AVOIDING FOOD POISONING

Chicken, many experts believe, is one of the commonest sources of food poisoning, largely because it is frequently served undercooked. Proper cooking is essential to get rid of the salmonella bacteria the chicken may contain. Otherwise, within 8–36 hours of eating the chicken, the characteristic symptoms of salmonella poisoning may appear – these include nausea, stomach pain, fever, vomiting and diarrhoea.

To avoid the risk of food poisoning, make sure that any frozen chicken or turkey is thawed out completely before you start to cook it and that the internal temperature of the meat – fresh or frozen – reaches at least 80°C/176°F during cooking. At the end of the cooking period, the meat should not be pink or bloody: a useful quick check, if practical, is to insert a meat skewer or the point of knife into the thickest part of the thigh. If the meat is cooked, the juices run clear.

You need to take extra precautions if you are stuffing a bird. This is because the stuffing can harbour bacteria that has spread from the raw meat and survived because the stuffing has not cooked at a high enough temperature. To avoid this, insert the stuffing only just before you are ready to start cooking, re-weigh the stuffed chicken and recalculate the cooking time upwards accordingly. For extra security, you should also test the stuffing's temperature with a meat thermometer after taking the bird out of the oven: it should have reached at least 75°C/167°F.

GOING FOR GAME

Like all meat, game and game birds are an excellent source of protein and rich in B vitamins and iron. They are also good sources of potassium, which the body needs to maintain its cells, and phosphorous, which helps to keep bones and teeth healthy. The recommended daily adult intake of phosphorous is 550 mg, and a single serving of roast venison will provide more than half of it. It will also provide almost the full daily requirement of iron.

Game is low in fat and calories, especially when compared with untrimmed beef, lamb and pork. Most of the game sold in Europe has been caught or shot in the wild, so any risk of contamination from pesticides, artificial growth hormones and other chemicals is minimal. In the US, on the other hand, most game available in the shops is farmed and consequently may not always be free of such chemicals.

As game meats tend to be tougher than that of domesticated animals, largely because the collagen in the muscles is more resistant, it is important to prepare the meats correctly. For example, hanging game helps to tenderize it, and also improves its flavour. How old the game is and how hot or cold the place is in which it is being hung can make a substantial difference: in cold conditions, pheasants may need hanging for as long as a fortnight, but, in warmer conditions, a day or two may suffice. Frozen game should not be hung after it has been thawed.

When it comes to cooking game, roasting is the best method of cooking young game birds; older, tougher ones taste better casseroled. Rabbit is best stewed, while venison can be casseroled or roasted. Whichever method is chosen, venison usually needs long, slow cooking to maximize the meat's tenderness and to make sure that it is full of flavour.

FOOD VALUES PER 100 G/3½ OZ

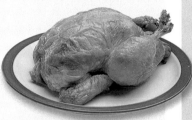

CHICKEN
(roasted with skin removed)

Protein:	25 g
Fat:	5 g
Calories:	148

Vitamins and minerals: good source of all B vitamins, particularly niacin, although only has trace amounts of Vitamin B_{12}, iron, zinc, phosphorus and potassium.

TURKEY
(roasted with skin removed)

Protein:	29 g
Fat:	3 g
Calories:	140

Vitamins and minerals: good source of Vitamin B12 and all other B vitamins, particularly niacin, potassium, zinc and phosphorous.

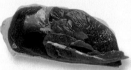

DUCK
(roasted with skin removed)

Protein:	25 g
Fat:	10 g
Calories:	189

Vitamins and minerals: good source of all B vitamins, particularly thiamin and riboflavin, iron, potassium and zinc.

GOOSE
(roasted with skin removed)

Protein:	29 g
Fat:	22 g
Calories:	319

Vitamins and minerals: good source of Vitamin B6, riboflavin, potassium, phosphorous and iron.

VENISON
(roasted)

Protein:	35 g
Fat:	6.4 g
Phosphorous:	290 mg
Potassium:	360 mg
Iron:	7.8 mg

RABBIT
(stewed)

Protein:	27.3 g
Fat:	7.7 g
Phosphorous:	200 mg
Potassium:	210 mg
Iron:	1.9 mg

HARE (JACK RABBIT)
(stewed)

Protein:	29.9 g
Fat:	8.0 g
Phosphorous:	250 mg
Potassium:	210 mg
Iron:	10.8 mg

PHEASANT
(roasted)

Protein:	32.2 g
Fat:	9.3 g
Phosphorous:	310 mg
Potassium:	410 mg
Iron:	8.4 mg

PIGEON
(roasted)

Protein:	27.8 g
Fat:	13.2 g
Phosphorous:	400 mg
Potassium:	410 mg
Iron:	19.4 mg

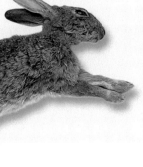

CHICKEN, COURGETTE (ZUCCHINI) AND MUSHROOM KEBABS (KABOBS)

(SERVES 2)

Ingredients
2 skinless, boneless chicken
breast portions
2 tbsp olive oil
juice ½ lemon
freshly ground black pepper
2 tsp chopped fresh thyme
2 courgettes (zucchini)
1 red (bell) pepper
50–85 g/2–3 oz/¾–1¼ cups button (white) mushrooms
6–10 cherry tomatoes

Preparation time: 10–15 minutes
Cooking time: 15–20 minutes

1. Dice the chicken into medium-size cubes.
2. Mix the oil with the lemon juice, season with black pepper and add the chopped thyme to make a marinade.
3. Pour the marinade over the chicken cubes, mix well and set aside in the refridgerator for 30 minutes.
4. Cut the courgettes (zucchini) into thick, round slices.
5. Deseed the (bell) pepper and chop it into squares.
6. Wipe the mushrooms clean.
7. Thread the chicken chunks, courgette (zucchini) slices, (bell) pepper cubes, mushrooms and tomatoes alternately on to six kebab (kabob) skewers.
8. Brush the kebabs (kabobs) with the marinade and place under a hot grill (broiler) for about 15–20 minutes, or until the chicken is tender and cooked through. Turn the skewers occasionally during the cooking time.
9. Remove the kebabs (kabobs) from the grill (broiler) and serve hot with a mixed salad.

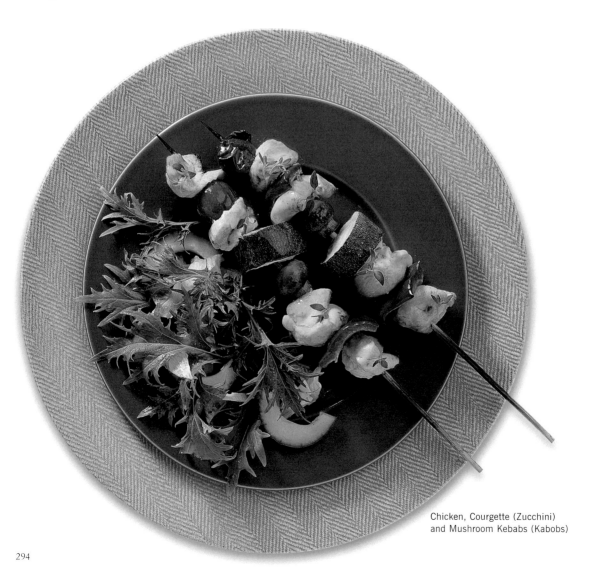

Chicken, Courgette (Zucchini)
and Mushroom Kebabs (Kabobs)

CHICKEN BAKED WITH TARRAGON

(SERVES 2)

Ingredients
2 boneless chicken breast portions
1 tbsp olive oil
2 fresh tarragon sprigs

Preparation time: 5 minutes
Cooking time: 40 minutes

1. Preheat the oven to 200°C/400°F/gas 6.
2. Brush the chicken all over with the olive oil and place in an ovenproof dish, topping each with a tarragon sprig.
3. Cover and bake for 30 minutes.
4. Baste with the juices and cook, uncovered for 10 minutes more, or until the chicken is cooked right through and tender. Serve with mixed side salad.

QUICK-COOK CHICKEN STIR-FRY

(SERVES 2)

Ingredients

2 boneless chicken breast portions
1 leek
2 carrots
1 red (bell) pepper
2 tbsp olive oil
mung beansprouts
cashew nuts
2 tbsp water
1 tsp soy sauce

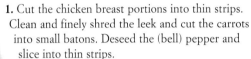

Preparation time: 10–15 minutes
Cooking time: 8–10 minutes

1. Cut the chicken breast portions into thin strips. Clean and finely shred the leek and cut the carrots into small batons. Deseed the (bell) pepper and slice into thin strips.
2. Heat the olive oil in a wok until it starts to smoke. Add the chicken strips and stir-fry rapidly until they are just tender. Remove the strips from the wok and put them to one side.
3. Add the shredded leek, carrot and red (bell) pepper slices to the wok and stir-fry for 2 minutes, before adding the beansprouts, cashews, water and soy sauce. Continue cooking for 2 minutes more.
4. Quickly stir in the chicken, heat through and serve piping hot.

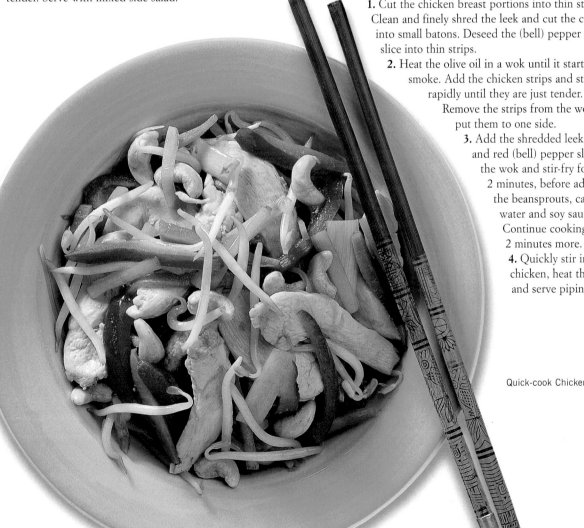

Quick-cook Chicken Stir-fry

295

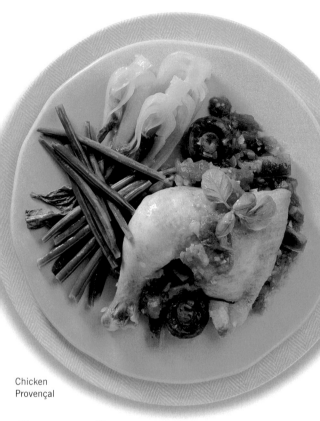

Chicken
Provençal

CHICKEN PROVENÇAL

(SERVES 2)

Ingredients
4 shallots
4 tomatoes
1 green (bell) pepper
2 garlic cloves
1 tbsp olive oil
8 brown mushrooms
2 chicken quarters
1 tbsp chopped fresh basil

Preparation time: 20–25 minutes
Cooking time: 1 hour 30 minutes

1. Preheat the oven to 190°C/375°F/gas 5.
2. Plunge the tomatoes into just boiled water for 2 minutes. Skin, deseed and chop them into pieces. Wash, deseed and slice the green (bell) pepper into strips.
3. Peel and finely chop the shallots, and peel and crush the cloves of garlic. Wipe the mushrooms clean and cut the larger ones in half.
4. Heat the oil in a frying pan (skillet). Add the shallots and garlic and gently sauté for 2–3 minutes.
5. Add the chopped tomatoes, the green (bell) pepper slices and the mushrooms. Stir-fry for 2–3 minutes.

6. Put the chicken quarters in a greased casserole, season with basil and cover with the vegetable mixture.
7. Bake for 1 hour 25 minutes, or until the chicken is cooked through and tender. Serve immediately with a selection of green vegetables.

TURKEY KEBABS (KABOBS) WITH TOMATO SALAD

(SERVES 2)

Ingredients
500 g/1 lb 2 oz tomatoes
3 onions
pinch herb salt
3½ tbsp olive oil
4–6 fresh basil leaves, chopped
1 red (bell) pepper
1 green (bell) pepper
6–8 button (white) mushrooms
6–8 cherry tomatoes
450 g/1 lb turkey breast fillet
2 tsp lemon juice
1 tsp chopped fresh thyme
pinch salt
pinch paprika
1 garlic clove

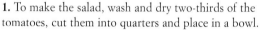

Preparation time: 25–30 minutes
Cooking time: 20–25 minutes

1. To make the salad, wash and dry two-thirds of the tomatoes, cut them into quarters and place in a bowl.
2. Peel and slice one onion, separate the slices into rings and add to the tomatoes in the bowl.
3. Season the salad with herb salt, sprinkle over 2 teaspoons of the olive oil and garnish with the chopped basil.
4. To make the kebabs (kabobs), wash and deseed the red and green (bell) peppers, then cut into squares. Wipe the mushrooms clean. Peel and slice the remaining onions. Wash the cherry tomatoes. Wash and chop the remaining tomatoes into pieces.
5. Rinse the turkey, pat dry and dice into cubes.
6. Arrange the turkey and vegetables alternately on kebab (kabob) skewers and sprinkle with lemon juice.
7. For the marinade, combine the remaining olive oil, thyme, salt and paprika. Peel and crush the garlic and add it to the mixture. Stir well.
8. Brush the kebabs (kabobs) with some of the marinade and cook under a hot grill (broiler) for 20–25 minutes, turning them frequently and brushing them with the remaining marinade. Serve hot with the tomato salad.

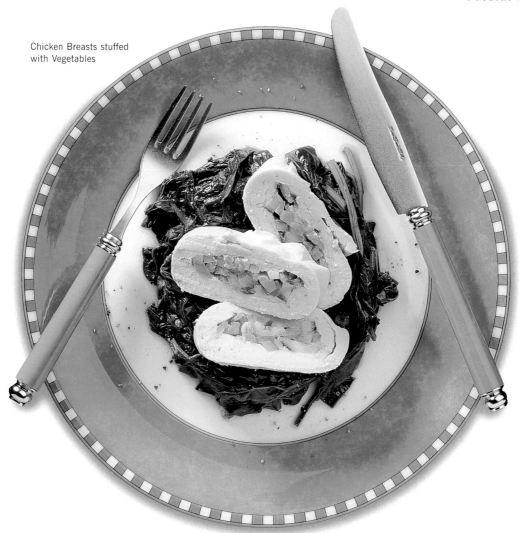

Chicken Breasts stuffed with Vegetables

CHICKEN BREASTS STUFFED WITH VEGETABLES

(SERVES 4)

Ingredients
1 shallot
1 carrot
1 courgette (zucchini)
2.5 cm/1 inch fresh ginger
2 tbsp olive oil
4 skinless, boneless chicken breast portions
salt
freshly ground black pepper
800 g/1 lb 12 oz fresh spinach

Preparation time: 12–15 minutes
Cooking time: 35–40 minutes

1. Preheat the oven to 200°C/400°F/gas 6.
2. Peel and finely chop the shallot. Wash and shred the carrot and the courgette (zucchini). Peel and grate the ginger.

3. Heat a little olive oil in a frying pan (skillet) and sauté the shallot over a low heat until soft. Add the carrot, courgette (zucchini) and ginger and mix well. Remove from the heat.
4. Sandwich the chicken portions between sheets of clingfilm (plastic wrap), then beat them to a 1 cm/½ inch thickness with a rolling pin.
5. Lightly oil four pieces of foil. Season the underside of each chicken portion and place each one in the centre of a piece of foil. Spread some of the vegetable stuffing down the centre of each portion. Pick up the edges of each piece of foil and roll each chicken portion around the stuffing to make a parcel, sealing the edges.
6. Cover a baking (cookie) sheet with greaseproof (waxed) paper. Place the parcels on the sheet and cook in the preheated oven for 30–35 minutes.
8. When the parcels are nearly ready, cook the spinach in a little water. Leave the parcels to rest for 5 minutes before opening, then serve with the spinach.

MEAT

Although beef has had a bad press recently, it is still a food that is packed with potential nutritional benefits. Lamb, too, is nutrient rich, although you should avoid the fattiest cuts or eat them only in moderation. Lean pork, however, is *probably the healthiest meat of them all: it contains only a little more fat than skinless chicken. In all three instances, organic cuts are the best buy, and all three foods combine well with non-starchy vegetables, salads, herbs and seeds.*

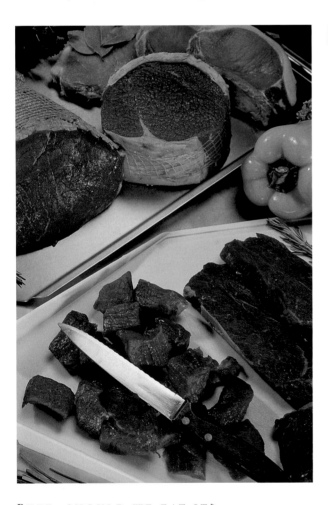

WHAT IS BSE?

BSE is a slow, but ultimately fatal illness that usually affects cattle when they are between three and five years old. It is believed to be passed on only through the consumption of infected offal, particularly the brain and the spinal cord. BSE is believed to have started when cattle in Britain were fed processed food derived from sheep carcasses. The sheep involved were suffering from a similar condition called scrapie. The problem was complicated by the fact that, up until 1989 when the practice was banned, the carcasses of cows that had died from BSE were also being processed into cattle feed and so were being reintroduced into the food chain.

One of the chief and lasting concerns people have about the condition is the possibility of a link between it and Creutzfeldt-Jakob Disease, a similar illness that affects the human central nervous system. Although, for some time it was confidently asserted that it was impossible for humans to catch BSE, there is now some evidence to show that this may not be the case. A new variant of Creutzfeldt-Jakob Disease, medically termed nvCJD (new variant CJD), appeared in the mid-1990s. In 1996, the British Spongiform Encephalopathy Advisory Committee concluded that 'the most likely explanation at present is that these cases are linked to exposure to BSE', although there is still no proof of a definite link.

One of the problems is the lengthy incubation period of nvCJD: it takes 5–15 years for symptoms to manifest themselves. Although effective action has been taken to eradicate BSE from British cattle, it will be some time before even tentative estimates can be made of the number of people likely to have contracted nvCJD from beef before 1989, assuming that such transmission did occur.

BEEF: SHOULD WE EAT IT?

Increasing concern that eating fatty red meat can contribute to heart disease plus the impact of BSE (bovine spongiform encephalopathy), more popularly known as 'mad cow disease', has led to a dramatic drop in beef consumption in the UK, the US and across much of Western Europe. Beef has also been linked with other diseases: for example scientific studies have associated excessive consumption of beef with an increased risk of cancer of the colon.

Despite this, beef's nutritional benefits are still manifold. Beef contains a wide range of valuable nutrients, plus many essential minerals, particularly zinc and iron. Thanks to a change in farming methods, beef is now much leaner than it used to be – a portion of lean rump (round) steak, for instance, on average, contains only 3 g/¹⁄₁₆ oz of fat. If you do buy a fatty cut, you can deal with the problem to a large extent by trimming off the visible fat before cooking. This is especially important when it comes to preparing casseroles and stews. Large cuts are best roasted, supported on a rack or trivet so that the fat can drip into a tray placed beneath the rack. Steaks and chops can be roasted, grilled (broiled) or dry-fried. The traditional method of cooking root vegetables under and around roast beef is best avoided.

LAMB: CUTTING DOWN THE FAT

When it comes to lamb, fat content varies with the cut and the way in which the meat is cooked. The leanest part is the leg, the fattiest parts are the shoulder and the rack (rib). These are high in saturated fat and calories and should be eaten only in moderation. Excessive consumption of saturated fat can lead to an increase in the level of cholesterol in the blood which, in turn, can contribute to an increased risk of eventually developing atherosclerosis and heart disease.

The meat itself, however, is protein-rich. As well as containing most of the B vitamins, which the body needs to maintain a healthy nervous system, lamb is also an excellent source of zinc and of iron.

PORK: THE HEALTHIEST RED MEAT

It may surprise some people, but pork is one of the healthiest of all meats, with the important exception of cured pork – bacon, gammon and smoked or cured ham – which contains high levels of sodium and nitrites, largely because of the ingredients the curing process employs. The main culprits, as far as levels of saturated fat is concerned, are streaky (fatty) bacon and processed pork products, such as salami, frankfurters and other sausage. As with all proteins, 25 g/1 oz is the minimum daily requirement but more than 100 g/3½ oz of meat is not utilized effectively. Pork is an excellent source of B vitamins and it also contains useful amounts of zinc.

The healthiest way to eat pork is to trim off any visible fat before cooking and then to roast or grill (broil) it. It is vital to make sure that any pork you eat is cooked thoroughly, so that bacteria or parasites that it may contain are destroyed. This is because if undercooked pork is eaten, there is a risk of contracting trichinosis (a parasitical worm infestation).

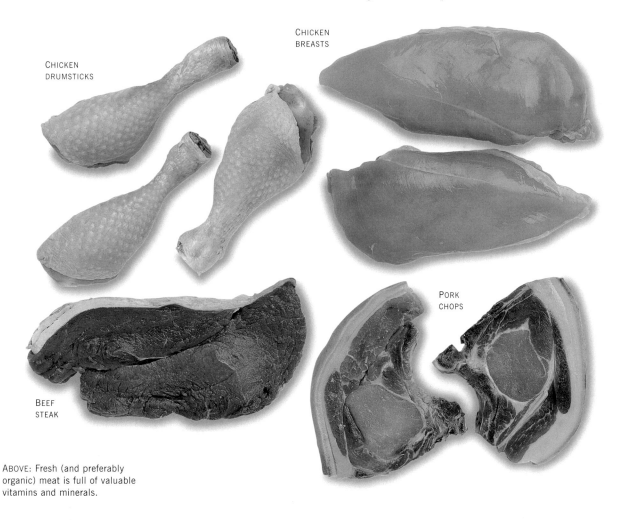

CHICKEN DRUMSTICKS

CHICKEN BREASTS

PORK CHOPS

BEEF STEAK

ABOVE: Fresh (and preferably organic) meat is full of valuable vitamins and minerals.

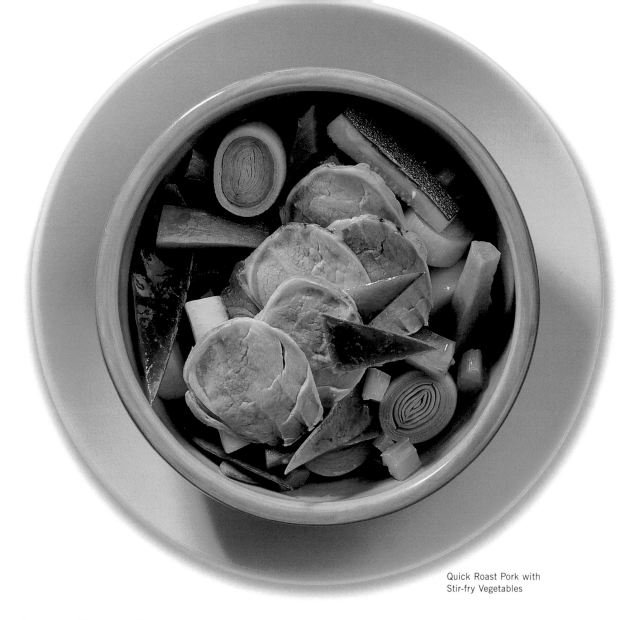

Quick Roast Pork with
Stir-fry Vegetables

QUICK ROAST PORK WITH STIR-FRIED VEGETABLES

(SERVES 4)

Ingredients
6 courgettes (zucchini)
6 carrots
175 g/6 oz/2¼ cups mangetouts (snow peas)
4 celery sticks (stalks)
2 leeks
450 g/1 lb pork fillet (tenderloin)
3–4 tbsp olive oil
1 garlic clove, peeled and crushed
salt and freshly ground black pepper

Preparation time: 15–20 minutes
Cooking time: 35–40 minutes

1. Preheat the oven to 220°C/425°F/gas 7.
2. Peel and cut the carrots and courgettes (zucchini) into narrow batons, trim and halve the mangetouts (snow peas), trim and dice the celery and clean and thinly slice the leek.
3. Trim any fat from the pork and brush liberally with 1 tbsp of the oil. Line a roasting tin (pan) with foil. Add the meat to the tin (pan) and roast for 15 minutes. Then reduce the oven temperature to 180°C/350°/gas 4 and roast for 20–25 minutes more, until the pork is thoroughly cooked. Baste the pork with the roasting juices several times during the cooking process. Once the pork is cooked, set it aside to rest for at least 5 minutes and then cut into slices.
4. Heat the remaining oil in a wok. Add the carrots, courgettes (zucchini) and mangetouts (snow peas). Stir-fry for 3 minutes before adding the rest of the vegetables, then stir-fry for 2–3 minutes more. Add the crushed garlic, season with salt and pepper, stir well and cook for 1 minute more.
5. Transfer the vegetables to four bowls with the pork slices and spoon any remaining vegetable liquid over each serving.

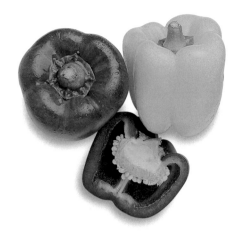

LAMB FILLET WITH RATATOUILLE

(SERVES 2)

Ingredients
1 onion
1 aubergine (eggplant)
1 courgette (zucchini)
1 green (bell) pepper
1 red (bell) pepper
4 tomatoes
4–5 tbsp olive oil
1 garlic clove, peeled and crushed
pinch mixed Mediterranean dried herbs
pinch salt
375 g/13 oz lamb fillet

Preparation time: 15 minutes
Cooking time: 17–20 minutes

1. Peel the onion, cut into slices and
then separate the slices into rings. Wash
and dry the aubergine (eggplant), courgette (zucchini) and
(bell) peppers. Deseed the (bell) peppers. Cut aubergine
(eggplant), courgette (zucchini) and (bell) peppers into
narrow strips.
2. Skin the tomatoes, deseed them and chop finely.
3. Heat half the olive oil in a frying pan (skillet), add the
onion rings and cook until transparent. Add the crushed
garlic, followed by aubergine (eggplant), courgette (zucchini)
and (bell) peppers. Continue stir-frying over a moderate heat
for 5–8 minutes.
4. Add the chopped tomatoes. Season to taste with mixed
Mediterranean herbs and salt, then cover and simmer the
ratatouille for 10–15 minutes.
5. Wash the lamb fillet, pat dry and season it lightly. Heat the
remainder of the olive oil in a second frying pan (skillet), add
the lamb and cook over a medium heat for about 4 minutes
on each side, then serve with the ratatouille.

STEAK CROQUETTES WITH SPICY (BELL) PEPPERS

(SERVES 2)

Ingredients
1 medium onion
2 red (bell) peppers
2 green (bell) peppers
4–5 tbsp olive oil
pinch paprika
125 ml/4 fl oz/½ cup water
1 small onion
1 garlic clove
300 g/10½ oz/2⅔ cups minced (ground) beef steak
1 egg, beaten
pinch salt
freshly ground cayenne pepper

Preparation time: 15 minutes
Cooking time: 17–20 minutes

1. Peel the medium onion and slice it into rings.
2. Wash and deseed the (bell) peppers and chop into strips.
3. Heat half the oil in a frying pan (skillet), add the onion
rings and the (bell) peppers and stir-fry for 2 minutes. Season
with the paprika, then add the water, cover and simmer over
a low heat for 5–8 minutes until the vegetables are cooked.
4. Peel and finely chop the small onion and peel and crush
the garlic clove. Put the onion and garlic in a bowl with the
steak and beaten egg, season with salt and cayenne pepper
and mix well. Divide the mixture into two portions and shape
into croquettes.
5. Heat the rest of the oil in a second frying pan (skillet), add
the croquettes and cook on a high heat, turning frequently,
for about 4 minutes until the croquettes are crispy brown all
over. Reduce the heat and cook for about 6 minutes more
until the croquettes are completely cooked through.
6. Serve each steak croquette topped with the spicy (bell)
pepper and onion ring mixture.

BEEF AND VEGETABLE HOT POT

(SERVES 2)

Ingredients
375 g/13 oz lean braising steak
2–3 tbsp olive oil
pinch paprika
1 bay leaf
freshly ground cayenne pepper
450 ml/16 fl oz/2 cups Vegetable Stock (see page 206)
2 leeks
1 onion
375 g/13 oz carrots
200 g/7 oz celeriac (celery root)
1 tbsp chopped fresh parsley, to garnish

Preparation time: 15–20 minutes
Cooking time: 1¼–2 hours

1. Rinse the steak, pat it dry with kitchen paper (paper towels) and cut it into small cubes.
2. Heat the oil in a large flameproof casserole, add the meat and cook briskly to brown it thoroughly. Add the paprika and bay leaf, season with cayenne pepper, pour in the vegetable stock and bring to the boil. Reduce the heat, cover and simmer for 1¼ hours, or until the meat is tender.
3. Clean the leeks and slice into rings. Peel and dice the carrots and celeriac (celery root).
4. When the meat is just cooked, add the vegetables to the pan and cover again. Simmer for 20 minutes more.
5. Remove the bay leaf and serve. Sprinkle each portion with chopped fresh parsley.

ITALIAN BEEF STIR-FRY

(SERVES 2)

Ingredients
1 aubergine (eggplant)
salt
2 courgettes (zucchini)
5 tomatoes
1 onion
1 garlic clove
1–2 tbsp olive oil
375 g/13 oz minced (ground) beef steak
6 tbsp water
pinch each dried rosemary and oregano

Preparation time: 15 minutes plus 20 minutes draining
Cooking time: 25–30 minutes

1. Wash and dry the aubergine (eggplant) and dice into cubes. Sprinkle with salt and set aside to drain for about 20 minutes. Rinse thoroughly and pat dry.
2. Wash the courgettes (zucchini), halve lengthways and chop into medium-size pieces. Skin and deseed the tomatoes and chop them coarsely. Peel the onion and garlic and chop them both finely.
3. Heat the oil in a large flameproof casserole. Add the steak, followed by the onion and garlic, and stir-fry until the meat is well browned all over.
4. Add the aubergine (eggplant) and courgettes (zucchini) and cook for 5 minutes more. Then stir in the tomatoes, together with the water.
5. Bring to the boil, cover and simmer for about 20 minutes, stirring occasionally. Remove from the heat and serve.

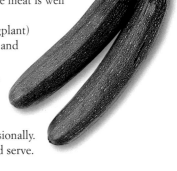

FILLET OF BEEF WITH LEEKS AND CREAM

(SERVES 2)

Ingredients
2 leeks
2–3 tbsp olive oil
150 ml/5 fl oz/⅔ cup Vegetable Stock (see page 206)
2 x 200–225 g/7–8 oz fillet steaks
salt and freshly ground black pepper
5 tsp sour cream
pinch paprika, to garnish

Preparation time: 10 minutes
Cooking time: 10 minutes

1. Wash and trim the leeks, halve each leek lengthways and then cut into slices.
2. Heat 1 tablespoon of the olive oil in a pan, add the leeks and cook gently until soft, stirring frequently. Add the vegetable stock, bring to the boil, then reduce the heat and cover. Simmer for 10 minutes.
3. Meanwhile, rinse the steaks, pat dry with kitchen paper (paper towels) and season with salt and pepper. Heat the rest of the oil in a frying pan (skillet), add the steaks and fry until well browned on both sides. Cover and cook over a gentle heat for 10–15 minutes.
4. Slice the beef and serve accompanied by the leeks. Just before you serve, top the leeks with a dash of sour cream dotted with paprika.

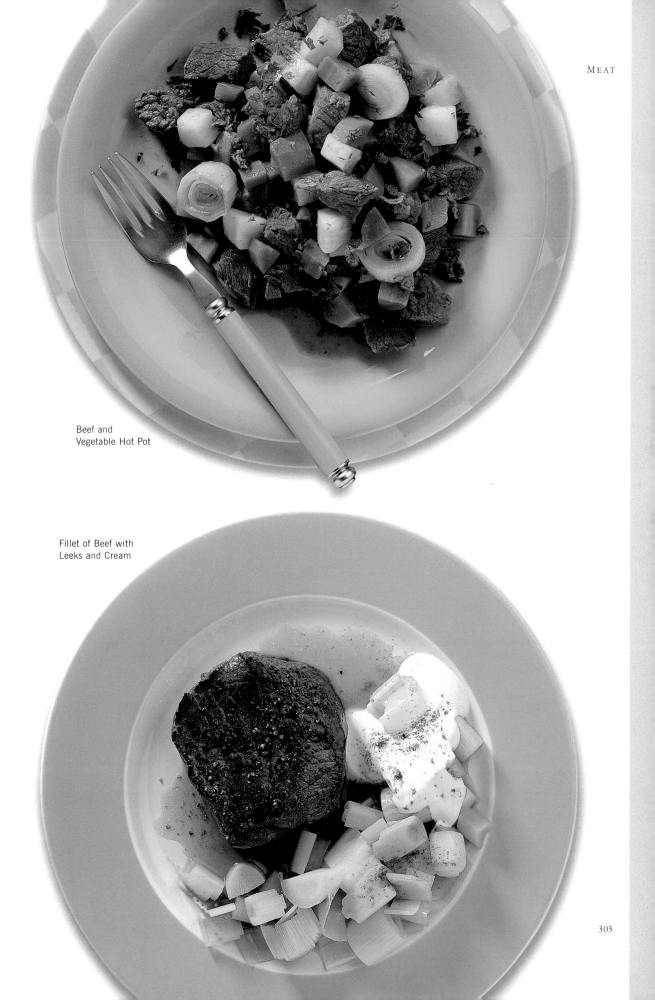

Beef and
Vegetable Hot Pot

Fillet of Beef with
Leeks and Cream

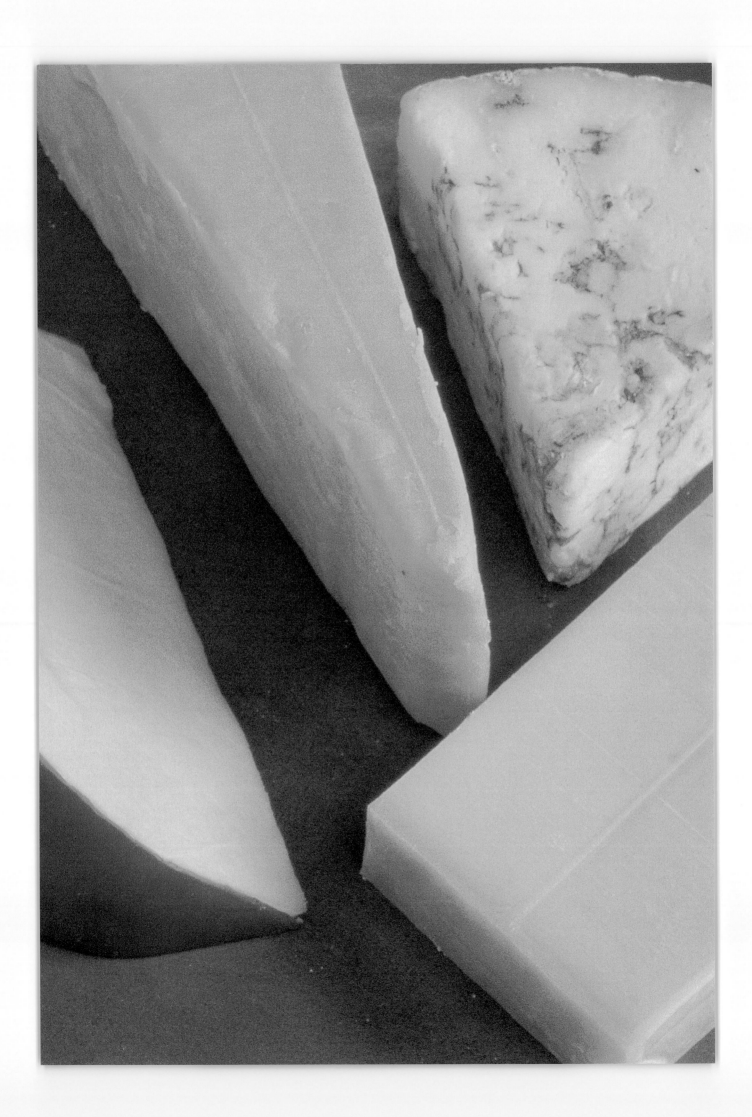

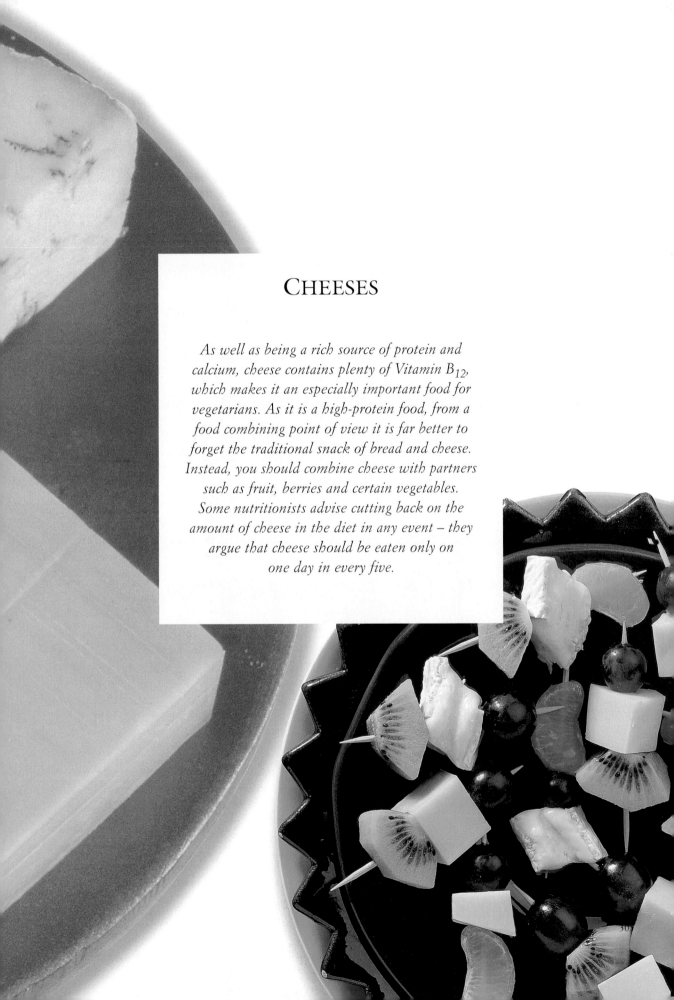

CHEESES

As well as being a rich source of protein and calcium, cheese contains plenty of Vitamin B$_{12}$, which makes it an especially important food for vegetarians. As it is a high-protein food, from a food combining point of view it is far better to forget the traditional snack of bread and cheese. Instead, you should combine cheese with partners such as fruit, berries and certain vegetables. Some nutritionists advise cutting back on the amount of cheese in the diet in any event – they argue that cheese should be eaten only on one day in every five.

CHEESE SALAD

(SERVES 1)

Ingredients
1 small handful of lettuce
4 heads lamb's lettuce (mâche)
1 tomato
1 spear of chicory (Belgian endive)
100 g/3½ oz medium-fat cheese,
such as Camembert, Gouda or Brie
4 fresh chives, chopped
1 radish, peeled and sliced

For the dressing:
100 g/3½ oz/scant ½ cup low-fat soft cheese
2–3 tsp chopped fresh mixed herbs

Preparation time: 10 minutes

1. Wash the lettuce and lamb's lettuce (mâche) and pat dry. Quarter the tomato and cut into chunks.
2. Cut the chicory (Belgian endive) in half, remove the bitter core and finely chop the remainder.
3. Mix the salad vegetables together, arrange on a plate with the cheese and garnish with the chives and the radish.
4. Mix the soft cheese with the herbs to make a dressing. Spoon it over the salad.

CHEESE CAUTIONS

One of the chief reasons for eating cheese only in moderation is the high levels of saturated fat in some varieties. Hard cheeses, such as Cheddar, Parmesan and Stilton, can contain up to 35 per cent fat, while soft cheeses, like Camembert and Brie, contain 26 per cent on average. Cottage cheese, on the other hand, can contain as little as four per cent fat. A second reason for limiting cheese intake is the propensity it has to trigger migraines in susceptible individuals. The culprit here is thought to be a chemical called tyramine, which causes nerve and blood vessels in the brain to constrict, so triggering an attack.

Nevertheless, cheese does have its value, particularly as an important source of calcium. The body finds it easier to absorb the calcium contained in cheese and other dairy foods than it does the calcium in other foodstuffs. In addition, chewing cheese has been proven medically to play a potentially important role in reducing tooth decay. It stops the formation of acids in the mouth, which occurs after eating sugary foodstuffs and which, if unchecked, will attack the tooth enamel and form cavities.

STUFFED CHERRY TOMATOES

(SERVES 4)

Ingredients
12–16 cherry tomatoes
4–6 fresh chives, finely chopped
150 g/5½ oz/scant ¾ cup cream cheese
pinch celery salt
2–3 shredded lettuce leaves, to garnish
cress, to garnish

Preparation time: 20 minutes

1. Wash and dry the tomatoes. Cut off the tops and scoop out the flesh with a sharp knife, taking care to leave the shells intact. Turn upside down to drain.
2. Combine the chopped chives with the cream cheese. Season with celery salt and mix well.
3. Stuff the tomatoes with the mixture. Arrange on a serving plate and garnish with lettuce strips and cress.

CHEESE-STUFFED MUSHROOMS

(SERVES 4)

Ingredients
20 medium-size mushrooms
200 g/7 oz/scant 1 cup Quark
1 tbsp grated Cheddar cheese
1 garlic clove, peeled and crushed
1 tsp finely chopped fresh parsley
4–6 chives, finely chopped
2 fresh basil leaves, finely chopped
freshly ground black pepper
pinch paprika

Preparation time: 10–15 minutes
Cooking time: 3–4 minutes

1. Wipe the mushrooms clean and remove the stalks (stems). (You can keep these for another dish.)
2. Blend the Quark with the grated Cheddar and the crushed garlic. Season this mixture with the finely chopped herbs, pepper and paprika.
3. Fill the mushroom caps with the Quark mixture and cook under a hot preheated grill (broiler) for 3–4 minutes or until brown. (Note: you can vary this recipe by using small tomatoes instead of the mushrooms.)

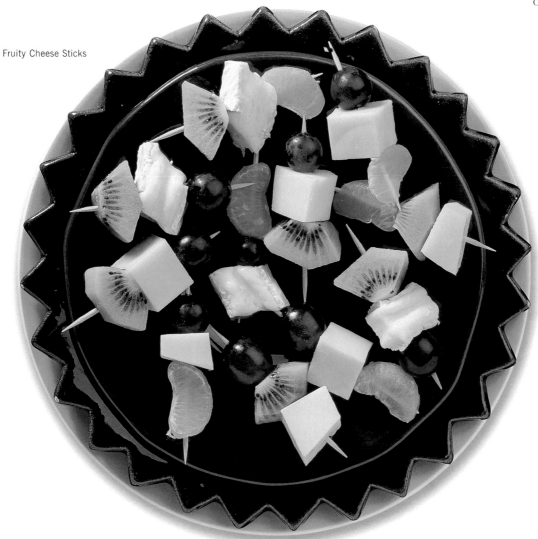

Fruity Cheese Sticks

FRUITY CHEESE STICKS

(MAKES 8 STICKS)

Ingredients
4 pieces of cheese of your choice (Camembert, Gouda,
Brie and Cheddar are all recommended)
2 kiwi fruit
1 bunch red or black, seedless grapes
2 seedless mandarins

Preparation time: 15 minutes

1. Dice the cheese into medium-size cubes.
2. Peel the kiwi fruit and cut into cubes that are roughly
the same size as the cheese cubes.
3. Wash the grapes and remove from their stems.
4. Peel the mandarin oranges and separate into segments.
5. Arrange cheese and fruit alternately on eight skewers.

MUSHROOMS IN BOURSIN

(SERVES 4)

Ingredients
500 g/1 lb 2 oz/7¼ cups mushrooms
1 tbsp butter
142 g/5 oz packet Boursin or any other
medium-fat herbed cream cheese
1 garlic clove, peeled and crushed

Preparation time: 5–10 minutes
Cooking time: 10–15 minutes

1. Wipe the mushrooms clean and slice thinly.
2. Melt the butter in a large pan. Add the mushrooms and
cook gently, stirring occasionally, for 10 minutes, or until
golden brown.
3. Add the Boursin and the garlic. Heat through gently until
the cheese has melted. Serve with a salad.

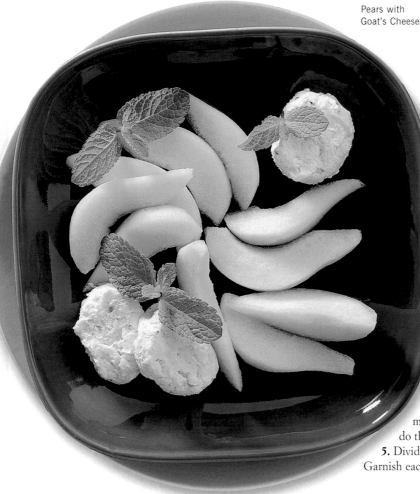

Pears with
Goat's Cheese

PEARS WITH GOAT'S CHEESE

(APPETIZER FOR 4)

Ingredients
2 ripe medium-size pears
150 g/5½ oz goat's cheese
100 g/3½ oz/scant ½ cup cream cheese
freshly ground black pepper
fresh mint leaves, to garnish

Preparation time: 10–15 minutes

1. Peel the pears, then remove and discard the cores. Slice the flesh and arrange on four plates.
2. Cut off the rind from the goat's cheese. Place in a bowl and mash the cheese with a fork.
3. Mix in the cream cheese and season the mixture with pepper.
4. Roll the cheese into a sausage shape – make sure that your hands are cool when you do this – and slice into 12 rounds.
5. Divide the cheese slices between the four plates. Garnish each portion with mint leaves.

STUFFED GOAT'S CHEESE

(APPETISER FOR 4)

Ingredients
4 x 90 g/3¼ oz fresh goat's cheeses
150 g/5½ oz/scant ¾ cup cream cheese
1 tbsp chopped fresh basil
1 fresh parsley sprig, finely chopped
3 chives, finely chopped
80 g/3 oz watercress, rinsed

Preparation time: 5–8 minutes

1. Cut the goat's cheeses in half horizontally.
2. Put the cream cheese in a bowl and combine it with the chopped basil, parsley and chives.
3. Spread the cream cheese mixture over four of the goat's cheese halves. Put the remaining halves on top. Serve on a bed of watercress.

GRILLED (BROILED) GOAT'S CHEESE

(APPETIZER FOR 4)

Ingredients
4 x 90 g/3¼ oz fresh goat's cheeses
½ head frisée lettuce, shredded
100 g/3½ oz lamb's lettuce (mâche), shredded
4 tomatoes, sliced
¼ cucumber, peeled and sliced

Preparation time: 5 minutes
Cooking time: 4–5 minutes

1. Preheat the grill (broiler) and toast the goat's cheeses until they begin to melt and brown.
2. Arrange the frisée lettuce, lamb's lettuce (mâche), tomatoes and cucumber on the four plates.
3. When the cheeses are ready, place one on each plate and serve immediately.

Italian Tomatoes

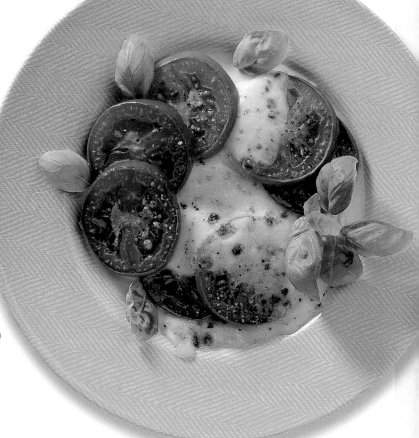

ITALIAN TOMATOES

(SERVES 4)

Ingredients
5 tomatoes
2 x 175 g/6 oz mozzarella cheeses
salt and freshly ground black pepper
fresh basil leaves, to garnish

Preparation time: 8–10 minutes
Cooking time: 6–8 minutes

1. Wash the tomatoes, pat dry, slice off the stalk ends and discard, then cut the remainder into even slices.
2. Slice the mozzarella evenly. Use an egg slicer for the best results.
3. Grease a shallow, flameproof dish. Place the cheese and tomato slices in the dish, layering them alternately. Season the slices with salt and black pepper and cook under a hot grill (broiler) until the cheese has melted.
4. Sprinkle the basil leaves over the dish. Serve hot.

CHEESE-FRUIT SALAD

(SERVES 4)

Ingredients
150 g/5½ oz young Edam or Gouda cheese
2 medium-size seedless oranges
1 kiwi fruit
1 apple

Preparation time: 15–20 minutes

1. Remove the rind from the cheese and discard. Dice the cheese into cubes and place in a bowl.
2. Peel the oranges and separate the fruit into segments. Add to the cheese cubes.
3. Peel the kiwi fruit, cut into small pieces and mix with the cheese and the orange.
4. Peel the apple, remove the core, dice into cubes and mix with the rest of the salad.
5. Serve with a salad dressing of your choice or mayonnaise (see pages 192–193).

GORGONZOLA MUSHROOMS

(SERVES 4)

Ingredients
250 g/9 oz/3⅔ cups mushrooms
150 g/5½ oz Gorgonzola cheese
4–6 chives, finely chopped

Preparation time: 10–15 minutes
Cooking time: 3–4 minutes

1. Wipe the mushrooms clean and remove the stalks (stems). (These may be saved for a soup.)
2. Put the Gorgonzola in a bowl and mash well with a fork. Fill the mushroom caps with the cheese.
3. Grease a shallow, flameproof dish. Add the mushrooms and cook under a hot grill (broiler) until the cheese has melted. Remove from the heat, sprinkle with the chopped chives and serve immediately.

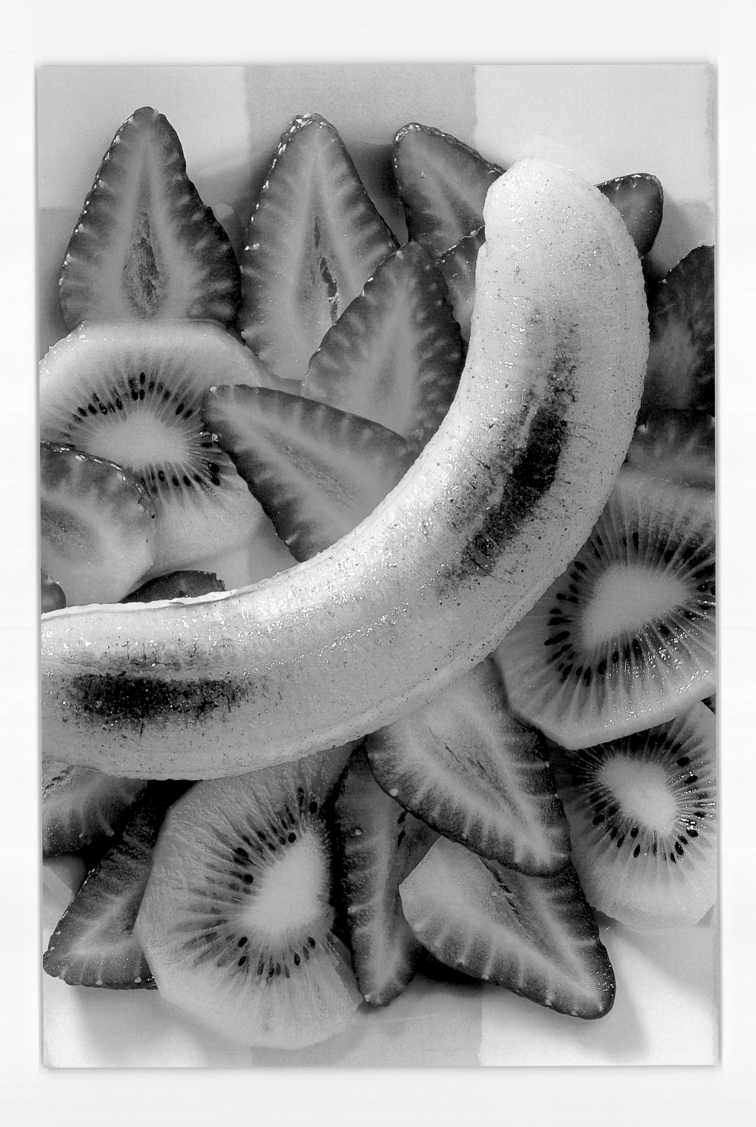

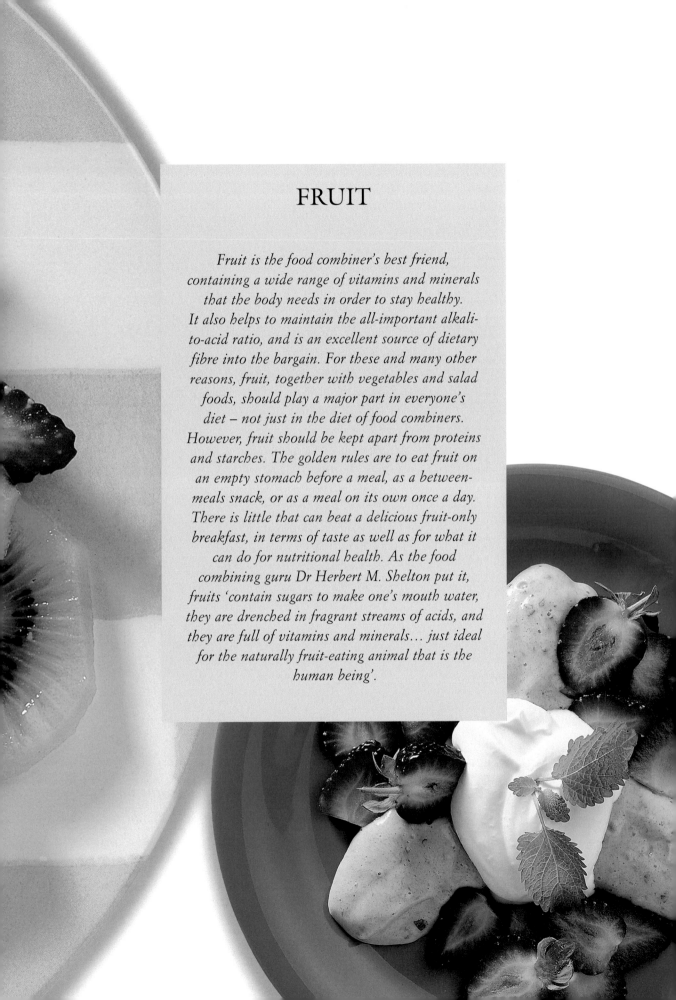

FRUIT

Fruit is the food combiner's best friend, containing a wide range of vitamins and minerals that the body needs in order to stay healthy. It also helps to maintain the all-important alkali-to-acid ratio, and is an excellent source of dietary fibre into the bargain. For these and many other reasons, fruit, together with vegetables and salad foods, should play a major part in everyone's diet – not just in the diet of food combiners. However, fruit should be kept apart from proteins and starches. The golden rules are to eat fruit on an empty stomach before a meal, as a between-meals snack, or as a meal on its own once a day. There is little that can beat a delicious fruit-only breakfast, in terms of taste as well as for what it can do for nutritional health. As the food combining guru Dr Herbert M. Shelton put it, fruits 'contain sugars to make one's mouth water, they are drenched in fragrant streams of acids, and they are full of vitamins and minerals… just ideal for the naturally fruit-eating animal that is the human being'.

FRUIT FACTS

Nutritionists everywhere agree that fruit is a vital dietary ingredient – the World Health Organization, for instance, recommends eating at least five portions of fruit and vegetables a day. Most fruit is low in calories and sweet-tasting, as well as being packed with health-giving nutrients, particularly Vitamin C, which is a powerful antioxidant, and helps to protect against cancer. Fruit is also a particularly rich source of potassium, which helps to regulate blood pressure.

BEST EATEN ALONE

Most modern food combining experts agree that fruit is best eaten on its own, rather than as part of a meal or combined with other foodstuffs. The reason for this is simple. On its own, fruit travels very quickly through the stomach, with fruit juices taking even less time to complete their journey. If this progress is hindered or blocked by slower-moving nutrients – notably proteins and starches, both of which take far longer to digest than fruit does – the fruit will start to ferment. The result is a build-up of intestinal gas, with discomfort and even pain as the inevitable consequences of the pressure this build-up causes.

Always eat fruit on its own.

Eat fruit on its own and it will pass through the stomach speedily, just as nature intended. A speedy progress also makes it much easier for the body to absorb and process the wealth of health-giving nutrients that fruit contains.

NUTRIENT SOURCES

Citrus fruit such as oranges, satsumas, tangerines, mandarins, lemons and grapefruit are rich in Vitamin C, and so are kiwi fruit, strawberries, blackcurrants and raspberries. A serving of any of these fruits each day will provide a substantial amount of the Vitamin C requirement. Apricots, mangoes and certain varieties of melon contain valuable amounts of beta-carotene, which the body converts into Vitamin A. All fruits are rich in potassium, especially bananas. As well as helping to regulate the blood pressure, potassium works in tandem with sodium to regulate the body's fluid levels.

Fruit also contains insoluble and soluble fibre. Both kinds of fibre can help to prevent constipation, while the latter can help to lower cholesterol levels in the blood. Citrus fruit and dried fruit, such as dried figs, dates, apricots and raisins, are particularly useful fibre sources.

ORANGES, LEMONS AND GRAPEFRUIT

Oranges, in particular, are packed with beneficial nutrients – it has been calculated, for instance, that just one medium-size orange contains nearly the entire daily Vitamin C requirement for an adult. Vitamin C is needed to make collagen, an essential element in keeping the skin healthy, and helps to maintain the body's defences against bacterial infection. Oranges also contain thiamine and folic acid, two important B vitamins. The membranes between the orange's segments (pith) are packed with pectin, a useful

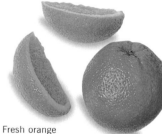

Fresh orange

source of soluble dietary fibre which, it is believed, helps to lower blood cholesterol levels, and substances called bioflavonoids, which have powerful antioxidant properties that help to protect the body against potential free-radical damage (free radicals are harmful particles that damage body cells).

Because of their sharp taste, lemons are usually reserved for flavouring sauces and drinks. They are an excellent source of Vitamin C, so it is well worth making freshly squeezed lemon juice a part of your diet, especially since it is thought that the juice contains an oil that may help to relieve the symptoms of rheumatism. It does this by encouraging the liver to expel harmful toxins that cause the complaint.

Grapefruits are also rich in Vitamin C – half a grapefruit provides more than half the daily adult requirement. Both pink and red grapefruit contain slightly more Vitamin C than other varieties.

BANANAS

Bananas are a good source of potassium. They are also rich in natural sugar, which they release quickly into the bloodstream. This is why people in need of a quick energy boost – notably athletes – often eat bananas as a fast convenient snack. However, unripe bananas should be

Banana

avoided. They contain what is termed 'resistant' starch, which, because it cannot be digested in the small intestine, starts fermenting in the large intestine, with troublesome wind (gas) as the result. As the fruit ripens, most of the starch turns to sugar, which is far easier for the body to digest.

PESTICIDE ALERT

Many fruits are coated with fungicides to stop mould from growing. Lemons, for instance, are normally treated with fungicide spray and wax. Although the use of such chemicals is strictly controlled by law, you should always wash any such fruit thoroughly in running water before you eat it. Alternatively buy organic fruit that has been left untreated.

FRUIT JUICE FACTS

There can be no doubt that drinking fruit juice is nutritious. Naturopaths believe that the drinking of such juices can help to cleanse the body by purging it of waste products and toxins. For best results, squeeze or juice your own; if you buy commercial juice, look for the following terms:

Freshly squeezed
This means exactly what it says – the only processing involved is the extraction of the liquid.

Freshly pressed
In the case of tomato juice, the fruit has been pulped and then pasteurized. Freshly pressed apple juice has a little ascorbic acid added to stop it from turning brown.

Concentrated
The squeezed fruit is heated to make the concentrate, which is then pasteurized before water is added.

Long-life
This has a substantially longer shelf-life than other juice varieties because it has been heated briefly to kill off bacteria.

Whichever type of juice you buy, carefully check the 'sell by' and 'use by' dates on the packaging.

DRIED FRUIT: NATURE'S HEALTH-GIVER

Generally recognized as being one of nature's most beneficial health foods, dried fruits contain lots of fibre and are concentrated sources of valuable minerals, notably iron and potassium. However, they are also sugar-rich and high in calories, so they should be eaten only in moderation.

Dried figs are useful for easing constipation, while a snack of dried apricots and raisins is an ideal energy booster because the drying process increases the concentration of the sugar, beta-carotene, potassium and iron that the fruit contains. For this reason, dried apricots were part of the diet of astronauts during the Apollo space missions.

A FRUIT FAST

A 24-hour fruit fast is a good way to give your digestive system a rest, while at the same time cleansing and refreshing it. Fruit is nature's original fast food: it is quick, easy and convenient to eat and healthy into the bargain. A serving can be a medium-size piece of fruit, 175 ml/6 fl oz of 100 per cent pure fruit juice, 125 g/4½ oz of cooked fruit, or 60 g/2¼ oz of the dried variety. You should remember that, according to the US Fruitarian Foundation, it can be counter-productive to mix different types of fruit. Their advice is to leave a gap of 1½–2 hours between eating different types of fruit.

As far as dried fruits are concerned, the advice is to eat only a small quantity of dried fruits at any one time and no more than the recommended amount: ideally, you should stop while you still feel like eating some more.

You can make your selection from the following, ringing the changes to make sure that it does not get monotonous.

ON WAKING
Freshly squeezed lemon juice
Melon or melon juice
Raisins

MORNING
Apples
Pineapple
Figs
Pears
White grapes
Yellow plums
Kiwi fruit

LUNCHTIME
Oranges
Tangerines
Peaches
Apricots
Papaya

AFTERNOON
Mangoes
Cherries
Strawberries
Red plums
Persimmons
Pomegranates
Watermelon
Tomatoes

EARLY EVENING
Black grapes
Blackberries
Raspberries

EVENING
Mangoes
Cherries
Strawberries
Red plums
Persimmons
Pomegranates
Water melon
Tomatoes

BEFORE BED
Passion fruit
Freshly squeezed lemon juice

You can eat the following fruits at any time of the day: bananas, coconuts, olives, avocados, cashews, raw chestnuts, hazelnuts, almonds and pine nuts – and drink as much lemon juice as you want, in addition to the amounts suggested here.

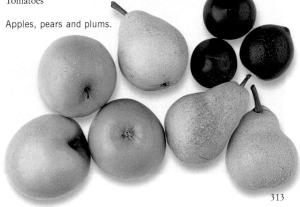

Apples, pears and plums.

313

STUFFED PINEAPPLE

(SERVES 2)

Ingredients
1 fresh pineapple
2 ripe pears
2 medium-size oranges
1 kiwi fruit
125 ml/4 fl oz/½ cup double (heavy) cream, whipped

Preparation time: 25 minutes

1. Cut the pineapple in half lengthways. Remove the hard core and scoop out the flesh with a grapefruit knife, taking care not to puncture the pineapple skin. Cut the flesh into bite-size pieces and put in a bowl. Reserve the pineapple halves for later.
2. Peel the pears, remove the cores, dice the flesh into cubes and add to the pineapple in the bowl.
3. Peel the oranges, removing all the pith. Separate out the flesh, segment by segment, using a sharp knife, and discard the rest.
4. Mix the prepared fruit together and use it to fill the hollow halves of the pineapple.
5. Peel the kiwi fruit, slice it thinly and use it to garnish the pineapple.
6. Top with the cream and serve.

PINEAPPLE POWER

Traditionally, pineapple has been thought to possess various healing powers, but modern nutritional science has concentrated on the fact that the fruit contains a powerful enzyme called bromelain, which acts to break down protein. Researchers believe that the substance may help to break up blood clots, while there is scientific evidence to suggest that it may help to relieve congested sinuses and infections of the urinary tract. Bromelain is thought to speed the repair of damaged tissues, so it is used to treat arthritis and many sports injuries.
Herbal practitioners advise gargling with the juice to relieve a sore throat and eating pineapple as part of the treatment of various disorders, including catarrh, bronchitis and indigestion.

* Unlike other fruit, pineapples do not become sweeter after they have been picked.
* To see whether a pineapple is ripe, hold it and check its leaves for colour. The fruit should feel heavy for its size, the leaves should be fresh and green and the pineapple should smell sweet and fragrant.
* Always eat fresh pineapple rather than canned, because the canning process destroys the bromelain.
* In rare instances, fresh pineapple can trigger allergic reactions. If these are severe, consult a doctor.

TROPICAL MANGO COCKTAIL

(SERVES 4)

Ingredients
1 ripe mango
6 lychees
1 ripe banana
1–2 tsp lemon juice
3 passion fruit
125 ml/4 fl oz/½ cup double (heavy) cream, whipped

Preparation time: 6–8 minutes

1. Wash and peel the mango, remove the stone (pit) and dice the flesh into cubes. Place in a bowl.
2. Wash and peel the lychees, remove the stones (pits), chop the flesh and add it to the mango pieces.
3. Peel the banana, slice thinly, sprinkle with lemon juice to prevent discoloration and add to the bowl.
4. Cut the passion fruit in half. Scoop out the flesh with a teaspoon and blend with the other fruit. Top with the whipped cream and serve.

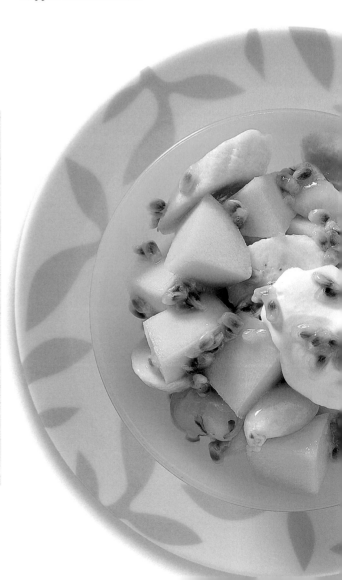

CINNAMON APPLES

(SERVES 2)

Ingredients
5 apples
½ lemon
2 tbsp chopped hazelnuts
½ tsp ground cinnamon, plus whole sticks, to decorate

Preparation time: 15 minutes
Cooking time: 5–7 minutes

1. Wash and dry the apples, then remove the cores. Steam four of them as follows. Make a shallow cut with a sharp knife around the widest part of the apple, about halfway up (this prevents the skin from bursting). Stand the apples in a colander over a pan of simmering water, then cover and steam for 5–7 minutes, until just tender. Remove from the heat.
2. Squeeze the lemon and rub some of the juice into the apple hollows to prevent discoloration. Shred the remaining apple roughly, sprinkle with a few more drops of lemon juice, and combine it with the ground hazelnuts and ground cinnamon.
3. Fill the apple hollows with the apple mixture and serve, garnished with cinnamon sticks.

Cinnamon Apples

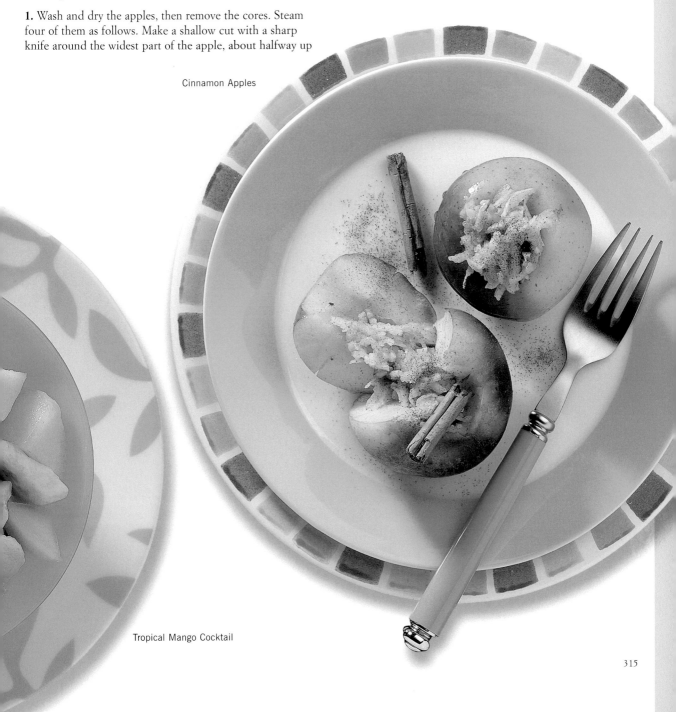

Tropical Mango Cocktail

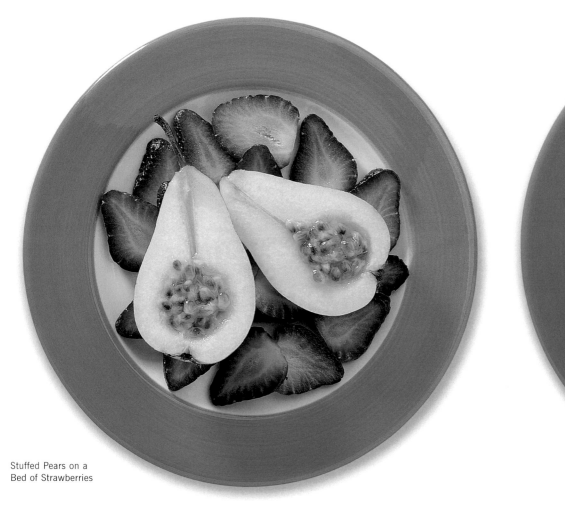

Stuffed Pears on a
Bed of Strawberries

WINTER PINEAPPLE

(SERVES 2)

Ingredients
1 pineapple
2 ripe apples
2 mandarin oranges
100 g/3½ oz/scant 1 cup toasted hazelnuts, chopped

Preparation time: 20 minutes

1. Cut the pineapple in half lengthways. Remove the hard core and scoop out the flesh with a grapefruit knife, taking care not to puncture the pineapple skin. Cut the flesh into bite-size pieces and put in a bowl.
2. Peel the apples, remove the cores, dice the flesh into cubes and mix with the pineapple pieces.
3. Peel the oranges, separate the segments, chop roughly and add to the bowl.
4. Mix the fruit salad well and fill the pineapple halves with it. Sprinkle with the chopped hazelnuts and serve.

STUFFED PEARS ON A BED OF STRAWBERRIES

(SERVES 2)

Ingredients
2 large ripe pears
2 tsp lemon juice
10 strawberries or 2 kiwi fruit
4 passion fruit

Preparation time: 12 minutes

1. Peel the pears and cut them in half. Remove the cores and sprinkle the flesh with lemon juice to prevent discoloration.
2. Wash the strawberries, remove the stalks and slice thinly. (You can use kiwi fruit as an alternative if strawberries are unavailable.) Arrange the slices neatly on two plates, taking care to overlap them.
3. Cut the passion fruit in half, scoop out the flesh and use it to fill the pear halves. Place the pears on top of the bed of strawberries and serve.

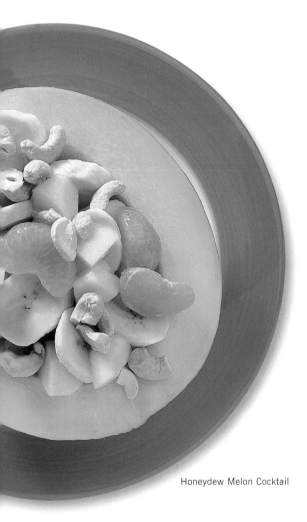

Honeydew Melon Cocktail

HONEYDEW MELON COCKTAIL

(SERVES 2)

Ingredients
1 melon, such as honeydew
1 apple
1 tbsp lemon juice
1 banana
1 mandarin
2 tbsp chopped cashew nuts

Preparation time: 15 minutes

1. Cut the melon in half and scoop out the seeds and core to form a hollow.
2. Peel the apple, remove the core, cut the flesh into pieces and place in a mixing bowl. Sprinkle with the lemon juice to prevent discoloration.
3. Peel and slice the banana into neat rounds and combine it with the apple pieces.
4. Peel the mandarin orange, separate into segments and add these to the fruit salad.
5. Mix well and fill the hollow of the melon with the cocktail. Decorate with the chopped cashews.

MELON MEDLEY

Popular varieties of melon include watermelon, honeydew, cantaloupe and charentais. The last two are small and particularly sweet and succulent. Cantaloupes are extremely nutritious – a single serving will supply the body with more than half the recommended daily Vitamin C intake, and it is also a rich source of beta-carotene. Melons with a lighter yellow or green flesh colour contain less Vitamin C and hardly any beta-carotene. All varieties are low in calories and their high water content is thought to help maintain healthy kidney function. Melon, however, does not combine well with other foods (see page 174).

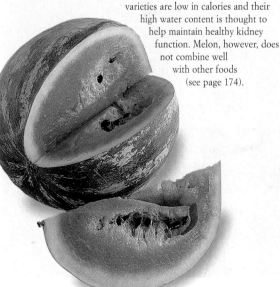

CITRUS SALAD

(SERVES 2)

Ingredients
2 oranges
1 pink grapefruit
2 mandarins
100 g/3½ oz seedless black grapes
2 tbsp almond flakes (slices)

Preparation time: 15 minutes

1. Peel the oranges, grapefruit and mandarins, removing all the pith with a sharp knife, divide into segments and place in a mixing bowl.
2. Wash the grapes, remove them from their stems, peel them and cut them in half.
3. Add the grapes to the bowl of citrus segments, mix the fruit together well, divide the salad among two bowls and sprinkle with the almond flakes (slices).

EXOTIC FRUIT SALAD

(SERVES 4)

Ingredients
1 pear
1 orange
100 g/3½ oz grapes
½ ripe pineapple
2 tbsp raisins, soaked in 2 tbsp water
whipped cream, to serve

Preparation time: 20 minutes

1. Peel the pear, remove the core and chop the flesh into bite-size pieces. Place in a large bowl.
2. Peel the orange and separate into segments.
3. Wash the grapes, remove the stems, cut them in half and remove the seeds.
4. Peel the pineapple, remove the hard core and cut the flesh into pieces. Add all the fruit to the bowl.
5. Add the soaked raisins and their liquid.
6, Mix all the ingredients together and serve the fruit salad in four bowls topped with whipped cream.

LAYERED FRUIT SALAD

(SERVES 4)

Ingredients
1 pomegranate
2 oranges
1 avocado
2 tsp lemon juice
½ pineapple
2 kiwi fruit
200 g/7 oz/1¼ cups strawberries
1 ripe mango
125 ml/4 fl oz/½ cup freshly squeezed orange juice
5–6 fresh lemon balm leaves

Preparation time: 25 minutes

1. Cut the pomegranate in half and remove the flesh with a spoon. Discard the shells and membrane.
2. Peel the oranges and separate into segments.
3. Peel the avocado, remove its stone (pit) and cut the flesh into slices, sprinkling with lemon juice to avoid discoloration.
4. Peel the pineapple, remove its hard core and cut the flesh into bite-size pieces.
5. Peel the kiwi fruit and slice.
6. Wash and hull the strawberries, then cut into slices.
7. Peel the mango, remove the stone (pit) and slice the flesh.
8. Arrange all the fruit in layers in a tall glass container. Start with a layer of pomegranate, then add layers of orange, avocado, pineapple, kiwi fruit, strawberry and mango.

9. Coat the fruit salad with the orange juice and garnish with lemon balm leaves.

FOREST BERRY COCKTAIL

(SERVES 2)

Ingredients
100 g/3½ oz/scant 1 cup blueberries
100 g/3½ oz/scant ¾ cup raspberries
100 g/3½ oz/scant 1 cup blackberries
100 g/3½ oz/scant 1 cup currants
4 tbsp Quark

1. Wash the fruit, pat dry and mix together.
2. Divide the fruits among four bowls and top with the Quark.

REFRESHING SUMMER SALAD

(SERVES 4)

Ingredients
2 peaches
2 plums
4 apricots
2 nectarines
4 tbsp sour cream
bay leaves, to decorate

Preparation time: 10 minutes

1. Wash all the fruit, cut in half, remove the stones (pits) and cut the flesh into bite-size pieces.
3. Mix all the fruit together, divide among four bowls and serve with the sour cream. Decorate with bay leaves.

BERRY FACTS

There are two main types of berry: soft ones, such as strawberries, raspberries and blackberries, and firm ones, such as blueberries and cranberries.
Both types are low in calories, and contain plenty of potassium, along with Vitamin C and other antioxidant substances. The potassium helps to maintain the body's mineral and fluid balances, while the Vitamin C supports the immune system and, with other antioxidants such as bioflavonoids, helps to protect the body against degenerative diseases such as cancer. The disadvantage of berries is that they contain salicylates – aspirin-like compounds, which can occasionally cause an allergic reaction in susceptible individuals.

Exotic Fruit Salad

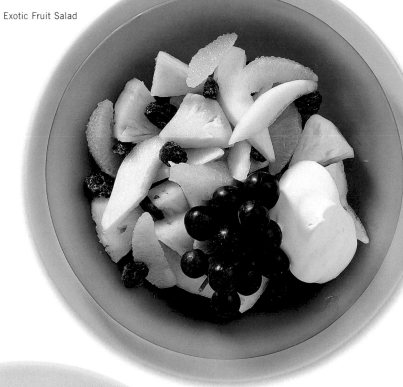

Refreshing Summer Salad

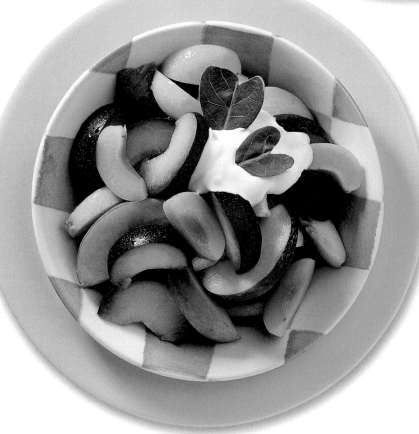

BERRY SALAD WITH QUARK

(SERVES 4)

Ingredients
150 g/5½ oz/scant 1 cup raspberries
150 g/5½ oz/scant 1½ cups blackberries
150 g/5½ oz/scant 1½ cups redcurrants
200 g/7 oz/scant 1 cup low-fat Quark
4 tbsp whipped cream, to decorate

Preparation time: 5 minutes

1. Wash and dry the berries.
2. Combine the Quark with the berries and decorate the mixture with whipped cream.

SWEET AVOCADO SALAD

(SERVES 2)

Ingredients
1 ripe avocado
1 mango
1 orange
1 kiwi fruit
1 apple
4 tbsp Greek (plain strained) yogurt

Preparation time: 20 minutes

1. Peel the avocado and mango, remove the stones (pits) and chop the flesh into bite-size pieces. Place in a large bowl.
3. Peel the orange. Separate into segments.
4. Peel and slice the kiwi fruit.
5. Peel the apple, remove the core and dice the flesh into cubes.
6. Add the rest of the fruit to the bowl, mix well, and serve with the Greek (strained plain) yogurt.

STUFFED APRICOTS

(SERVES 2)

Ingredients
8 fresh apricots
2 dried, no-soak apricots
150 ml/5 fl oz/⅔ cup sour cream
8 fresh mint leaves, to decorate

Preparation time: 15 minutes

1. Wash the fresh apricots, cut them in half and remove the stones (pits).
2. Finely chop the dried apricots, place them in a bowl and stir in the sour cream.
4. Fill one half of each apricot with the sour cream mixture. Place the other apricot half on top.
5. Decorate with mint leaves.

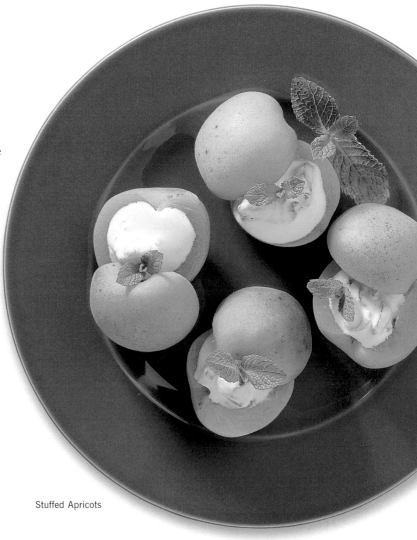

Stuffed Apricots

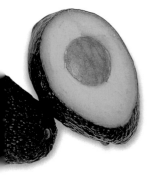

FRIED BANANAS WITH GINGER

(SERVES 4)

Ingredients
4 bananas
2 tbsp safflower oil
1 tsp ground ginger
20 g/¾ oz/scant ¼ cup strawberries
1 kiwi fruit, sliced

Preparation time: 8–10 minutes
Cooking time: 3 minutes

1. Peel the bananas, but keep them whole.
2. Heat the oil in a pan over a low heat. Add the bananas and sprinkle with the ginger. Fry the bananas gently for 3 minutes.
3. Wash and hull the strawberries and cut into slices.
4. Divide the strawberry slices between 4 plates and put the fried bananas on top, one to each plate.
5. Decorate with slices of kiwi fruit.

GINGER'S HEALING POWERS

Nutritionists believe that ginger aids digestion and helps to improve the circulation. It is also a popular remedy for nausea, notably for travel and morning sickness, while, in traditional herbal medicine, the spice is also prescribed to combat respiratory and digestive infections. Ginger is considered to be a useful aid in easing of flatulence and treating stomach gripes. Taken at the first signs of a cold, ginger tea may help to clear a blocked nose. To make a cup of ginger tea, mix a teaspoon of freshly grated ginger with the same amount of honey and the juice of half a lemon, and top up with boiling water to create a potent brew.

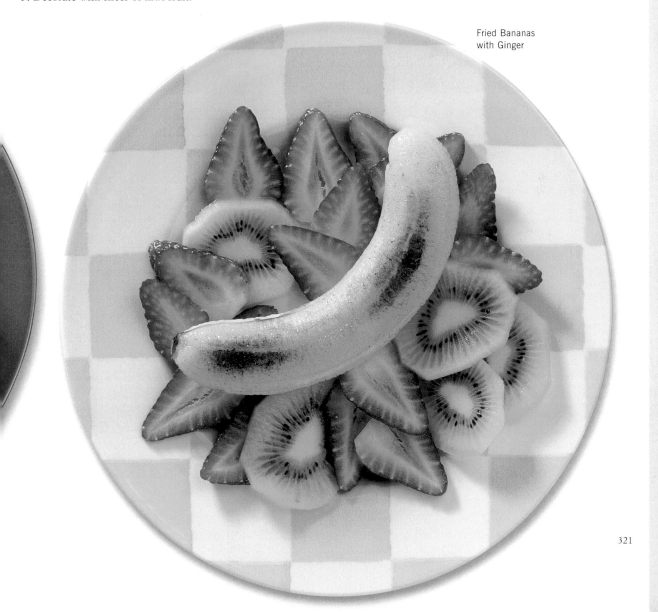

Fried Bananas
with Ginger

UGLI-GRAPEFRUIT SALAD WITH THYME HONEY

(SERVES 4)

Ingredients
1 ugli fruit
1 grapefruit
1 orange
1 mandarin
5 kumquats
1 tbsp thyme honey
125 ml/4 fl oz/½ cup freshly squeezed orange juice
2 tbsp lemon juice
1 tsp dried thyme

Preparation time: 10–15 minutes plus cooling time
Cooking time: 2–3 minutes

1. Peel the ugli fruit, grapefruit, orange and mandarin and separate into segments. Mix together in a bowl.
2. Wash the kumquats, slice and add to the citrus fruit.
3. Put in the thyme honey, orange and lemon juices and thyme in a small pan and warm gently. Pour the honey sauce over the citrus salad, set aside to cool, stir and serve.

SHARON FRUIT SALAD

(SERVES 2)

Ingredients
2 sharon fruit
1 banana
1 tsp lemon juice
2 kiwi fruit
4 passion fruit
2–4 tbsp whipped cream

Preparation time: 10 minutes

1. Wash the sharon fruit, dry and cut into pieces.
2. Peel the banana, slice and sprinkle the slices with lemon juice to prevent discoloration.
3. Peel and slice the kiwi fruit.
4. With the exception of the passion fruit, put all the fruit in a bowl and mix together thoroughly.
5. Cut the passion fruit in half, remove the flesh, mash with a fork and blend with the salad.
6. Serve with whipped cream.

PINEAPPLE SALAD WITH COCONUT

(SERVES 4)

Ingredients
½ pineapple
200 g/7 oz/generous 1 cup raspberries
100 g/3½ oz/¾ cup raisins or dried cranberries, soaked in 2 tbsp water
1 banana
3 tbsp shredded coconut

Preparation time: 10–15 minutes

1. Peel the pineapple, remove the hard core and cut the flesh into pieces. Place in a bowl.
2. Wash the raspberries, remove any stalks and add the fruit to the pineapple pieces.
3. Add the raisins or cranberries and their soaking liquid to the salad.
4. Peel the banana, slice and combine with the salad.
5. Sprinkle the coconut over the pineapple salad and serve.

SUMMER FRUITS IN BERRY SAUCE

(SERVES 4)

Ingredients
400 g/14 oz/3½ cups mixed berries (blueberries, blackberries, raspberries and strawberries)
2 peaches
2 apricots
4 slices fresh pineapple
2 tbsp blueberries
4 fresh mint leaves
2–4 tbsp whipped cream

Preparation time: 10–15 minutes

1. Wash the berries, remove the stalks and purée together. Strain the fruit purée on to four dessert plates.
2. Wash the peaches, dry them, cut into four pieces, removing the stones (pits), and slice.
3. Wash and dry the apricots, then cut them in half and remove the stones (pits). Cut the flesh into slices.
4. Arrange the sliced peaches, apricots and pineapple on top of the berry sauce.
5. Decorate with blueberries, mint and whipped cream.

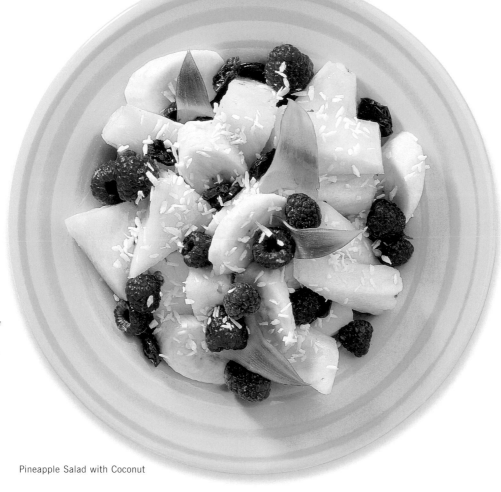

Pineapple Salad with Coconut

Ugli-grapefruit Salad
with Thyme Honey

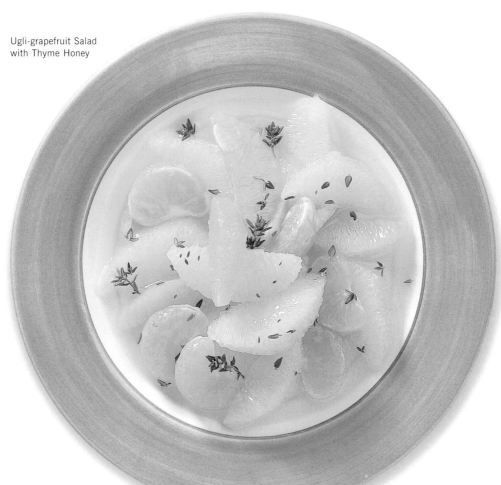

MELON COCKTAIL WITH MINT SYRUP

(SERVES 4)

Ingredients
3 tbsp finely chopped fresh mint
125 ml/4 fl oz/½ cup water
1 tbsp honey
1 lemon
1 orange
1 honeydew melon
4–8 fresh mint leaves, to decorate

Preparation time: 15 minutes plus cooling time
Cooking time: 5 minutes

1. Put the chopped mint in a small bowl.
2. Put the water and honey in a small pan. Bring to the boil on a low heat, then simmer for 5 minutes. Add the chopped mint leaves, set aside to cool, then strain.
3. Squeeze the juice from the lemon and the orange and add it to the mint syrup.
4. Scoop out the flesh from the melon with a melon baller or teaspoon.
5. Fill four cocktail glasses with melon balls and coat the melon with the mint syrup.
6. Decorate with the mint leaves.

APPLE COCKTAIL

(SERVES 4)

Ingredients
2 apples
125 ml/4 fl oz/½ cup freshly squeezed orange juice
6 fresh apricots
½ tsp ground ginger
2–3 tbsp whipped cream
½ tsp ground cinnamon

Preparation time: 10 minutes

1. Peel the apples, remove the cores, and cut the flesh into segments. Place in a bowl.
2. Coat the apples with orange juice.
3. Wash the apricots, quarter them, remove the stones (pits) and add the apricot quarters to the apple.
4. Sprinkle with the ginger and mix well.
5. Serve the salad in four cocktail glasses, topped with whipped cream and sprinkled with the cinnamon.

FIG COCKTAIL WITH LEMON CREAM

(SERVES 2–3)

Ingredients
5 fresh figs
2 peaches
1 banana
125 ml/4 fl oz/½ cup whipped cream
2 tsp lemon juice
1 tbsp grated lemon rind
2–3 fresh lemon balm sprigs

Preparation time: 15 minutes

1. Wash the figs and cut into quarters.
2. Wash the peaches, cut in half, remove the stones (pits) and slice the flesh.
3. Peel and slice the banana, and sprinkle the slices with a little lemon juice to prevent discoloration. Mix with the sliced figs and peaches.
4. Blend the whipped cream with a teaspoon of lemon juice and the lemon rind.
5. Divide the fruit cocktail between two or three plates, serve with lemon cream and decorate with the lemon balm leaves.

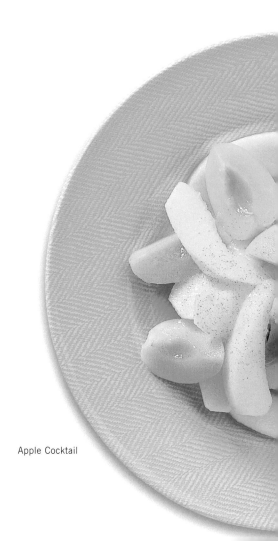

Apple Cocktail

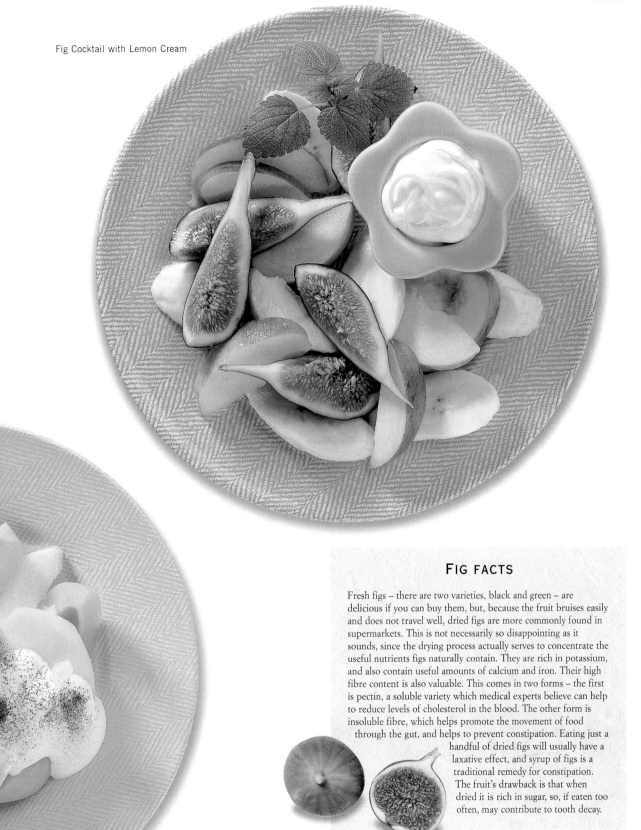

Fig Cocktail with Lemon Cream

FIG FACTS

Fresh figs – there are two varieties, black and green – are
delicious if you can buy them, but, because the fruit bruises easily
and does not travel well, dried figs are more commonly found in
supermarkets. This is not necessarily so disappointing as it
sounds, since the drying process actually serves to concentrate the
useful nutrients figs naturally contain. They are rich in potassium,
and also contain useful amounts of calcium and iron. Their high
fibre content is also valuable. This comes in two forms – the first
is pectin, a soluble variety which medical experts believe can help
to reduce levels of cholesterol in the blood. The other form is
insoluble fibre, which helps promote the movement of food
through the gut, and helps to prevent constipation. Eating just a
handful of dried figs will usually have a
laxative effect, and syrup of figs is a
traditional remedy for constipation.
The fruit's drawback is that when
dried it is rich in sugar, so, if eaten too
often, may contribute to tooth decay.

325

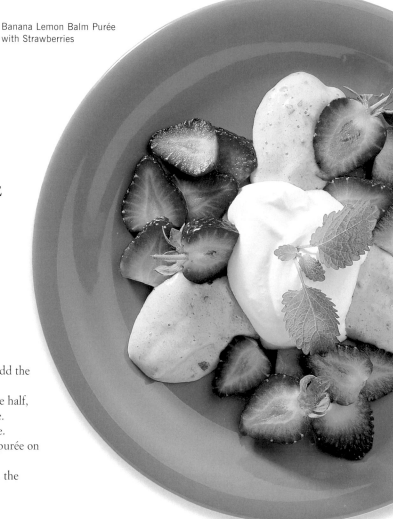

Banana Lemon Balm Purée
with Strawberries

BANANA LEMON BALM PURÉE WITH STRAWBERRIES

(SERVES 4)

Ingredients
2 bananas
juice of ½ lemon
8 fresh lemon balm sprigs
125 g/4½ oz/generous 1 cup strawberries
3–4 tbsp whipped cream

Preparation time: 10–15 minutes

1. Peel the bananas, chop into pieces and purée. Add the lemon juice to the purée.
2. Wash the lemon balm leaves and pat dry. Reserve half, chop the rest finely and mix with the banana purée.
3. Wash and hull the strawberries, pat dry and slice.
4. Arrange the sliced strawberries and the banana purée on four dessert plates.
5. Decorate with a spoonful of whipped cream and the remaining lemon balm.

PEACH AND APRICOT SALAD WITH CINNAMON

(SERVES 4)

Ingredients
2 peaches
6 apricots
4 plums
2 nectarines
1 orange
½ tsp ground cinnamon

Preparation time: 10–15 minutes

1. With the exception of the orange, wash all the fruit, cut into quarters, remove the stones (pits), slice, and arrange in a bowl.
2. Squeeze the orange and pour the juice over the sliced fruit. Add the cinnamon and mix together well.

POACHED PEARS WITH MARJORAM

(SERVES 4)

Ingredients
4 pears
125 ml/4 fl oz/½ cup grape or apple juice
2 tbsp lemon juice
2 fresh marjoram sprigs

Preparation time: 10 minutes
Cooking time: 15 minutes

1. Peel the pears, cut in half and remove the cores.
2. In a pan, gently heat the grape or apple juice, adding the lemon juice and marjoram sprigs. Bring the liquid to the boil, then add the pear halves and poach them gently for about 15 minutes, or until tender. Serve hot or cold.

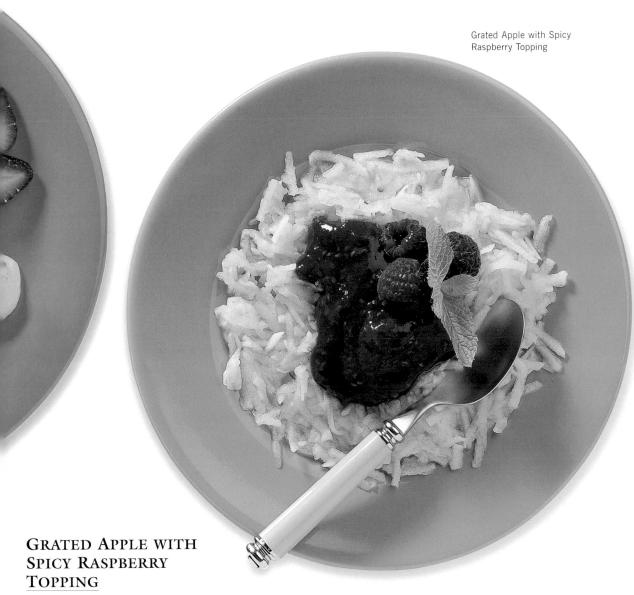

Grated Apple with Spicy
Raspberry Topping

GRATED APPLE WITH SPICY RASPBERRY TOPPING

(SERVES 4)

Ingredients
6 apples
juice of ½ lemon
125 g/4½ oz/¾ cup raspberries
¼ tsp ground ginger
few drops of vanilla essence (extract)
¼ tsp grated nutmeg
4 fresh mint leaves

Preparation time: 15 minutes

1. Peel the apples, remove the cores and grate the flesh.
Mix in the lemon juice to prevent discoloration.
2. Wash the raspberries and remove their stalks, reserving a
few raspberries for decoration. Purée the remainder.
3. Stir the ginger, vanilla, and grated nutmeg into the purée.
4. Divide the apple among four small bowls and pour some of
the topping over each serving.
5. Decorate each bowl with a few raspberries and a mint leaf.

327

NON-ALCOHOLIC DRINKS

If you drink alcohol, cutting back on the amount you drink makes good food combining sense. Although it is loaded with calories that supply almost instant energy, alcohol lacks most nutrients and vitamins. Also, if you drink heavily, you run *the risk of developing serious long-term health problems. If you drink alcohol regularly, you should adjust your lifestyle to allow for some alcohol-free days to give the digestive system a rest and boost the immune system. Try these drinks instead.*

ORANGE-GINGER DRINK

(MAKES 4 GLASSES)

Ingredients
10 oranges
1 grapefruit
½ tsp ground ginger or shredded fresh ginger

Preparation time: 10–15 minutes

Orange-Ginger Drink (left),
Banana Drink (centre), and
Yogurt Drink (right)

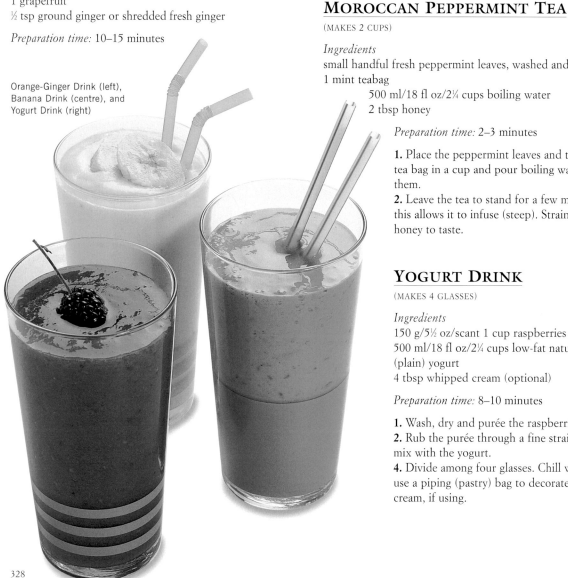

1. Squeeze the juice from the oranges and grapefruit.
2. Add the ginger, mix well and chill in the refrigerator.
3. Pour into tall glasses and serve.

MOROCCAN PEPPERMINT TEA

(MAKES 2 CUPS)

Ingredients
small handful fresh peppermint leaves, washed and torn
1 mint teabag
500 ml/18 fl oz/2¼ cups boiling water
2 tbsp honey

Preparation time: 2–3 minutes

1. Place the peppermint leaves and the mint tea bag in a cup and pour boiling water over them.
2. Leave the tea to stand for a few minutes – this allows it to infuse (steep). Strain and add honey to taste.

YOGURT DRINK

(MAKES 4 GLASSES)

Ingredients
150 g/5½ oz/scant 1 cup raspberries
500 ml/18 fl oz/2¼ cups low-fat natural (plain) yogurt
4 tbsp whipped cream (optional)

Preparation time: 8–10 minutes

1. Wash, dry and purée the raspberries.
2. Rub the purée through a fine strainer and mix with the yogurt.
4. Divide among four glasses. Chill well and use a piping (pastry) bag to decorate with cream, if using.

BANANA DRINK

(MAKES 2 GLASSES)

Ingredients
2 bananas
250 ml/8 fl oz/1 cup natural (plain) yogurt
125 ml/4 fl oz/½ cup cream

Preparation time: 3–5 minutes

1. Peel, chop and purée the bananas, then
put in a bowl.
2. Add the yogurt and cream to the purée.
3. Process in a blender until the mixture is
creamy. Serve in tall glasses.

APRICOT MILK

(MAKES 2 GLASSES)

Ingredients
6 dried apricots
500 ml/18 fl oz/
2¼ cups buttermilk

Preparation time: 3–5 minutes
plus 2–3 hours soaking

1. Soak the apricots in water for
2–3 hours.
2. Place 1 tbsp of the soaking liquid
in a blender. Add the apricots and
buttermilk.
3. Blend until smooth and serve chilled.

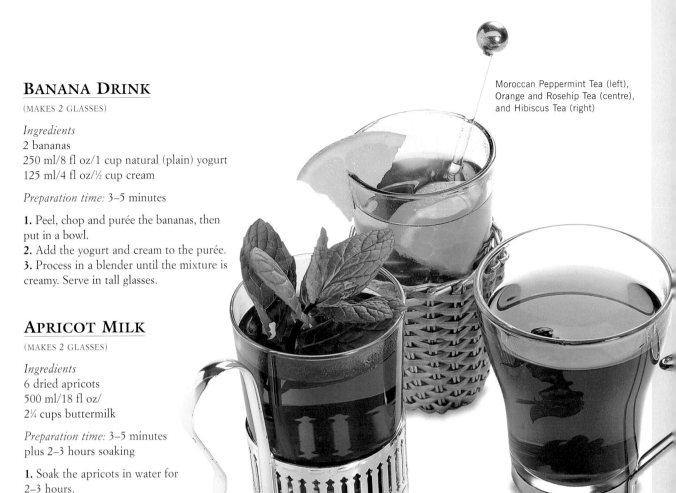

Moroccan Peppermint Tea (left),
Orange and Rosehip Tea (centre),
and Hibiscus Tea (right)

HIBISCUS TEA

(MAKES 4 CUPS)

Ingredients
2 hibiscus teabags
500 ml/18 fl oz/2¼ cups boiling water
500 ml/18 fl oz/2¼ cups apple juice
whipped cream (optional)
½ tsp ground cinnamon

Preparation time: 8–10 minutes

1. Put the teabags in a teapot or jug (pitcher). Pour in the
boiling water and leave to infuse (steep) for 5 minutes.
2. Remove the teabags from the water, pour the liquid into a
pan and add the apple juice.
3. Heat the liquid again and pour it into cups.
4. If using, add a spoonful of whipped cream to each cup,
then sprinkle with cinnamon.

ORANGE AND ROSEHIP TEA

(MAKES 4 CUPS)

Ingredients
2 rosehip teabags
1 orange blossom teabag
500 ml/18 fl oz/2¼ cups boiling water
½ orange
honey, to sweeten (optional)

Preparation time: 2–3 minutes

1. Put the tea bags in a teapot or jug (pitcher). Pour the
boiling water over the tea bags and leave to infuse (steep)
for 5 minutes.
2. Wash and slice the orange. Divide the slices among four
cups and pour the tea over them.
3. Add honey to taste, if using.

GLOSSARY

A

Acidosis – condition in which there is excessive acid in the blood, for instance diabetes or kidney disease.

Adaptogen – substance taken for medical reasons which will affect takers differently, depending on their needs.

Allergen – usually harmless substance that causes an allergic reaction.

Allergic reaction – occurs when the immune system attacks a usually harmless substance, an allergen, that accesses the body.

Amines – potentially harmful organic compounds which cause pungent intestinal gas. They can pass through the wall of the intestines and travel through the bloodstream to the brain.

Amino acid – one of the building blocks of protein.

Anaphylactic shock – a sudden and severe allergic reaction which causes the respiratory and circulatory systems to stop functioning. It can be fatal.

Antibiotics – drugs that fight infections.

Antibody – protein which is a vital part of the body's immune response.

Antigen – something potentially capable of inducing an immune response.

Antioxidant – food additive which slows down the oxidation process – that is, the reaction with oxygen. Oxidation in foodstuffs causes the food to spoil.

Antiseptic – substance which kills or inhibits the growth of bacteria and other micro-organisms, without harming the skin.

Artery – vessel along which blood travels from the heart. See also Vein.

Astringent – anything which causes cells to shrink is an astringent. For example, they are used to stop bleeding from minor cuts.

B

Bacteria – organisms responsible for infectious disease. However, some bacteria are 'friendly'. They are present at the end of the small intestine and throughout the large intestine, and continue the digestive breakdown of protein and sugars.

Bile – see gall bladder.

Bioflavenoid – vitamin that regulates the permeability of capillary walls. It occurs in citrus fruit, blackcurrants and rosehips, and is responsible for most of the red, pink and purple colours in plants. Also called flavenoid or citrin.

C

Calorie – unit of energy. The higher the calorie content of a foodstuff, the more energy is required to 'burn it' or use it up. Exercise uses more calories than, for instance, watching television does.

Carcinogen – cancer-causing substance.

Carotenoid – group of plant pigments that absorb light during photosynthesis; have antioxidant properties.

Catalyst – substance which affects the rate of a reaction, but which itself remains unchanged by the reaction.

Cholesterol – important constituent of all membranes, but when present at high levels in the blood it can thicken the artery walls.

Chyme – partially digested food that passes from the

stomach to the duodenum and the small intestine.

Coenzyme – organic molecule which must be present for a particular biochemical reaction to take place between enzymes, but which remains unaffected by the reactions.

Colic – severe spasmodic abdominal pain, caused by constipation or an obstruction in the intestine.

Craving – selective desire to eat that is triggered by an emotion, rather than real hunger. Cravings can also be caused by hormones, for instance, during pregnancy.

D

Dietetics – scientific study of diet and its relation to health.

Digestion – the process by which food is taken in and broken down, to provide the raw materials for growth and energy.

Diuretic – substance that increases the amount of urine that is produced and excreted.

Diverticular disease – diverticula are small bulging sacs pushing outward from the colon wall. If they become inflamed or infected, the condition is called diverticulitis. While most patients have few or no symptoms. they can include abdominal cramping, constipation, diarrhoea and bloating.

Dominant nutrient – the nutrient in a particular food which governs the digestive process.

Duodenum – first part of the small intestine.

Dyspepsia – see indigestion.

E

E numbers – identification codes consisting of the letter E, for European, followed by a number used to denote all food additives, except flavourings, that have been approved by the European Union. Not all E-numbers are bad.

Emetic – substance which induces vomiting.

Emulsifier – substance that enables two liquids to form an emulsion, that is, a stable mixture in which the drops of one liquid are dispersed uniformly throughout the other. Salad cream and low-fat spreads are such.

Endorphins – so-called 'feel-good' chemicals naturally occurring in the brain with pain-relieving properties similar to those of morphine. They are thought to be involved in the control of emotional responses.

Enzyme – a specialised protein molecule that acts as a catalyst for biochemical reactions in living cells.

Essential oils – mixture of volatile oils obtained from certain aromatic plants which have distinctive and characteristic odours. These are the oils used in aromatherapy.

Expectorant – substance which causes the coughing-up of phlegm.

F

Fatty acid – group of acids which can irritate the wall of the intestine, causing diarrhoea and tummy upsets.

Fermentation – bio-chemical process in which micro-organisms are used to break down an organic compound, usually a carbohydrate, in the absence of oxygen.

GLOSSARY

Flatulence – uncomfortable build-up of gas formed during digestion in the stomach or intestine.

Flavenoid – see Bioflavenoid.

Food intolerance – this is an unpleasant reaction to certain foods. The cause is often unknown, although it is sometimes caused by problems with the metabolism. It differs from an allergic reaction.

Free radical – a group of atoms containing at least one unpaired electron that is capable of initiating a wide range of chemical reactions.

G

Gall bladder – bile is stored in the gall bladder. Bile flows into the intestine to aid digestion of fatty foods.

Gastric juices – acids and enzymes produced by the stomach lining to break down food chemically and dissolve its nutrients.

Gluten – protein in wheat flour which gives bread dough its elasticity. Some people are sensitive to it, and may suffer from coeliac disease, caused by the lining of the small intestine being abnormally sensitive to gluten, leading to improper digestion or absorption of food.

H

Heartburn – indigestion caused by excess acid in the stomach being forced back into the oesophagus, characterized by a 'hot' feeling and discomfort in the chest.

Hormone – substance secreted by an endocrine gland and carried in the bloodstream to organs and tissues elsewhere in the body. Hormones perform specific physiological actions.

I

Immune response – The way in which the immune system responds to the introduction of an antigen.

Immune system – a complex system that is responsible for recognizing and attacking antigens and protecting against infections and foreign substances.

Indigestion – uncomfortable feeling caused by excessive acid in the stomach. It can be triggered by eating particular foods, but can also be caused by stress, eating too quickly and not chewing properly before swallowing. Sometimes called dyspepsia. See also Heartburn and Colic.

Intestine, Large – part of the digestive system in which useful substances such as water and minerals are absorbed through the walls, back into the blood. The remains become faeces.

Intestine, Small – part of the digestive system in which enzymes break down food, until the nutrients are small enough to pass through the lining of the small intestine and into the blood where they are carried away to the liver and elsewhere to be processed, stored and distributed.

Irritable bowel syndrome (IBS) – abnormal gut contractions, which are characterized by abdominal pain, bloating, mucous in stools, and irregular bowel habits with alternating diarrhoea and constipation, symptoms that tend to be chronic and come and go over time. Although uncomfortable, it does not lead to any serious organ problems. Also called spastic colitis, mucus colitis or nervous colon syndrome.

L

Lactose intolerance – inability to digest milk, caused by a shortage of lactase, the enzyme that is required to digest milk sugar.

Laxative – medicine or food which induces movement of the bowels.

Legumes – family of vegetables, which comprises peas, beans and lentils. They are difficult to digest.

M

Metabolism – the sum of all the chemical reactions that occur within the cells of a living organism.

N

Neurotransmitter – chemical that is released from a nerve fibre and allows an impulse to pass to a muscle or nerve.

Nutrient – any substance which provides nourishment. Food combining recognises five main nutrients: protein, fat, sugar, starch and acid.

O

Oesophagus – narrow tube through which food passes to the stomach.

Osteoporosis – thinning of the bones with reduction in bone mass due to depletion of calcium and bone protein, predisposing them to fractures.

P

Pancreas – organ behind the stomach which produces digestive enzymes.

Pasteurisation – method of sterilisation of food by heating it to a specific temperature for a short period before rapidly cooling it.

Peptide – short chain of amino acids that can be converted into amines, which cause dysfunction in the intestine.

pH value – measure of relative acidity. pH7 is neutral. Anything below this is acid, anything above this is alkaline.

Physiology – branch of biology concerned with the internal processes and functions of living organisms.

Phytochemical – any chemical derived from a plant.

Platelet aggregation – platelets are responsible for starting the formation of a clot when bleeding occurs. Platelet aggregation is the formation of blood clots where the platelets combine for other reasons, and can obstruct circulation.

S

Saturated fats – group of fats said to be harmful. Unsaturated fats can be important in maintaining good health and helping to prevent disease.

Sedative – drug or other agent that has a calming effect.

T

Trace element – chemical element that is only needed in very small amounts for growth, development and general health. In fact, they can be toxic if absorbed in large quantities.

U

Unsaturated fats – see saturated fats.

V

Vein – vessel which returns blood to the heart. See also artery.

Volatile oil – see essential oil.

USEFUL ADDRESSES AND WEBSITES

The following addresses and websites are useful for general nutritional information as well as more specific information on the practice of food combining.

ENGLAND

British Allergy Association
Deepdene House
30 Bellegrove Road
Welling
Kent
DA16 3PY
England

Tel: + 44 (0) 208 303 8583
Email: info@allergy
foundation.com
Website: www.allergy
foundation.com

Diabetes UK
10 Queen Anne Street
London
W1M 0BD
England

Tel: + 44 (0) 207 323 1531
Fax: + 44 (0) 207 637 3644
Email: info@diabetes.org.uk
Website: www.diabetes.org.uk

Eating Disorders Association
First Floor Wensum House
103 Prince of Wales Road
Norwich
NR1 1DW
England

Tel: + 44 (0) 1603 621 414
(helpline)
Tel: +44 (0) 1603 610 090
(administration)
Email: info@edauk.com
Website: www.edauk.com

Institute for Optimum Nutrition
Blades Court
Deodar Road
London
SW15 2NU
England

National Association for Colitis and Crohn's Disease
4 Beaumont House
Sutton Road
St Albans
Herts
AL1 5HH
England

Tel: + 44 (0) 1727 844 296
(information line)
Tel: +44 (0) 1727 830 038
(administration)
Fax: +44 (0) 1727 862 550
Email: nacc@nacc.org.uk
Website: www.nacc.org.uk

NORTH AMERICA

American Anorexia and Bulimia Association
293 Central Park West
Suite 1R
New York
NY 10024
USA

Tel: 1 212 501 8351

American Diabetes Association
1660 Duke Street
Alexandria
Virginia 22314
USA

Tel: 1 800 232 3472

The Crohn's and Colitis Association of America
386 Park Avenue South
17th Floor
New York
NY 10616-8804
USA

Tel: 1-800-932-2423 or
212-685-3440
Fax: 212-779-4098
Email: info@ccfa.org
Website: www.ccfa.org

Eating Disorders Awareness and Prevention
603 Steward Street
Suite 8013
Seattle
Washington 98101
USA

Tel: 1 206 382 3587

WEBSITES

www.rawfood.com/ shelton.com
Website about Shelton, the founder of food combining, and bibliography of his well-known books.

http:detox.org/ foodcombining.html
The basic techniques of food combining, with useful hints and tips.

www.realfood4thought.com
Describes the basic techniques of food combining, suggestions for replacing snacks with healthy alternatives and a selection of healthy recipes.

www.kelownahealth.com/ properfood.html

PICTURE CREDITS AND ACKNOWLEDGMENTS

The publishers would like to thank the following for permission to use copyright material: **Bridgeman Art Library**: pp:20TR; **British Museum, London**: 32BR; **Palazzo della Ragione, Padua**: 33TL; **Guildhall Library, Corporation of London**; **Cephas Picture Library**: p. 292; **Garden Picture Library**: p. 22, 32BL, 129L; **GettyOneStone**: pp. 23, 48, 60T, 61B, 70T, 76, 79T, 82, 84B, 86L, 88, 89B, 103, 104, 106, 110C, 123T, 148B, 158B, 161, 164, 165, 166, 174T; **Image Bank**: pp. 12, 14, 17, 59, 65T, 72, 75, 107, 128T, 152, 156, 179, 298; **Science Photo Library**: pp. 61R, 85T, 91TL, 95T, 158L.

(T=top, B=bottom, L=left, R=right, C=center)

Cover photograph: GettyOneStone.

FURTHER READING

BINGHAM, R.
Food Combining. Better Health –
The Natural Way
(Natural Meals Publishing: 1998)

BROSTOFF, J. AND GAMLIN, L.
The Complete Guide to Food Allergy
and Intolerance
(Bloomsbury: 1992)

CARPER, J.
Food: Your Miracle Medicine
(Simon and Schuster: 1993)

DANIEL, R.
Healing Foods: How to Nurture
Yourself and Fight Illness
(Thorsons: 1996)

DAVIES, S. AND STEWART, A.
Nutritional Medicine
(Pan: 1987)

DRIES, I.
200 New Food Combining Recipes:
Tasty Dishes from Around the World
(Element: 1995)

GRANT, B.
A–Z of Natural Healthcare
(Optima: 1993)

GRANT, D.
Food Combining For Health: Get Fit
with Foods That Don't Fight
(Inner Traditions: 1990)

HABGOOD, J.
Get Well with the Hay Diet: Food
Combining and Good Health with
More Help for Medically
Unrecognised Diseases
(Souvenir Press: 2000)

The Hay Diet Made Easy: A
Practical Guide to Food Combining
(Souvenir Press: 1997)

HARTVIG, K. AND ROWLEY, N.
You Are What You Eat
(Piatkus: 1996)

JOICE, J. AND LE TISSIER, J.
Food Combining Cookbook
(Thorsons: 2000)

LAZARIDES, L.
Principles of Nutritional Therapy
(Thorsons: 1996)

LE TISSIER, J.
Food Combining for Vegetarians
(Thorsons: 1998)

LIDOLT, E.
Food Combining Cookbook
(Thorsons: 1998)

LOVE, G.
Food Combining
(Lorenz Books: 2001)

MARSDEN, K.
Food Combining: A
Step-by-Step Guide
(Element: 1999)

MEYEROWITZ, S.
Food Combining and Digestion:
A Rational Approach to Combining
What You Eat to Maximise Digestion
and Health
(Sprout House: 1996)

MINDELL, E.
The Vitamin Bible
(Arrow: 1993)

NELSON, D.
Food Combining Simplified:
28 Recipes Included
(Dennis Nelson: 1998)

POLUNIN, M.
Healing Foods
(Dorling Kindersley: 1997)

READER'S DIGEST
Foods That Harm, Foods That Heal
(Reader's Digest Association: 1996)

SHARON, M.
Complete Nutrition
(Prion: 1997)

STRATEN, M. VAN AND GRIGGS, B.
Superfoods: Superfoods Diet Book
and Superfast Foods
(Dorling Kindersley: 1994)

SHELTON, HERBERT M.
Food Combining Made Easy
(Willow Publishing: 1940)

SMYTH, A.
Gentle Medicine
(Thorsons: 1994)

TAYLOR, B.
The Balanced Diet Cookbook: Easy
Menus and Recipes for Combining
Carbohydrates, Proteins and Fats
(Crossing Press: 1997)

TENNY, L.
Louise Tenny's Nutritional Guide
with Food Combining
(Woodland Publishing: 1994)

WERBACH, M.R.
Healing through Nutrition
(Thorsons: 1995)

INDEX